Antimicrobial Activity of Natural Products and Plants Extracts

Antimicrobial Activity of Natural Products and Plants Extracts

Guest Editors

Mihaela Niculae
Daniela Hanganu

MDPI

Basel • Beijing • Wuhan • Barcelona • Belgrade • Novi Sad • Cluj • Manchester

Guest Editors
Mihaela Niculae
Faculty of Veterinary Medicine
University of Agricultural Sciences and Veterinary Medicine of Cluj-Napoca
Cluj-Napoca
Romania

Daniela Hanganu
Faculty of Pharmacy
Iuliu Hațieganu Medicine and Pharmacy University
Cluj-Napoca
Romania

Editorial Office
MDPI AG
Grosspeteranlage 5
4052 Basel, Switzerland

This is a reprint of the Special Issue, published open access by the journal *Antibiotics* (ISSN 2079-6382), freely accessible at: https://www.mdpi.com/journal/antibiotics/special_issues/HOV59S2740.

For citation purposes, cite each article independently as indicated on the article page online and as indicated below:

Lastname, A.A.; Lastname, B.B. Article Title. *Journal Name* **Year**, *Volume Number*, Page Range.

ISBN 978-3-7258-4891-1 (Hbk)
ISBN 978-3-7258-4892-8 (PDF)
https://doi.org/10.3390/books978-3-7258-4892-8

Contents

About the Editors

Mihaela Niculae

Mihaela Niculae is currently a Senior Lecturer in the Department of Clinics, Discipline of Infectious Diseases, Faculty of Veterinary Medicine at University of Agricultural Sciences and Veterinary Medicine Cluj-Napoca, Romania. Her research interests span from animal infectious diseases, epidemiology, zoonosis, one health, and animal welfare to the therapeutic potential of natural products. Her multidisciplinary approach is highlighted by a relevant number of peer-reviewed publications and oral and poster contributions at international scientific conferences worldwide. She is also the holder of two patents. She has obtained recognition for her activity as an active reviewer for many scientific publishers (*Frontiers in Veterinary Science, Frontiers in Microbiology, BMC Veterinary Research, Journal of Applied Research on Medicinal and Aromatic Plants, Journal of Traditional and Complementary Medicine, Evidence-Based Complementary and Alternative Medicine, Chemistry and Biodiversity, Fitoterapia, European Journal of Integrative Medicine*), as well as the Biomolecules 2023 Outstanding Reviewer Award. She is serving as Guest Editor for Special Issues in *Antibiotics, Animals,* and *International Journal of Molecular Sciences.*

Daniela Hanganu

Daniela Hanganu is currently Associated Professor in the Department of Pharmacognosy at Faculty of Pharmacy, Iuliu Hațieganu Medicine and Pharmacy University, Romania. Her research lies in the field of phytochemistry, methods for the chemical analysis and separation of compounds in plants (eg. chromatography), as well as methods testing the biological activities of plant-origin extracts and bioactive compounds (antioxidant, hepatoprotective, antitumoral). Her scientific activity consists of obtaining phytopreparations standardized in active principles to further assess their chemical characterization and their bioactivity. Her constant dedication is widely recognized within the academic community and this aspect is highlighted not only by a numerous peer-reviewed publications, but also by a high number of citations and invitations to speak at national and international scientific conferences. She has obtained recognition for her activity as an active reviewer for many scientific publishers and has been serving as Guest Editor for Special Issues in *Separations, Antibiotics, Animals.*

antibiotics MDPI

Review

Phytochemistry, Mechanisms, and Preclinical Studies of Echinacea Extracts in Modulating Immune Responses to Bacterial and Viral Infections: A Comprehensive Review

Fatemeh Ahmadi [1,2]

[1] UWA School of Agriculture and Environment, The University of Western Australia, Perth 6009, Australia; fatemeh.ahmadi@uwa.edu.au
[2] Tasmanian Institute of Agriculture, University of Tasmania, Hobart 7001, Australia

Abstract: Background: Echinacea species, particularly *Echinacea purpurea, Echinacea angustifolia,* and *Echinacea pallida,* are renowned for their immunomodulatory, antibacterial, and antiviral properties. Objectives: This review explores the mechanisms by which echinacea herbal extracts modulate immune responses, focusing on their effects on both innate and adaptive immunity in bacterial and viral infections. Results: Key bioactive compounds, such as alkamides, caffeic acid derivatives, flavonoids, and polysaccharides, contribute to these effects. These compounds enhance immune cell activity, including macrophages and natural killer cells, stimulating cytokine production and phagocytosis. The antibacterial activity of echinacea against respiratory pathogens (*Streptococcus pneumoniae, Haemophilus influenzae, Legionella pneumophila*) and skin pathogens (*Staphylococcus aureus, Propionibacterium acnes*) is reviewed, as well as its antiviral efficacy against viruses like herpes simplex, influenza, and rhinovirus. Echinacea's potential as a complementary treatment alongside conventional antibiotics and antivirals is discussed, particularly in the context of antibiotic resistance and emerging viral threats. Conclusions: Challenges associated with variability in phytochemical content and the need for standardized extraction processes are also addressed. This review provides a comprehensive overview of echinacea's therapeutic potential and outlines future directions for research, including clinical trials and dosage optimization.

Keywords: alkamides; caffeic acid derivatives; COVID-19; immune system; medicinal plant; phytochemistry

1. Introduction

Herbal and botanical products have been utilized for disease prevention and treatment for thousands of years. Many Native Indian tribes and Asian cultures across the globe are recognized for their significant role in advancing botanical medicine [1]. It is estimated that more than 30,000 herbs and botanicals have been explored for medicinal purposes, though fewer than 300 are actively incorporated into Western medicine today [2]. The genus Echinacea (Asteraceae) includes a small group of hardies, herbaceous perennial species indigenous to parts of North America [3]. *Echinacea purpurea*, derived from a flowering plant, is a popular herbal medicine. This plant is native to the United States, particularly in regions east of the Rocky Mountains, and the Atlantic drainage area, including the Great Plains, and extends to the central U.S. and nearby areas of Canada [4]. According to the Royal Botanic Kew Gardens' "Plants of the World Online", native Echinacea species range from Western Europe to Southeastern Asia [5]. There are at least nine species of echinacea, each potentially varying in medicinal properties. Three species—*Echinacea angustifolia* (DC.) Hell., *Echinacea pallida* (Nutt.) Nutt., and *Echinacea purpurea* (L.) Moench—are commonly used for therapeutic purposes [6]. Some vernacular names for echinacea species include black Sampson, coneflower, pale purple coneflower (*E. pallida*), purple coneflower (*E. purpurea, E. angustifolia*), narrow-leaf purple coneflower (*E. angustifolia*), and Kansas snakeroot (*E. angustifolia*) [7]. The medicinal parts include the fresh or dried roots and rhizomes of all three species, with *E. purpurea* also using its fresh or dried flowering tops and fresh-pressed juice [8]. Commercial echinacea products, which may contain one or more of these raw materials from different regions, are available in various forms such as tinctures, tablets, teas, capsules, and parenteral preparations [9]. Echinacea has a long-standing history in medicine for treating diverse conditions, including infections such as syphilis and septic wounds, and has been historically utilized as an "anti-toxin" for snakebites and blood poisoning [10].

Historically, echinacea was regarded as an "anti-infective" agent, commonly used to address bacterial and viral infections, mild septicemia, furunculosis (frequent painful skin nodules), and a range of skin conditions, such as boils, carbuncles, and abscesses [11]. It was also traditionally employed in the treatment of nasopharyngeal catarrh, pyorrhoea (periodontitis), and tonsillitis, as well as a supportive remedy for flu-like symptoms, recurring respiratory tract infections, and urinary tract infections. Externally, it was applied to poorly healing superficial wounds [12]. In recent efforts to substantiate these traditional uses, numerous studies have investigated the effects of standardized *E. purpurea* formulations on pathogens, inflammatory processes, and gene expression in both infected and healthy human cells and animal models [13]. Today, echinacea is primarily recognized as an over-the-counter herbal remedy for colds and flu and is also used for pain, inflammation, migraines, and other health conditions. However, in some regions, echinacea is regulated as a licensed medicinal product and is even prescribed by doctors, although such prescriptions are not always required [14]. The belief that echinacea should be avoided in autoimmune diseases assumes that boosting any aspect of immune function could be harmful [15]. However, the immune system is highly complex, and substances primarily enhancing phagocytic activity may be safe or beneficial in autoimmune disorders [16,17]. A case study on the long-term use of echinacea in chronic lymphocytic leukemia found no negative effects and underscored its benefits for immune function [18].

Echinacea species, now commonly recognized as immune stimulants, were historically used by North American Indigenous Peoples to treat throat infections, wounds, and pain. In the past, echinacea was also employed in eclectic medicine to treat septic conditions [19]. Ongoing research continues to investigate its pharmacological properties and potential therapeutic applications, including anti-inflammatory, analgesic, anxiolytic, and antimicrobial effects [20]. Echinacea is generally considered safe, with severe side effects being rare. Most users experience few adverse effects, with mild reactions such as gastrointestinal discomfort or skin irritation occurring infrequently [21]. However, like any herbal supplement, there is a potential for allergic reactions, particularly in individuals allergic to members of the Asteraceae family, which includes ragweed, chrysanthemums, marigolds, and daisies [13]. The morphology of the echinacea is depicted in Figure 1.

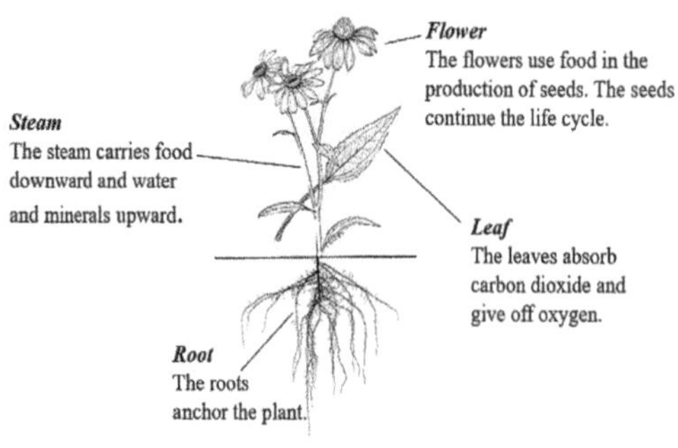

Figure 1. Botanical illustration of *E. purpurea*, depicting the aerial and root structures (Figure drawn by F. Ahmadi).

2. Methodology

Multiple academic databases were utilized to conduct a comprehensive literature search, including Web of Knowledge, Scopus, ScienceDirect, Google Scholar, Web of Science Core Collection by Clarivate Analytics, and ResearchGate. The search focused on publications from 1989 to 2024. Several keywords were employed to obtain a wide range of search results. These keywords encompassed various aspects related to echinacea species, phytochemistry, medicinal plants, echinacea biology, biochemistry, bioactive compounds, antibacterial properties, antivirus, viral infections, immune response, traditional medicine, biological models, and antibacterial mechanisms. In addition to the initial search, the references cited within the obtained publications were collected to ensure a comprehensive literature review. The chosen keywords were combined using operators like "OR" and "AND" to refine the search and obtain more precise results. Including quotation marks around specific terms, such as "echinacea", ensured accurate retrieval of relevant records. All the keywords were used in all six databases to maximize search coverage and gather a comprehensive collection of literature on the subject. The keywords and topics that are trending in each specific review section were identified. To address the research question and achieve the review objective, a thorough search for peer-reviewed studies was conducted specifically focused on echinacea's medicinal properties and mechanisms. The search was primarily centered on journal articles, excluding grey literature such as books, book chapters, and conference papers, except in rare cases where they provided valuable insights. The author screened and evaluated titles and abstracts from over 255 articles, employing a rigorous selection process to identify relevant papers. A key criterion for inclusion was the presence of quantitative information within the study. Specifically targeted studies addressed the following topics: (i) echinacea species phytochemistry, physiology, and medicinal properties; and (ii) the mechanisms of echinacea bioactive compounds on bacterial and viral infections. After comparing and analyzing the remaining articles, we categorized them based on relevant keywords. Additionally, the author summarized the conducted research, critically evaluated the content of over 192 studies, extracted essential features, and identified key challenges that warrant further investigation. By following this rigorous methodology, the author aimed to provide a comprehensive review that synthesizes the current state of knowledge, highlights significant findings, and identifies areas that require additional research attention within the context of echinacea phytochemistry and medicinal properties.

3. Phytochemistry

The composition of echinacea varies between species and their different plant parts [12]. It is commonly believed that no single compound or group of compounds is solely responsible for the effects of echinacea [22]. Rather, several classes of compounds—including alkamides, caffeic acid derivatives, polysaccharides, and alkenes (such as polyenes)—are thought to collectively contribute to its activity [23]. Below is a summary of the key constituents found in various echinacea species, compiled from several references, along with the structural formulas of some of these components [24].

3.1. *Alkamides*

Alkamides are plant-derived, lipophilic compounds characterized by a combination of various amines and aliphatic acids connected via an amine linkage [25]. These amine residues, which can be either aromatic or aliphatic, are produced through the decarboxylation of amino acids [26]. The main alkamides found in different echinacea species are depicted in Figure 2, including the isomeric dodeca-2E, 4E, 8Z, and 10E/Z-tetraenoic acid isobutylamide (8a/8b) (Figure 2). Isobutylamine originates from the amino acid valine and is the most common amine present in alkamides [27]. Other frequent amine residues include piperidine—derived from lysine, pyrrolidine—derived from ornithine, N-2-methylbutyl—whose precursor is isoleucine, and N-phenethyl—derived from phenylalanine [28]. A characteristic feature of echinacea alkamides is the attachment of isobutyl or 2-methylbutyl amines to an unsaturated fatty acid chain, which contains one or more double or triple bonds [29]. However, two alkamides isolated from hydroalcoholic extracts of *E. purpurea* roots possess a hydroxyl group and a carboxylic acid at the terminal end of the fatty acid chain [30]. Alkamide concentrations vary significantly between the roots, stems, and flowers of *E. purpurea*, with higher levels of dodeca-2,4-diene-8,10-diyne alkamides in the roots, while dodecatetraene alkamides and nonadeca-2,4-diene-8,10-diynes are more prevalent in the stems [31]. A distribution study found that the root bark and secondary roots of *E. angustifolia* lacked alkamides. High-quality *E. purpurea* root material contains up to 6 mg/g of alkamides [32].

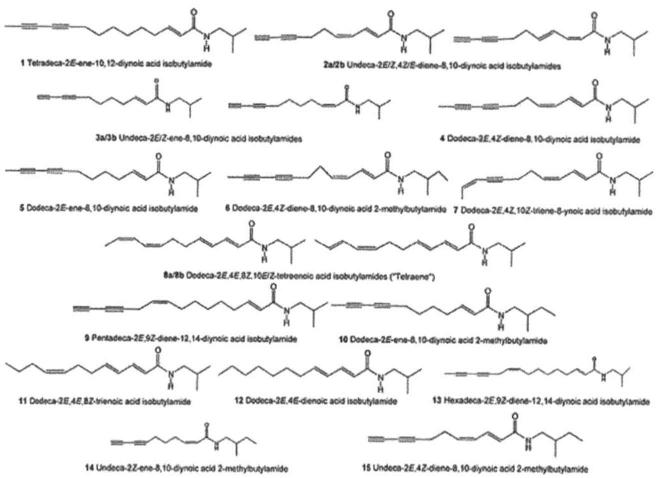

Figure 2. Structure of the main echinacea alkamides (Figure drawn by F. Ahmadi).

3.2. *Flavonoids*

There are only three documented reports of flavonoids in echinacea species. Previous research [33] identified the main anthocyanin pigments in the flowers of *E. purpurea* and *E. pallida* as cyanidin 3-glucoside and cyanidin 3-(6″-malonylglucoside) (Figure 3). Earlier studies [34] also produced anthocyanin-containing callus and suspension cultures from the stem of *E. purpurea*. From these suspension cultures, three anthocyanins were isolated: cyanidin 3-glucoside and two additional acylated cyanidin glycosides that were not fully characterized [35]. The only other report comes from unpublished data in a doctoral thesis, which noted trace amounts of quercetin and kaempferol glycosides, including the 3-rutinosides (rhamnosyl (1→6) glucosides, 56, 57), in the aerial parts of *E. purpurea* [36].

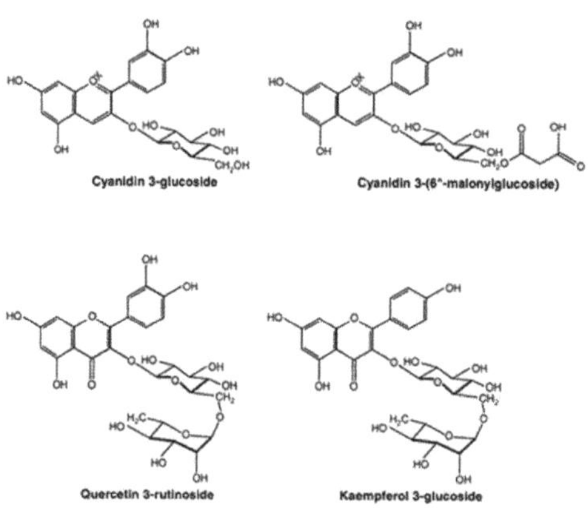

Figure 3. Flavonoids found in echinacea species (Figure drawn by F. Ahmadi).

3.3. Hydrocarbons

Hydrocarbons are key root constituents of *E. pallida*, with approximately 11 derivatives identified, primarily ketoalkenes and ketoalkynes (polyacetylenes). The major compounds include the ketoalkenes—(Z)-pentadec-8-en-2-one, (8Z,11Z)-pentadeca-8,11-dien-2-one [37], (8Z,11Z,13E)-pentadeca-8,11,13-trien-2-one, and (8Z,11E,13Z)-pentadeca-8,11,13-trien-2-one [38]—and the ketoalkenynes—(8Z,13Z)-pentadeca-8,13-dien-11-yn-2-one, (Z)-tetradeca-8-diene-11,13-diyn-2-one [39], and (Z)-pentadeca-8-ene-11,13-diyn-2-one [40]. Additionally, two notable alkenes, pentadec-1-ene [41] and (Z)-pentadeca-1,8-diene [42], have been detected in the roots of *E. angustifolia* [43]. In contrast, the only hydrocarbon reported from *E. purpurea* roots is dodeca-2,4-dien-1-yl isovalerate, which is also found in the roots of *E. angustifolia* [44]. The absence of polyacetylenes in the roots of *E. angustifolia* and *E. purpurea* serves as a distinguishing factor between these species and *E. pallida*. Research has demonstrated that commercially available *E. pallida* root preparations are often contaminated with *E. angustifolia* [45]. This suggests that some early reports of hydrocarbons in *E. angustifolia* roots may have been due to misidentification or contamination with *E. pallida*. The hydrocarbons identified in the rhizomes of echinacea species are listed in Table 1.

Table 1. Hydrocarbons from Rhizomes [a] of echinacea species [46].

Species	Hydrocarbon
E. angustifolia	Dodeca-2,4-dien-1yl isovalerate (Z)-Pentadeca-1,8 diene Pentadec-1-ene
E. pallida	(Z)-Pentadec-8-en-2-one (Z)-Pentadeca-1,8-diene Pentadec-1-ene (8Z,11Z)-Pentadeca-8,11-dien-2-one (8Z,13Z)-Pentadeca-8,13-dien-11-yn-2-one (Z)-Tetradeca-8-diene-11,13-diyn-2-one (E)-10-Hydroxy -4,10-dimethydodeca-4, 11-dien-2-one (echinolone) (Z)-Pentadeca-8-ene-11,13-diyn-2-one (8Z,11Z,13E)-Pentadeca-8,11,13-trien-2-one (8Z,11E,13Z)-Pentadeca-8,11-trien-2-one
E. purpurea	Dodeca-2,4-dien-1-yl isovalerate

[a] Referred to as roots in most references.

3.4. Polysaccharides

Two immunostimulatory polysaccharides, PS I and PS II, have been isolated from the aerial parts of *E. purpurea*. PS I is identified as 4-O-methyl-glucuronoarabinoxylan with an average molecular weight of 35,000, while PS II is an acidic arabinorhamnogalactan with a molecular weight of 50,000. Both of these polysaccharides exhibited significant activity in various in vitro and in vivo immunological tests [47]. A crude polysaccharide extract from the roots of *E. purpurea* has not been fully analyzed, though it seems to have a similar composition to that of the aerial parts [48]. Additionally, from cell cultures of *E. purpurea*, three homogeneous polysaccharides were obtained: two neutral fucogalactoxyloglucans, with molecular weights of 10,000 and 25,000, and an acidic arabinogalactan, with a molecular weight of 75,000 [49]. The fucogalactoxyloglucan with a molecular weight of 25,000 was found to enhance phagocytosis in both in vitro and in vivo assays, while the arabinogalactan specifically triggered macrophages to secrete tumor necrosis factor (TNF) [50,51]. The acidic arabinorhamnogalactan from *E. purpurea* is now produced biotechnologically on an industrial scale and is being considered for clinical trials [52]. Previous research classified this polysaccharide as a type II arabinogalactan, characterized by a (1→3)-linked β-D-galactan backbone, which is likely attached to rhamnogalactan and arabinan chains [53,54]. The polysaccharides produced through tissue culture differ structurally from those found in the aerial parts, as they are components of the primary cell walls in cultured cells. As a result, the polysaccharides derived from the aerial parts of *E. purpurea* show little resemblance to those produced by tissue cultures [55].

3.5. Caffeic Acid Derivatives (CADs)

Another important group of phytochemicals contributing to echinacea's pharmacological effects is CADs (Figure 4). Unlike alkylamides, which are more limited in their distribution across taxa, phenolic metabolites like CADs are widely distributed among plants. Although echinacea has a unique collection of CADs, these compounds are found across many plant families [56,57]. Two of the most extensively studied CADs in *E. purpurea* are caftaric acid and chicoric acid, as they represent the dominant polyphenols in this species [58]. In addition to their role in plant defenses, such as deterring herbivores and providing interspecies protection, CADs are associated with echinacea's immunostimulatory and antioxidant properties [59]. However, oral administration studies indicate that these compounds have poor bioavailability, raising questions about their effectiveness in humans [60]. Chicoric acid is particularly abundant in *E. purpurea*, making up as much as 20% of total CADs in the roots, while the flowers, stems, and leaves contain approximately 35%, 10%, and 35%, respectively [61]. For natural health products, this distribution suggests that products should prioritize flowers and leaves, which contain higher concentrations of CADs. Some natural health products reflect this, whereas others focus on alkylamides, which are mainly concentrated in the roots and found in smaller amounts in the aerial parts [62].

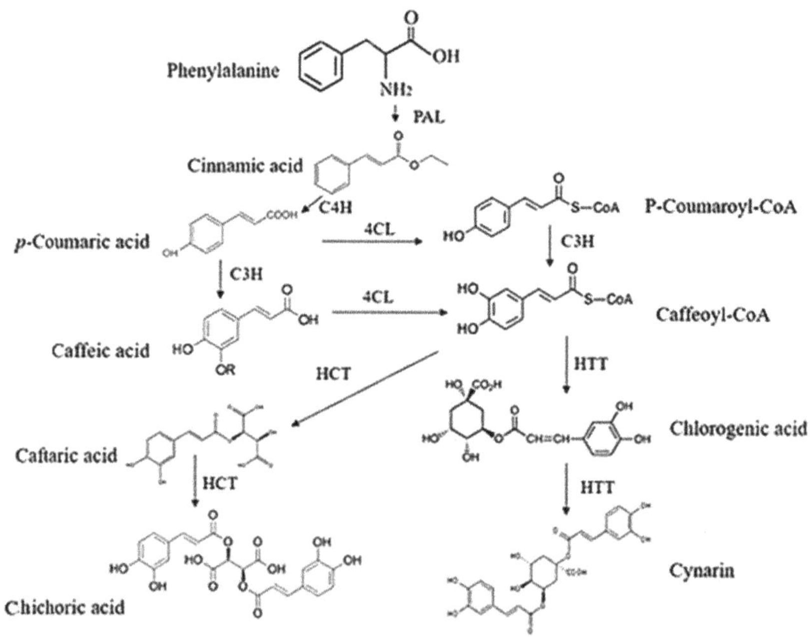

Figure 4. A possible biosynthesis pathway for chicoric acid and caffeic acid is derived via the phenylpropanoid pathway in echinacea species. PAL: phenylalanine ammonia-lyase, C4H: cinnamate-4-hydroxylase, C3H: coumarate 3-hydroxylase, 4CL: 4-coumarate-CoA ligase, HCT: shikimate o-hydroxycinnamoyl transferase (Figure drawn by F. Ahmadi).

4. Antibacterial Activities of Echinacea Species

There are numerous reports detailing the traditional use of echinacea species in treating bacterial infections [63]. Three species in particular, *E. purpurea*, *E. angustifolia*, and *E. pallida*, have historically been used as antibacterial remedies. Research [64] has also discussed the application of *E. purpurea* in Brazil, where a leaf infusion is applied topically to infected areas [65]. Several studies have since been conducted to validate the antibacterial properties traditionally attributed to echinacea species and their preparations [66]. One such study investigated the antibacterial activity of a fermented extract of *E. purpurea* (5% w/v, fermented with Lactobacillus plantarum) [67]. Using disc diffusion and broth microdilution assays, the extract was tested on a range of bacterial strains, including *E. coli*, *Enterobacter aerogenes*, *Enterococcus durans*, *Yersinia enterocolitica*, *Weissella confusa*, *Leu-*

conostoc lactis, *Propionibacterium jensenii*, *Lactobacillus sakei*, and *Bacillus megaterium*. The results demonstrated that the fermented extract inhibited the growth of most of the strains tested, with the greatest inhibition seen in *B. megaterium* and *L. lactis*, where inhibition halos measured over 3.5 mm and between 2.5–3.5 mm, respectively. No inhibitory effect was observed for *L. sakei* [68].

A previous study [69] investigated the bactericidal effects of a 65% ethanol extract from freshly harvested aerial parts and roots of *E. purpurea* at concentrations of 40 and 120 mg of dry mass/mL. The microdilution method, using both light and dark assays, was applied to test the extract against strains responsible for respiratory infections, including *L. pneumophila*, *Streptococcus pyogenes*, *Mycobacterium smegmatis*, and *H. influenzae*. Results showed that *S. pyogenes*, *H. influenzae*, and *L. pneumophila* were sensitive to the higher concentration of the extract. Another study [70], employing agar diffusion tests, assessed the antibacterial activity of hydroethanol extracts (prepared via conventional and ultrasonic extraction) from the aerial parts of *E. purpurea* (20 mg/mL). The extracts were tested against standard strains such as *E. coli*, *P. aeruginosa*, *Bacillus subtilis*, and *S. aureus*. The conventional extraction method produced larger inhibition zones for all strains, with *E. coli* (11.2 $\pm$ 0.2 mm) and *B. subtilis* (10.9 $\pm$ 0.1 mm) showing the most significant inhibition. In another study [71], the antibacterial activity of *E. angustifolia* extracts was evaluated using solvents of increasing polarity (petroleum ether, methanol, and water) at concentrations of 0.5, 1.5, and 1.5 mg/mL, respectively, against *B. subtilis*, *S. aureus*, *E. coli*, and *Staphylococcus epidermidis*. The study did not specify the plant parts used for extraction, and the aqueous extracts were less effective than those prepared with other solvents.

Respiratory infections can be caused by various pathogenic bacteria, including *Streptococcus pneumoniae*, *H. influenzae*, *Moraxella catarrhalis*, *S. pyogenes*, *Bordetella pertussis*, *Mycoplasma pneumoniae*, *S. aureus*, *P. aeruginosa*, and *Burkholderia cepacia* [72], among others. In this context, plants from the echinacea genus have shown promising antibacterial activity against microorganisms involved in these infections, as demonstrated by previous studies [73]. Additionally, *E. purpurea* has been found to inhibit *L. pneumophila*, the bacterium responsible for pneumonia [74]. However, the results for *S. aureus* have been inconsistent, possibly due to variations in the echinacea species used, plant parts, extraction methods, and thus their chemical compositions. Earlier research [75] suggested that neither alkylamides nor polysaccharides alone were responsible for the reported bactericidal effects. Furthermore, no clear link was found between bactericidal activity and caffeoyl derivatives [76]. Conversely, other studies [77] have correlated antimicrobial activity with total phenolic and flavonoid content.

Several bacteria, including *P. acnes*, *S. aureus*, *S. pyogenes*, *P. aeruginosa*, *Pasteurella multocida*, *Capnocytophaga canimorsus*, *Bartonella* spp., *Klebsiella rhinoscleromatis*, and *Vibrio vulnificus*, are key pathogens involved in skin infections [78]. Studies have shown that echinacea plants possess active compounds with antimicrobial properties that target these skin pathogens, supporting their traditional use in ethnomedicine for treating skin infections [79]. Additionally, recent research has demonstrated the potential of *E. purpurea* in addressing throat and mouth conditions (Oto-rhino-laryngological, OTO). One study [80] revealed that extracts from *E. angustifolia* and its primary alkylamide isomers, dodeca-2E, 4E, 8Z, and 10Z/E-octadecenoic acid (alkylamide 8/9, which is also found in *E. purpurea*), inhibited the growth of *Candida albicans*, a leading cause of fungal throat infections [81]. These findings align with ethnobotanical evidence supporting the use of echinacea for OTO-related conditions. Moreover, echinacea has been reported to inhibit microorganisms responsible for respiratory infections, including *Legionella pneumophila*, *Streptococcus pyogenes*, and *Mycobacterium smegmatis* [82]. However, despite being a well-studied respiratory pathogen, *Pseudomonas* has not been thoroughly investigated concerning echinacea treatments [83].

Purple coneflower (*E. purpurea*) is known to counteract proinflammatory cytokine stimulation, regardless of the bacterial or viral source of infection [84]. Several studies have examined the effects of *E. purpurea* on the activation of lipopolysaccharide, an inflammatory mediator typically produced by *E. coli*, in various human cell cultures and animal models, as well as research involving live bacteria [85]. While these models do not always fully replicate live bacterial infections, they provide useful insights for testing potential anti-inflammatory agents. The findings suggest that *E. purpurea* acts as a general anti-inflammatory agent, capable of reducing several symptoms associated with respiratory infections [86]. Extracts obtained from the aerial parts of *E. purpurea* have shown stronger antibacterial and antioxidant properties compared to those derived via ultrasonic extraction methods [87]. Currently, antibiotics and vaccines are the main treatments for bacterial infections, used both therapeutically and prophylactically. However, managing respiratory infections remains a challenge due to the variety of microorganisms involved. In this context, the use of phytopreparations could offer a promising alternative [88]. To better understand the synergistic interactions between echinacea extracts and antibiotics, further research is necessary to elucidate the mechanisms of their antimicrobial effects and identify potential pathways that could be targeted [83].

5. Mechanism of Antibacterial Activity of Polyphenols

Echinacea species exhibit antimicrobial activity through several distinct mechanisms, which together enhance their effectiveness against a wide range of pathogens [89]. A key mechanism is the disruption of microbial cell membranes, primarily due to the hydrophobic compounds like alkamides present in echinacea [90]. These compounds can integrate into the lipid bilayers of microbial membranes, leading to structural instability and increased permeability, ultimately causing cell lysis and death [90]. Another important mechanism is the inhibition of microbial enzymes essential for survival and replication. Compounds such as caffeic acid derivatives inhibit enzymes responsible for processes like cell wall synthesis and nucleic acid production, thereby hindering microbial growth and reproduction [91]. Additionally, echinacea has immunomodulatory effects, stimulating immune cells like macrophages and natural killer cells, enhancing phagocytosis, and increasing cytokine production, which helps coordinate the body's immune response to infections [92]. Furthermore, echinacea extracts have been shown to prevent biofilm formation—protective layers bacteria form to evade immune responses and resist antibiotics—making bacteria more vulnerable to immune defenses and antimicrobial treatments [93]. The antioxidant properties of echinacea also contribute by neutralizing free radicals generated during infections, reducing oxidative stress, and protecting host tissues from damage, which further supports its antimicrobial action [89]. Together, these multiple mechanisms position echinacea as a versatile antimicrobial agent, capable of combating a variety of pathogens through both direct antimicrobial activity and indirect immune system modulation [90].

5.1. Reactions with Proteins

The antibacterial activity of flavonoids may be attributed to their ability to form complexes with proteins through nonspecific interactions, such as hydrogen bonding and hydrophobic forces, as well as through covalent bond formation [94]. The binding of polyphenols to proteins results in the formation of soluble or insoluble complexes, which affects the functions of both polyphenols and proteins [95]. This interaction can cause certain amino acids in proteins to be blocked or lead to conformational changes, altering the protein's structure, solubility, hydrophobicity, thermal stability, and isoelectric point [96]. As a result, protein–phenolic complexation can modify their physicochemical and biological properties, influencing the digestibility of food proteins, the activity of digestive enzymes, and nutrient availability [94]. It has been shown that polyphenols, such as condensed tannins, can inhibit several digestive enzymes, including α-glycosidase, α-amylase, lipase, pepsin, trypsin, and chymotrypsin, thereby modulating nutrient availability, and altering microbiota composition [95]. Additionally, polyphenols can bind to crucial bacterial proteins, such as adhesins and enzymes, and transport proteins in the bacterial cell envelope, inactivating them and exerting an antimicrobial effect. However, the complexation of polyphenols with proteins may also impact the bioaccessibility and activity of phenolic compounds [97].

Some flavones have shown activity against *E. coli* by forming complexes with extracellular and soluble proteins [94]. Flavonoids are also known to influence the activity of bacterial enzymes essential for cell survival, including those involved in synthesizing cell wall components, membrane fatty acids, or adenosine triphosphate (ATP). Fatty acid synthase II (FAS-II) is a critical enzyme in bacterial membrane fatty acid synthesis, catalyzing the elongation of fatty acid chains from 16–24 carbons produced de novo by FAS-I to longer chains of 36–48 carbons, as well as mycolic acids [97]. Flavonoids such as isoliquiritigenin, butein, fisetin, and4′-trihydroxy chalcone have been found to inhibit FAS-II, thus hindering the growth of Mycobacterium smegmatis [98].

5.2. Inhibition of Bacterial DNA Synthesis and Interaction with Nucleic Acids

Flavonoids derived from *Elaeagnus glabra* were tested for antibacterial effects against *Proteus vulgaris* and *Staphylococcus aureus* [99]. The presence of a free 3′, 4′, and 5′-trihydroxy B-ring, along with a free 3-OH group, was found to be necessary for antibacterial activity. In *P. vulgaris*, DNA synthesis was primarily inhibited by active flavonoids, while in *S. aureus*, RNA synthesis was inhibited [100]. Robinetin, myricetin, and (−)-epigallocatechin were identified as the most potent inhibitors of DNA synthesis. It is suggested that the B-ring of these flavonoids may interact with nucleic acid bases by forming hydrogen bonds or intercalating, leading to the inhibition of bacterial nucleic acid synthesis. A previous study [101] found that p-coumaric acid exhibited dual bactericidal actions: disrupting the bacterial cell membrane and binding to bacterial genomic DNA, which inhibited essential cellular functions and caused cell death [102]. In *S. aureus*, membrane depolarization and the inhibition of DNA, RNA, and protein synthesis were observed when treated with flavonoids from *Dorstenia* species, such as 6,8-diprenyleriodictyol, isobavachalcone, and 4-hydroxylonchocarpin. At higher concentrations, cell lysis occurred.

There is also evidence that flavonoids can inhibit bacterial type II topoisomerases, including DNA gyrase and topoisomerase II (also known as topoisomerase IV) [101]. These enzymes, which regulate DNA topology, are specific to prokaryotes, making them attractive targets for antibacterial drugs. DNA gyrase consists of two key subunits: DNA gyrase subunit A (GyrA), responsible for DNA cleavage and rejoining, and DNA gyrase subunit B (GyrB), which contains the ATP-binding site. Natural compounds like coumarins and cyclothialidines inhibit ATPase activity in DNA gyrase by blocking ATP binding to the GyrB subunit. Research [99] demonstrated that quercetin inhibits the supercoiling activity of bacterial gyrase and induces DNA cleavage, likely through interaction with DNA. Quercetin binds to the 24 kilodalton fragment of GyrB in *E. coli* with a dissociation constant of 15 μM, inhibiting ATPase activity by competing with ATP for the binding site. Quercetin's binding site overlaps with the ATP-binding pocket and can be competitively displaced by either ATP or novobiocin [101]. The proposed mechanism suggests that quercetin inhibits gyrases by interacting with either the DNA or the ATP-binding site [101]. Other polyphenols, such as catechins, have also been found to inhibit bacterial DNA gyrase by binding to the ATP site on the GyrB subunit, with epigallocatechin gallate being the most active, followed by epicatechin gallate and epigallocatechin [102]. Flavonoids such as quercetin, apigenin, and 3,3′,4′,6,7-pentahydroxyflavone have also shown inhibitory activity against *E. coli* DNA gyrase [102].

5.3. Interaction with the Bacterial Cell Wall or Inhibition of Cell Wall Formation

Differences in antimicrobial activity between Gram-negative and Gram-positive bacteria may result from variations in their cell surface structures [103]. The main function of the bacterial cell wall is to provide shape, maintain cell integrity, and serve as an osmotic barrier. Gram-negative bacteria are known to be resistant to many antibacterial agents due to the hydrophilic nature of their outer membrane and the presence of enzymes in the periplasmic space, which can break down external molecules [104]. Additionally, the negatively charged lipopolysaccharide layer in the outer membrane acts as a protective shield against catechins. In contrast, Gram-positive bacteria, which lack an outer membrane, tend to be more vulnerable to the action of phenolic acids. This lack of an outer membrane allows phenolic acids to diffuse more easily through the cell wall and reach the intracellular environment [105]. It is suggested that one potential mechanism behind the antimicrobial action of phenolic acids involves hyperacidification at the plasma membrane interface, caused by the dissociation of these acids. This process disrupts the cell membrane potential, increases membrane permeability, and causes irreversible changes to the sodium-potassium ATPase pump, ultimately leading to cell death [104].

Flavones form complexes with cell wall components, which can inhibit bacterial adhesion and further microbial growth. Flavonoids with a C-7-modified naringenin core have been shown to inhibit bacterial enzymes, such as tyrosyl-tRNA synthetase. These compounds have also demonstrated inhibitory effects on the growth of *S. aureus*, *E. coli*, and *P. aeruginosa*. Baicalein, in particular, was found to be an effective bactericidal agent, and when combined with cefotaxime, it exhibited synergistic effects by inhibiting the expression of extended-spectrum β-lactamase beta-lactamase messenger RNA [105]. Another mechanism contributing to antibacterial activity is the inhibition of bacterial efflux pumps, which enhances the susceptibility of bacteria to existing antibiotics by causing membrane depolarization. Artonin, derived from *Morus mesozygia*, was effective against *S. aureus* by blocking efflux mechanisms and inducing membrane depolarization [103]. Furthermore, artonin was able to reverse multidrug resistance, lowering the minimum inhibitory concentrations of antibiotics and increasing their potency.

5.4. Alteration of Cytoplasmic Membrane Function

The bacterial cell membrane is essential for multiple vital functions, including osmoregulation, respiration, transport, biosynthesis, and the cross-linking of peptidoglycan and lipids [106]. Any disruption to its structure or function can result in metabolic failure and cell death, making membrane disruption a key mechanism in the antibacterial action of polyphenols. For example, catechins have been shown to damage bacterial membranes by binding to the lipid bilayer, inhibiting the synthesis of both intracellular and extracellular enzymes [107]. Apigenin was observed to cause dysfunction in fungal membranes, increasing permeability and triggering the release of small intracellular components such as ions and sugars, but not proteins [107]. Epicatechin-3-gallate and caffeic acid were found to target both the cell wall and cytoplasmic membrane of *P. aeruginosa*, leading to membrane destruction, increased permeability, and the enhanced entry of hydrophobic antibiotics. This process also caused the release of potassium ions and the leakage of nucleotides. Due to their partially lipophilic properties, phenolic acids can penetrate the cell membrane via passive diffusion, increasing permeability, reducing intracellular pH, and causing protein denaturation [108]. A methanol extract from Coriolus versicolor, rich in polyphenols, inhibited cell division in *S. aureus* by interfering with septum formation and causing the accumulation of peptidoglycan and teichoic acid precursors in the cytoplasm [107]. In *Salmonella enteritidis*, the extract damaged the cell envelope. Furthermore, at higher concentrations, catechins have been shown to induce the generation of reactive oxygen species, leading to oxidative stress, altered membrane permeability, and subsequent membrane damage.

Flavonoids and flavonol have been shown to destabilize membrane structures by disrupting and disorienting membrane lipids, leading to leakage from vesicles [106]. An inverse relationship was observed between the number of hydroxyl groups in flavonoids and their ability to induce leakage. Previous research [93] suggested that flavonoids lacking hydroxyl groups on their B rings were more effective at inhibiting microbial growth compared to those with –OH groups. On the other hand, previous research found that the presence of hydroxyl groups in the phenyl rings A and B generally did not affect the antibacterial activity level of flavones [107]. A notable increase in activity was observed for hydroxy derivatives of flavones, specifically against *S. aureus*. Interestingly, in contrast to other studies, the compounds tested showed greater effectiveness against Gram-negative bacteria such as *E. coli* and *P. aeruginosa* than against Gram-positive bacteria like *Enterococcus faecalis* and *Staphylococcus aureus* [108].

6. Antiviral Activities of Echinacea Species

In vitro studies have demonstrated that aqueous extracts of *E. purpurea* Moench are effective against both acyclovir-resistant and acyclovir-susceptible strains of HSV-1 and HSV-2 (herpes simplex virus) [109]. Specifically, HSV-1 was inhibited by chicoric acid, and a hexane extract derived from the plant's roots [110]. Additionally, chicoric acid was shown to inhibit the integrase enzyme of human immunodeficiency virus type 1 (HIV-1) [111]. Mouse embryonic fibroblasts incubated with alcoholic root extract and plant juice for 24 h were resistant to infection by herpes, influenza A2, and the vesicular stomatitis virus [112]. Various influenza virus strains, including avian (H7N7 and H5N1), influenza A (H1N1 and H3N2), and the pandemic swine-origin H1N1, were significantly inhibited by direct contact with standard echinacea preparations [113]. Hemagglutination (HA) assays revealed that these preparations suppressed HA activity, suggesting they may block viral entry into cells [114]. In influenza A H1N1-infected mice, administration of a polysaccharide extract from the plant resulted in weight loss, although lung virus titers remained similar between treated and untreated animals [115]. However, treated mice exhibited reduced levels of keratinocyte chemoattractant, interleukin-10 (IL-10), and systemic interferon-gamma, indicating that *E. purpurea* may modulate cytokines to reduce the clinical symptoms of influenza [116]. Recent studies suggest that different plant components may positively impact influenza patients through various mechanisms [117]. To establish *E. purpurea* as a biological agent, further research—especially in vivo studies and assessments of potential toxicity—is needed [118]. Ongoing clinical trials related to SARS-CoV support the use of *E. purpurea* against coronaviruses. Due to structural similarities among coronaviruses, preparations of *E. purpurea* (L.) Moench could serve as a preventative treatment for all coronaviruses, although additional studies are required [119].

A randomized, double-blind, placebo-controlled clinical trial was conducted to assess the efficacy of *E. purpurea* in preventing infections caused by rhinovirus type 39 (RV-39) [120]. It was reported that 59% of the 48 participants who were infected and treated with pressed juice from the aerial parts of *E. purpurea* in a 22% alcohol base developed a cold, compared to 86% of the placebo group ($p = 0.0883$, according to Fisher's exact test) [121]. Meanwhile, *E. pallida* var. *angustifolia* exhibited significant anti-rhinovirus activity. Root extracts of *E. pallida* var. *angustifolia* in ethanol 70%, hexane, and ethyl acetate demonstrated anti-RV activity, with MIC100 (the minimum concentration required to inactivate 100% of the virus) values of 62, 69, and 85 μg/mL, respectively. The study concluded that alkamide-rich hexane fractions were more effective against rhinovirus due to their lower MIC100 compared to ethyl acetate fractions, which contained fewer alkamides [122]. Treatment with echinaforce, a standardized preparation from freshly harvested *E. purpurea* including root extracts in a 65% *v*/*v* ethanol solution, showed a slight reduction in viral titers at the highest dose of 50 μg/mL in post-infection cell lines with HCoV-229E [123]. When exposed to echinaforce, HCoV-229E was irreversibly inactivated, with a 50% inhibitory concentration (IC50) of 3.2 μg/mL, as demonstrated through 3-(4,5-dimethylthiazol-2-yl)-2,5-diphenyltetrazolium bromide assays conducted on Huh-7, Vero, and Vero E6 cells [124]. Additionally, it is reported that [121] the efficacy of *E. purpurea* for the prevention of rhinovirus colds, further supporting its potential clinical applications.

The aqueous fraction of *E. purpurea* roots has been reported to show potent antiviral activity against the influenza virus, whereas the ethyl acetate fraction from *E. angustifolia* root extracts demonstrated moderate activity against the herpes simplex virus, influenza, and rhinovirus [125]. In contrast, extracts from *E. pallida* roots exhibited no antiviral activity [126]. The minimum concentration of *E. purpurea* needed to inactivate 100% of the virus (MIC100) in tablet or capsule form was found to be 2.5 μg/mL. Interestingly, *E. purpurea* tea brewed at 80 °C showed a MIC100 of 2.2 μg/mL, indicating that the tea preparation of *E. purpurea* may offer superior antiviral activity compared to capsules or tablets. Among several extracts of *E. pallida* var. *angustifolia* roots (55% ethanol extract at 40 °C, water extracts at 40 °C and 80 °C, 70% ethanol extract at 40 °C, hexane, and ethyl acetate extracts), only the 55% ethanol extract at 40 °C and the ethyl acetate extract displayed anti-influenza effects [127]. Notably, the ethyl acetate extract of *E. pallida* var. *angustifolia* exhibited the strongest antiviral activity against influenza, with a MIC100 of 33.5 μg/mL, significantly outperforming the ethanol extract, which had a MIC100 of 348 μg/mL [128].

Research has been conducted on the antiviral effects of echinacea extract against the SARS-CoV-2 virus [129]. SARS-CoV-2 enters host cells by interacting with ACE2 receptors, and the virus's pathogen-associated molecular patterns (PAMPs) activate innate immune cells, including antiviral effectors like CD8+ T cells, neutrophils, monocytes, and macrophages, in response to the infection [130]. Innate immune cells, equipped with pattern recognition receptors (PRRs) such as Toll-like receptors (TLRs), retinoic acid-inducible gene I (RIG-I)-like receptors (RLRs), and nucleotide-binding oligomerization domain (NOD)-like receptors (NLRs), detect PAMPs and trigger an immune response against the invading pathogen [131]. The interaction between PRRs and PAMPs stimulates phagocytosis and leads to the production of proinflammatory cytokines, including type I interferons (IFNα/β), type II interferons (IFN-γ), and chemokines like interferon gamma-induced protein 10 and monocyte chemoattractant protein-1, generating an antiviral response [132]. The immunomodulatory properties of echinacea induce an antiviral response by influencing the activity of PRRs, PAMPs, and damage-associated molecular patterns (DAMPs). Echinacea has demonstrated efficacy against rhinoviruses [133], influenza [134], respiratory syncytial virus (RSV) [135], herpes virus [136], adenoviruses [137], and coronaviruses [138]. Additionally, chicoric acid, a compound found in echinacea, has shown potent antiviral activity against herpes simplex, influenza, enterovirus, hepatitis B, vaccinia virus, and vesicular stomatitis virus-Ebola [139]. In HIV-1, chicoric acid and its derivatives inhibit the enzyme integrase, which is responsible for integrating viral DNA into the host genome, a crucial step in viral replication [140] (Figure 5). Treatment with echinacea has also been shown to preserve the activity of natural killer cells and monocytes, providing nonspecific immunity, and helping to eliminate virus-infected cells [141].

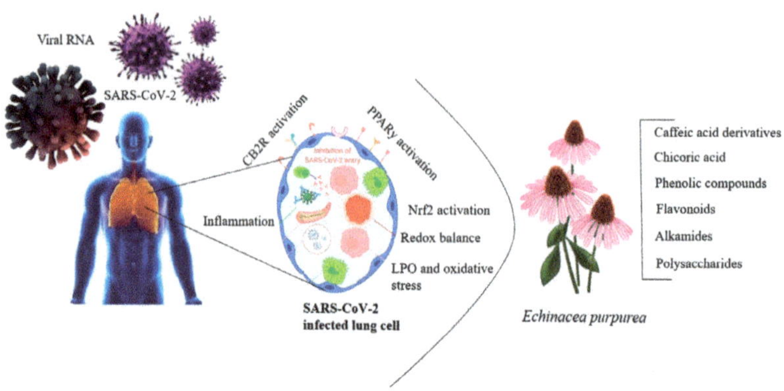

Figure 5. Antiviral activity of echinacea extract against SARS-CoV-2 virus (Figure drawn by F. Ahmadi).

In other in vitro studies, the antiviral effects of an aqueous solution of *E. purpurea* herb were tested against aciclovir-susceptible and aciclovir-resistant strains of HSV-1 and HSV-2 [142]. For aciclovir-susceptible strains of HSV-1 and HSV-2, the median effective dose (ED50) values for the echinacea preparation were 1:100 (ranging from 1:25 to 1:400) and 1:200 (ranging from 1:50 to 1:1600), respectively. Similarly, for aciclovir-resistant HSV-1 and HSV-2, the median ED50 values were 1:100 (ranging from 1:50 to 1:400) and 1:200 (ranging from 1:50 to 1:3200), respectively [143]. In light-activated antiviral activity studies, an n-hexane extract of *E. purpurea* root, an ethanolic extract of *E. pallida* var. *sanguinea* herb, and the isolated compound chicoric acid were the most potent inhibitors of HSV-1, with minimum inhibitory concentrations of 0.12, 0.026, and 0.045 mg/mL, respectively [144]. Additional in-vitro studies using mouse fibroblasts demonstrated that pre-incubation with *E. purpurea* herb juice and methanolic and aqueous extracts of *E. purpurea* root provided 24-h resistance to infections caused by influenza A2, herpes, and the vesicular stomatitis virus [145].

7. Mechanism of Antiviral Activity of Polyphenols

7.1. Inhibition of Virus Entry

Echinacea demonstrates antiviral activity through several key mechanisms, starting with the inhibition of viral entry into host cells [146], a vital step in halting the infection process. Compounds such as caffeic acid derivatives (including chicoric acid and echinacoside) and flavonoids (like quercetin and kaempferol) in echinacea can bind to viral surface proteins or host cell receptors [147]. This interaction effectively blocks the virus from attaching to host cells, which is an essential initial phase in the viral replication cycle [148]. Additionally, these compounds can interfere with the viral envelope or disrupt the host cell membrane, particularly in enveloped viruses, preventing the fusion process needed for the virus to release its genetic material into the host cell. By obstructing both attachment and fusion, echinacea compounds substantially reduce the likelihood of viral entry and subsequent infection.

7.2. Inhibition of Viral Replication

Another key mechanism by which echinacea exerts its antiviral effects is through the inhibition of viral replication [149]. Once a virus successfully enters a host cell, it must replicate its genetic material to produce new viral particles. Polyphenols found in echinacea, such as chicoric acid and rosmarinic acid, can disrupt this process by inhibiting viral RNA and DNA polymerases—enzymes that are essential for replicating viral genetic material [150]. By blocking these polymerases, these compounds effectively stop the virus from replicating its genome, thereby preventing the production of new viral particles. Moreover, echinacea extracts can interfere with viral protein synthesis by binding to viral mRNA or the host's ribosomes. This disruption of protein translation is crucial, as it hinders the assembly of new virions, ultimately reducing the viral load within infected cells [151].

7.3. Modulation of Host Immune Response

Echinacea also influences the host's immune response, which is crucial for its antiviral effectiveness. The plant's compounds can boost the activity of immune cells like macrophages, dendritic cells, and natural killer cells, all of which play vital roles in identifying and eliminating virus-infected cells [152]. Alkamides, caffeic acid derivatives, and polysaccharides found in echinacea activate these immune cells, enhancing their capacity to detect and destroy infected cells early in the infection process [153]. Moreover, echinacea compounds stimulate the production of cytokines, particularly interferons, which are key signaling molecules involved in antiviral defense. Interferons induce an antiviral state in nearby cells and strengthen the adaptive immune system, making it more effective in fighting viral infections [154].

7.4. Antioxidant and Anti-Inflammatory Effects

Echinacea's antiviral effects are also supported by its antioxidant and anti-inflammatory properties. Viral infections often trigger oxidative stress, which can result in damage to host cells and tissues [155]. Polyphenols, such as chicoric acid and rosmarinic acid, possess potent antioxidant capabilities, helping to neutralize reactive oxygen species and mitigate oxidative stress, thereby protecting host cells from harm [156]. This protective action not only aids the immune system but also strengthens the body's capacity to fend off viral infections [156]. Beyond their antioxidant properties, echinacea compounds have notable anti-inflammatory effects, which are especially beneficial during viral infections. Excessive inflammation can be harmful and lead to tissue damage. Polyphenols like flavonoids and caffeic acid derivatives can suppress the production of pro-inflammatory cytokines, such as TNF-alpha and IL-6, along with enzymes like cyclooxygenase-2, thus helping to regulate the inflammatory response [157]. By controlling inflammation, echinacea promotes a balanced immune reaction, enabling viral clearance while minimizing tissue damage [157].

7.5. Inhibition of Virus Release

Echinacea can inhibit the release of viruses from infected cells, a critical step in the viral life cycle that allows the infection to propagate [158]. Some studies indicate that echinacea compounds disrupt the later stages of viral replication, particularly the assembly and release of new viral particles [159]. This interference may result from interactions between polyphenols and viral proteins or host cell membranes, preventing the formation of mature virions or hindering their ability to bud off from the host cell surface [160]. By blocking these processes, echinacea helps to limit viral spread within the host, enhancing its overall antiviral effectiveness.

8. Immunomodulatory Activity

The term "immunomodulatory" is increasingly seen as more appropriate than "immunostimulatory" to describe echinacea's immunological effects, although the latter remains widely used in earlier scientific discussions on the plant [161]. It has been suggested that broadly stimulating the highly complex immune system may not always be beneficial, as some immune responses can be detrimental [162]. Numerous studies, both in vitro and in vivo, have explored the immunological effects of various echinacea preparations, covering different species, plant parts, and extraction methods. Collectively, the findings suggest that echinacea preparations do impact certain immune functions, though there is no consensus on which specific preparations have the strongest effects [163]. Enhanced macrophage function has been observed in response to different echinacea formulations, as demonstrated by in vitro and in vivo studies using methods like the carbon-clearance test and cytokine measurement to assess macrophage activity [164]. In vitro studies on human macrophages found that fresh-pressed juice and dried juice from the aerial parts of *E. purpurea* stimulated the production of cytokines such as interleukin (IL)-1, IL-10, and tumor necrosis factor (TNF-α) [165].

Other research has reported that purified polysaccharides from *E. purpurea* triggered macrophages to produce IL-1 [166], while an arabinogalactan polysaccharide, isolated from *E. purpurea* plant cell cultures, was found to induce the production of TNF-α and interferon-2 in murine macrophages [167]. Polysaccharides from *E. purpurea* plant cell cultures have also been previously shown to exhibit immunological activity in vitro [168]. In another series of in vitro experiments, *E. purpurea* promoted macrophage activation, as indicated by TNF-α production, following simulated digestion (incubation with gastric fluid) to replicate the potential effects of oral consumption [169]. Further studies demonstrated that *E. purpurea* dry root powder (containing 1.5% total polyphenols, calculated as chlorogenic acid) enhanced the resistance of splenic lymphocytes to apoptosis. This effect was seen in splenic lymphocytes from mice that received the echinacea preparation orally at doses of 30 or 100 mg/kg daily for 14 days [170].

In an in vitro study, peripheral blood mononuclear cells from healthy individuals, as well as from patients with chronic fatigue syndrome, were exposed to increasing concentrations of *E. purpurea* extracts, which resulted in enhanced natural killer cell function [171]. Similarly, in vivo studies have shown that oral administration of *E. purpurea* root extract increases natural killer cell numbers in normal [172], leukemic [173], and aging mice [174]. A subsequent in-vivo study using a randomized, double-blind design examined the effects of an echinacea supplement (Nature's Resource; CVS Pharmacy, USA; containing 1.05 g of echinacea aerial parts and 10.5 mg of chicoric acid) in 16 aging male rats [175]. The animals received 50 mg/kg body weight of echinacea (potentially *E. purpurea*), equivalent to 0.5 mg/kg of chicoric acid, or a placebo administered in peanut butter daily for 8 weeks. During the first two weeks, echinacea-treated rats showed significantly higher mean circulating white blood cell counts compared to the control group ($p < 0.05$) [176]. IL-2 concentrations were significantly higher in the echinacea group compared to the control for the last five weeks of the study (P<0.05). Additionally, differential white cell counts changed markedly over the 8 weeks: lymphocyte and monocyte levels increased, while neutrophil and eosinophil levels decreased in the echinacea group compared to placebo [177].

No changes in the phagocytic activity of circulating leukocytes, measured by their ability to ingest latex particles, were observed in either group. Other in-vivo studies in rats demonstrated that water-ethanol extracts of *E. purpurea* roots and aerial parts, containing chicoric acid, polysaccharides, and alkamides, increased macrophage phagocytic activity, with greater concentrations of these components leading to enhanced activity [178]. Moreover, spleen macrophages from echinacea-treated rats displayed increased nitric oxide release when stimulated with lipopolysaccharide. In a similar experiment, alkamides were shown to stimulate alveolar macrophage function in healthy rats [179].

A proprietary preparation combining *E. purpurea* root extract and licorice root extract [180] has been found to stimulate phagocytosis both in vitro and in vivo, as evidenced by the carbon-clearance test following oral administration in mice [181] (Figure 6). This combination demonstrated a more potent immunostimulatory effect compared to either extract used independently. Another blend, consisting of aqueous ethanol extracts from *E. purpurea* and *E. pallida* roots, *Baptisia tinctoria* root, and *Thuja occidentalis* herb, was administered orally to mice through their diet or drinking water for 7 days, resulting in an enhanced antibody response to sheep red blood cells [182]. However, despite the substantial research supporting the immunostimulatory properties of echinacea preparations, some recent studies have reported no such effects [183]. For example, no evidence of natural killer cell activity or antibody production was observed in studies where rats were fed various echinacea formulations, including alcoholic extracts of *E. purpurea* root and alcoholic extracts of the roots of *E. angustifolia*, *E. purpurea*, and *E. pallida*, in their diet [184].

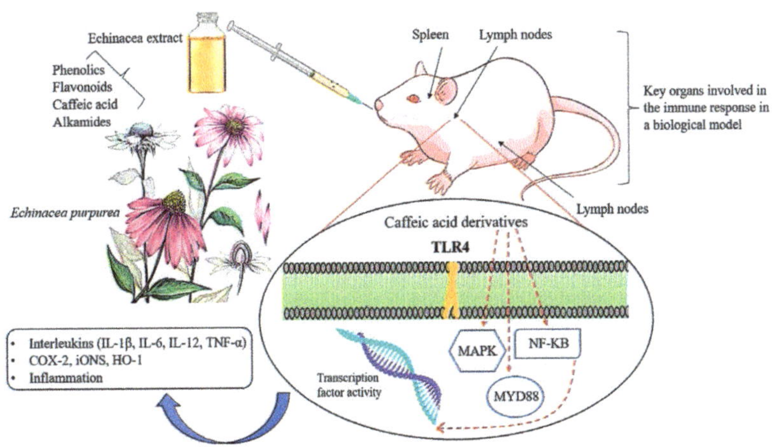

Figure 6. A schematic representation of the main molecular pathways linked to inflammatory and immunomodulatory activities modulated by echinacea. The solid red line indicates the pathway's activation, whereas the truncated red line indicates inhibition of the pathway. TLR-4: Toll-like Receptor-4; MyD88: Myeloid Differentiation Primary Response 88; NF-KB: Nuclear Factor kappa B; MAPK: Mitogen-Activated Protein Kinase; COX-2: cyclooxygenase-2; iNOS: inducible Nitric Oxide Synthase; HO-1: Heme Oxygenase-1; IL: Interleukin; TNF: Tumor Necrosis Factor (Figure drawn by F. Ahmadi).

9. Conclusions and Future Perspective on Echinacea Research

Echinacea's phenolic and flavonoid compounds, including caffeic acid derivatives and alkamides, are known for their antimicrobial properties [185]. Studies have shown that the phytochemicals in *E. purpurea* significantly reduce inflammatory swelling in mice and rats and lower blood levels of cytokines such as IL-2, IL-6, and TNF-α [186]. These effects are similarly observed with the administration of alkylamides in animal models. With continued research and the establishment of standardized extraction methods, echinacea extract has the potential to become a successful product line in the echinacea industry [187]. Currently, echinacea is predominantly marketed in the US as an immune-boosting supplement [188]. Echinacea alkylamides have been shown to disrupt bacterial cell walls and membranes, with one structural class, the diynoic alkylamides, demonstrating the greatest cell wall disruption [189,190]. The natural variation in phytochemical profiles across echinacea species provides the opportunity to selectively propagate cultivars with unique metabolic profiles for specific purposes, such as producing antimicrobial compounds. Alternatively, echinacea cultivars could be bred to increase the production of caffeic acid derivatives in the flowers, which could be used in dietary supplements. Roots and flowers rich in alkylamides and chicoric acid could be used to produce antibacterial face washes, shampoos, or creams. Although echinacea, like other members of the Asteraceae family, contains some phototoxic polyacetylene compounds, these are unstable and can be easily deactivated by minimal processing [187]. Additionally, the leaves of echinacea, which are rich in vitamin C and phenolic compounds, could be marketed as natural health products. However, the full potential of echinacea's diverse applications remains largely untapped. The development of new biotechnologies presents significant opportunities for improving echinacea-based products [190,191]. Moving forward, it is important to weigh the benefits and drawbacks of different approaches, such as improving yields, optimizing phytochemical profiles, enhancing propagation efficiency, managing costs, addressing public perception, and ensuring scalability. A combination of tissue culture, chemical treatments, and traditional field cultivation will likely be used to achieve higher production standards and improved phytochemical quality. These advancements will allow the industry to expand the range of echinacea products and meet the growing market demand.

Funding: This research received no external funding or grants.

Data Availability Statement: Data are available upon request.

Conflicts of Interest: The author declares no conflicts of interest.

References

1. Ahmadi, F.; Kariman, K.; Mousavi, M.; Rengel, Z. Echinacea: Bioactive compounds and agronomy. *Plants* **2024**, *13*, 1235. [CrossRef] [PubMed]
2. Xu, W.; Zhu, H.; Hu, B.; Cheng, Y.; Guo, Y.; Yao, W.; Qian, H. Echinacea in hepatopathy: A review of its phytochemistry, pharmacology, and safety. *Phytomedicine* **2021**, *87*, 153572. [CrossRef] [PubMed]
3. Kligler, B. Echinacea. *Am. Fam. Physician* **2003**, *67*, 77–80. [PubMed]
4. Manayi, A.; Vazirian, M.; Saeidnia, S. *Echinacea purpurea*: Pharmacology, phytochemistry and analysis methods. *Pharmacogn. Rev.* **2015**, *9*, 63.
5. Karg, C.A.; Wang, P.; Vollmar, A.M.; Moser, S. Re-opening the stage for Echinacea research-Characterization of phylloxanthobilins as a novel anti-oxidative compound class in *Echinacea purpurea*. *Phytomedicine* **2019**, *60*, 152969. [CrossRef] [PubMed]
6. Miroshina, T.; Poznyakovskiy, V. *Echinacea purpurea* as a medicinal plant: Characteristics, use as a biologically active component of feed additives and specialized foods. *E3S Web Conf.* **2023**, *380*, 01005. [CrossRef]
7. Ng, J.Y.; Chiong, J.D.; Liu, M.Y.M.; Pang, K.K. Characteristics of the *Echinacea* spp. research literature: A bibliometric analysis. *Eur. J. Integr. Med.* **2023**, *57*, 102216. [CrossRef]
8. Hanifah, W.N.; Yunus, A.; Widiyastuti, Y. Morphological, agronomic characteristics, and flavonoid content of *Echinacea purpurea* at various gamma ray doses. *Bulg. J. Agric. Sci.* **2024**, *30*, 451.
9. Freeman, C.; Spelman, K. A critical evaluation of drug interactions with *Echinacea* spp. *Mol. Nut. Food Res.* **2008**, *52*, 789–798. [CrossRef]
10. Kakouri, E.; Talebi, M.; Tarantilis, P.A. *Echinacea* spp.: The cold-fighter herbal remedy? *Pharmacol. Res.-Mod. Chin. Med.* **2024**, *10*, 100397. [CrossRef]
11. Saema, S.; Shaheen, N.; Pandey, V. Immunostimulatory properties of *Echinacea purpurea* and conservation strategy. In *Plants for Immunity and Conservation Strategies*; Springer Nature: Singapore, 2023; pp. 153–168.
12. Petrova, A.; Ognyanov, M.; Petkova, N.; Denev, P. Phytochemical characterization of purple coneflower roots (*Echinacea purpurea* (L.) Moench.) and their extracts. *Molecules* **2023**, *28*, 3956. [CrossRef]

13. İduğ, T. Herbal food supplements usage awareness of university students: Example of *Echinacea* and St. John's Wort. *Int. J. Agric. Environ. Food Sci.* **2023**, *7*, 792–797. [CrossRef]
14. Toselli, F.; Matthias, A.; Gillam, E.M. Echinacea metabolism and drug interactions: The case for standardization of a complementary medicine. *Life Sci.* **2009**, *85*, 97–106. [CrossRef] [PubMed]
15. Williams, M.; Jenks, A.; Brinckmann, J. Echinacea purpurea. *HerbalGram* **2023**, *138*, 13569.
16. Shahrajabian, M.H.; Sun, W. Seed biology and pharmacological benefits of fennel, lavender, thyme, and echinacea Species. *Seeds* **2023**, *2*, 290–308. [CrossRef]
17. Kesar, V.; Ahmad, J.; Odin, J.; Kesar, V. Echinacea-induced acute hepatitis transitioning to autoimmune hepatitis. *J. Am. Coll. Gastroenterol. ACG* **2015**, *110*, S397. [CrossRef]
18. Missenda, M.; Morris, D.; Nault, D. Herbal supplement Use for evidence-based indications in US aadults: An analysis of national survey data. *J. Integr. Complement. Med.* **2023**, *29*, 584–591. [CrossRef]
19. Ghutke, T.D.; Parvin, K.; Rashida Banu, A.M.; Bansal, S.; Srivastava, A.; Rout, S.; Ramzan, U. A comprehensive review on the therapeutic properties of medicinal plants. *Acta Tradit. Med.* **2023**, *V2i01*, 13–18.
20. Chaughule, R.S.; Barve, R.S. Role of herbal medicines in the treatment of infectious diseases. *Vegetos* **2024**, *37*, 41–51. [CrossRef]
21. Imtiaz, I.; Schloss, J.; Bugarcic, A. Traditional and contemporary herbal medicines in management of cancer: A scoping review. *J. Ayurveda Integr. Med.* **2024**, *15*, 100904. [CrossRef]
22. Ahmadi, F.; Samadi, A.; Sepehr, E.; Rahimi, A.; Shabala, S. Morphological, phytochemical, and essential oil changes induced by different nitrogen supply forms and salinity stress in *Echinacea purpurea* L. *Biocatal. Agric. Biotechnol.* **2022**, *43*, 13932. [CrossRef]
23. Ahmadi, F.; Samadi, A.; Rahimi, A. Improving morphological properties and phytochemical compounds of *Echinacea purpurea* (L.) medicinal plant using novel nitrogen slow-release fertilizer under greenhouse conditions. *Sci. Rep.* **2020**, *10*, 13842. [CrossRef] [PubMed]
24. Ahmadi, F.; Samadi, A.; Sepehr, E.; Rahimi, A.; Shabala, S. Perlite particle size and NO_3^-/NH_4^+ ratio affect the growth and chemical composition of purple coneflower (*Echinacea purpurea* L.) in hydroponics. *Ind. Crops Prod.* **2021**, *162*, 113285. [CrossRef]
25. Micheli, L.; Maggini, V.; Ciampi, C.; Gallo, E.; Bogani, P.; Fani, R.; Firenzuoli, F. *Echinacea purpurea* against neuropathic pain: Alkamides versus polyphenols efficacy. *Phytother. Res.* **2023**, *37*, 1911–1923. [CrossRef] [PubMed]
26. Vieira, S.F.; Fonseca-Rodrigues, D.; Mendanha, D.; Castro, V.I.B.; Pires, R.A.; Reis, R.L.; Pinto-Ribeiro, F. *Echinacea purpurea* roots extracts. *Plant-Deriv. Bioact. Compd. Inflamm. Dis.* **2023**, *447*, 56–63.
27. AghaAlikhani, M.; Iranpour, A.; Naghdi Badi, H. Changes in agronomical and phytochemical yield of purple coneflower (*Echinacea purpurea* (L.) moench) under urea and three biofertilizers application. *J. Med. Plants* **2013**, *12*, 121–136.
28. Chopra, H.; Bibi, S.; Gupta, S.K.; Hasan, M.M.; Zeb, M.A.; Khan, M.S.; Yousafi, Q. Alkamides as metabolites in plants. In *Strigolactones, Alkamides and Karrikins in Plants*; CRC Press: Boca Raton, FL, USA, 2023; pp. 177–193.
29. Cai, F.; Wang, C. Comprehensive review of the phytochemistry, pharmacology, pharmacokinetics, and toxicology of alkamides (2016–2022). *Phytochemistry* **2024**, *220*, 114006. [CrossRef]
30. Lee, S.K.; Lee, D.R.; Kim, H.L.; Choi, B.K.; Kwon, K.B. A randomized, double-blind, placebo-controlled study on immune improvement effects of ethanolic extract of *Echinacea purpurea* (L.) Moench in Korean adults. *Phytother. Res.* **2024**, *5*, 38–45. [CrossRef]
31. Jose, A.; Karthika, C.; Athira, K.V.; Rahman, M.H.; Sweilam, S.H. Pharmacological potential of plant-derived alkylamides. In *Strigolactones, Alkamides and Karrikins in Plants*; CRC Press: Boca Raton, FL, USA, 2023; pp. 195–205.
32. Wang, W.; Jiang, S.; Zhao, Y.; Zhu, G. Echinacoside: A promising active natural products and pharmacological agents. *Pharmacol. Res.* **2023**, *197*, 106951. [CrossRef]
33. Vergun, O.; Svydenko, L.; Shymanska, O.; Hlushchenko, L.; Sedlačková, V.H.; Ivanišová, E.; Brindza, J. Accumulation of total content of polyphenol compounds and antioxidant activity of Echinacea moench species. *Agrobiodivers. Improv. Nutr. Health Life Qual.* **2024**, *8*, 63–71. [CrossRef]
34. Karadağ, A.E.; Baydar, R.; Kırcı, D. Phytochemical quality analysis of commercial preparations containing *Echinacea purpurea*. *Eur. J. Life Sci.* **2024**, *3*, 45–54. [CrossRef]
35. Choirunnisa, J.P.; Widiyastuti, Y.; Sakya, A.T.; Yunus, A. Morphological characteristics and flavonoid accumulation of Echinacea purpurea cultivated at various salinity. *Biodiversitas: J. Biol. Divers.* **2021**, *22*, 156–163. [CrossRef]
36. Clifford, L.J.; Nair, M.G.; Rana, J.; Dewitt, D.L. Bioactivity of alkamides isolated from *Echinacea purpurea* (L.) Moench. *Phytomedicine* **2002**, *9*, 249–253. [CrossRef] [PubMed]
37. Coelho, J.; Barros, L.; Dias, M.I.; Finimundy, T.C.; Amaral, J.S.; Alves, M.J.; Ferreira, I.C. *Echinacea purpurea* (L.) Moench: Chemical characterization and bioactivity of its extracts and fractions. *Pharmaceuticals* **2020**, *13*, 125. [CrossRef] [PubMed]
38. Dennehy, C. Need for additional, specific information in studies with Echinacea. *Antimicrob. Agents Chemother.* **2001**, *45*, 369–370. [CrossRef]
39. Soltanbeigi, A.; Maral, H. Agronomic yield and essential oil properties of purple coneflower (*Echinacea purpurea* L. Moench) with different nutrient applications. *Chil. J. Agric. Anim. Sci.* **2022**, *38*, 164–175. [CrossRef]
40. Maggini, V.; Bandeira Reidel, R.V.; De Leo, M.; Mengoni, A.; Rosaria Gallo, E.; Miceli, E.; Pistelli, L. Volatile profile of *Echinacea purpurea* plants after in vitro endophyte infection. *Nat. Prod. Res.* **2020**, *34*, 2232–2237. [CrossRef]
41. Rousseaux, C.G. Herbal remedies. In *Haschek and Rousseaux's Handbook of Toxicologic Pathology*; Academic Press: Cambridge, MA, USA, 2023; pp. 183–303.

42. Pretorius, T.R.; Charest, C.; Kimpe, L.E.; Blais, J.M. The accumulation of metals, PAHs, and alkyl PAHs in the roots of *Echinacea purpurea*. *PLoS ONE* **2018**, *13*, e0208325. [CrossRef]
43. Harborne, J.B.; Williams, C.A. Phytochemistry of the genus Echinacea. In *Echinacea*; CRC Press: Boca Raton, FL, USA, 2004; pp. 71–88.
44. Mirjalili, M.H.; Salehi, P.; Badi, H.N.; Sonboli, A. Volatile constituents of the flowerheads of three Echinacea species cultivated in Iran. *Flavour Fragr. J.* **2006**, *21*, 355–358. [CrossRef]
45. Woelkart, K.; Xu, W.; Pei, Y.; Makriyannis, A.; Picone, R.P.; Bauer, R. The endocannabinoid system as a target for alkamides from *Echinacea angustifolia* roots. *Planta Medica* **2005**, *71*, 701–705. [CrossRef]
46. Perry, N.B.; Wills, R.B.; Stuart, D.L. Factors affecting echinacea quality: Agronomy and processing. In *Echinacea*; CRC Press: Boca Raton, FL, USA, 2004; pp. 127–142.
47. Cozzolino, R.; Malvagna, P.; Spina, E.; Giori, A.; Fuzzati, N.; Anelli, A.; Impallomeni, G. Structural analysis of the polysaccharides from *Echinacea angustifolia* radix. *Carbohydr. Polym.* **2006**, *65*, 263–272. [CrossRef]
48. Bone, K. Echinacea: What makes it work. *Altern. Med. Rev.* **1997**, *2*, 87–93.
49. Melchart, D.; Clemm, C.; Weber, B.; Draczynski, T.; Worku, F.; Linde, K.; Saller, R. Polysaccharides isolated from *Echinacea purpurea* herba cell cultures to counteract undesired effects of chemotherapy—A pilot study. *Phytother. Res. Int. J. Devoted Pharmacol. Toxicol. Eval. Nat. Prod. Deriv.* **2002**, *16*, 138–142. [CrossRef] [PubMed]
50. Lee, T.T.; Huang, C.C.; Shieh, X.H.; Chen, C.L.; Chen, L.J.; Yu, B.I. Flavonoid, phenol and polysaccharide contents of *Echinacea purpurea* L. and its immunostimulant capacity in vitro. *Int. J. Environ. Sci. Dev.* **2010**, *1*, 5. [CrossRef]
51. Li, Q.; Yang, F.; Hou, R.; Huang, T.; Hao, Z. Post-screening characterization of an acidic polysaccharide from *Echinacea purpurea* with potent anti-inflammatory properties in vivo. *Food Funct.* **2020**, *11*, 7576–7583. [CrossRef]
52. Roesler, J.; Steinmüller, C.; Kiderlen, A.; Emmendörffer, A.; Wagner, H.; Lohmann-Matthes, M.L. Application of purified polysaccharides from cell cultures of the plant *Echinacea purpurea* to mice mediates protection against systemic infections with Listeria monocytogenes and Candida albicans. *Int. J. Immunopharmacol.* **1991**, *13*, 27–37. [CrossRef]
53. Raso, G.M.; Pacilio, M.; Di Carlo, G.; Esposito, E.; Pinto, L.; Meli, R. In-vivo and in-vitro anti-inflammatory effect of *Echinacea purpurea* and *Hypericum perforatum*. *J. Pharm Pharmacol.* **2002**, *54*, 1379–1383. [CrossRef] [PubMed]
54. Wang, X.; Shi, Q.; Zhang, Y.; Gao, G.; Shen, P.; Gao, G.; Wu, N. Effects of *Echinacea purpurea* polysaccharide on IEC-6 cell proliferation. *Agric. Sci. Technol.* **2014**, *15*, 1876.
55. Schöllhorn, C.; Schecklies, E.; Wagner, H. Immunochemical investigations of polysaccharides from *Echinacea purpurea* cell suspension cultures. *Planta Medica* **1993**, *59*, A662–A663. [CrossRef]
56. Lee, J. Caffeic acid derivatives in dried *Lamiaceae* and *Echinacea purpurea* products. *J. Funct. Foods* **2010**, *2*, 158–162. [CrossRef]
57. Kim, H.O.; Durance, T.D.; Scaman, C.H.; Kitts, D.D. Retention of caffeic acid derivatives in dried *Echinacea purpurea*. *J. Agric. Food Chem.* **2000**, *48*, 4182–4186. [CrossRef] [PubMed]
58. Tsai, Y.L.; Chiou, S.Y.; Chan, K.C.; Sung, J.M.; Lin, S.D. Caffeic acid derivatives, total phenols, antioxidant and antimutagenic activities of *Echinacea purpurea* flower extracts. *LWT-Food Sci. Technol.* **2012**, *46*, 169–176. [CrossRef]
59. Wu, C.H.; Murthy, H.N.; Hahn, E.J.; Lee, H.L.; Paek, K.Y. Efficient extraction of caffeic acid derivatives from adventitious roots of Echinacea purpurea. *Czech J. Food Sci.* **2008**, *26*, 254–258. [CrossRef]
60. Erkoyuncu, M.T.; Yorgancilar, M. Optimization of callus cultures at *Echinacea purpurea* L. for the amount of caffeic acid derivatives. *Electron. J. Biotechnol.* **2021**, *51*, 17–27. [CrossRef]
61. Rady, M.R.; Aboul-Enein, A.M.; Ibrahim, M.M. Active compounds and biological activity of in vitro cultures of some *Echinacea purpurea* varieties. *Bull. Natl. Res. Cent.* **2018**, *42*, 1–12. [CrossRef]
62. Paek, K.Y.; Murthy, H.N.; Hahn, E.J. Establishment of adventitious root cultures of *Echinacea purpurea* for the production of caffeic acid derivatives. *Protocols for In Vitro Cult. Second. Metab. Anal. Aromat. Med. Plants* **2009**, *547*, 3–16.
63. Sharifi-Rad, M.; Mnayer, D.; Morais-Braga, M.F.B.; Carneiro, J.N.P.; Bezerra, C.F.; Coutinho, H.D.M.; Sharifi-Rad, J. Echinacea plants as antioxidant and antibacterial agents: From traditional medicine to biotechnological applications. *Phytother. Res.* **2018**, *32*, 1653–1663. [CrossRef]
64. Chiellini, C.; Maida, I.; Maggini, V.; Bosireeman, E.; Mocali, S.; Emiliani, G.; Fani, R. Preliminary data on antibacterial activity of *Echinacea purpurea*-associated bacterial communities against Burkholderia cepacia complex strains, opportunistic pathogens of Cystic Fibrosis patients. *Microbiol. Res.* **2017**, *196*, 34–43. [CrossRef]
65. Zaushintsena, A.V.; Milentyeva, I.; Babich, O.; Noskova, S.Y.; Kiseleva, T.F.; Popova, D.G.; Lukin, A. Quantitative and qualitative profile of biologically active substances extracted from purple echinacea (*Echinacea purpurea* L.) growing in the Kemerovo region: Functional foods application. *Foods Raw Mater.* **2019**, *7*, 84–92. [CrossRef]
66. Burlou-Nagy, C.; Bănică, F.; Negrean, R.A.; Jurca, T.; Vicaș, L.G.; Marian, E.; Pallag, A. Determination of the bioactive compounds from *Echinacea purpurea* (L.) Moench leaves extracts in correlation with the antimicrobial activity and the in vitro wound healing potential. *Molecules* **2023**, *28*, 5711. [CrossRef]
67. Barnes, J.; Anderson, L.A.; Gibbons, S.; Phillipson, J.D. Echinacea species (*Echinacea angustifolia* (DC.) Hell., *Echinacea pallida* (Nutt.) Nutt., *Echinacea purpurea* (L.) Moench): A review of their chemistry, pharmacology and clinical properties. *J. Pharm. Pharmacol.* **2005**, *57*, 929–954. [CrossRef] [PubMed]

68. Aksoy, H.; Arslanoglu, S.; Edbeib, M.; Kaya, Y.; Marakli, S. Antibacterial activity of *Calendula officinalis* and *Echinacea purpurea* extracts against the causal agent of tomatoes' bacterial canker: *Clavibacter michiganensis* subsp. michiganensis. *Boletín Latinoam. Y Del Caribe De Plantas Med. Y Aromáticas* **2021**, *20*, 496–502. [CrossRef]
69. Daley, E. A Phytochemical and Antibacterial Analysis of Echinacea purpurea (L.) Moench throughout Seasonal Development. Doctoral Dissertation, Université d'Ottawa/University of Ottawa, Ottawa, ON, Canada, 2019.
70. Taghizadeh, M.; Jarvandi, S.; Yasa, N. A review of Echinacea. *J. Med. Plants.* **2002**, *1*, 13–26.
71. Vaverková, L.B.P.O.Š. Antimicrobial and antimutagenic activities of extracts from different organs of *Echinacea angustifolia* DC (Asteraceae). *J. Food Nutr. Res.* **2012**, *51*, 201–206.
72. Zazharskyi, V.V.; Davydenko, P.; Kulishenko, O.; Borovik, I.V.; Brygadyrenko, V.V. Antimicrobial activity of 50 plant extracts. *Biosyst. Divers.* **2019**, *27*, 163–169. [CrossRef]
73. Kerem, S.; Özbek, Ö. Antimicrobial activities of some species in Asteraceae and Lamiaceae families from Türkiye. *Int. J. Second. Metab.* **2024**, *11*, 277–291. [CrossRef]
74. Gotti, R.; Pomponio, R.; Bertucci, C.; Cavrini, V. Simultaneous analysis of the lipophilic and hydrophilic markers of Echinacea plant extracts by capillary electrophoresis. *J. Separation Sci.* **2002**, *25*, 1079–1086. [CrossRef]
75. Sharma, S.M.; Anderson, M.; Schoop, S.R.; Hudson, J.B. Bactericidal and anti-inflammatory properties of a standardized Echinacea extract (*Echinaforce*®): Dual actions against respiratory bacteria. *Phytomedicine* **2010**, *17*, 563–568. [CrossRef]
76. Garzoli, S.; Maggio, F.; Vinciguerra, V.; Rossi, C.; Donadu, M.G.; Serio, A. Chemical Characterization and Antimicrobial Properties of the Hydroalcoholic Solution of *Echinacea purpurea* (L.) Moench. and Propolis from Northern Italy. *Molecules* **2023**, *28*, 1380. [CrossRef]
77. Rehman, F.; Sudhaker, M.; Roshan, S.; Khan, A. Antibacterial activity of *Eachinacia angustfolia*. *Pharmacogn. J.* **2012**, *4*, 67–70. [CrossRef]
78. Giles, J.T.; Palat III, C.T.; Chien, S.H.; Chang, Z.G.; Kennedy, D.T. Evaluation of echinacea for treatment of the common cold. *Pharmacotherapy: J. Hum. Pharmacol. Drug Ther.* **2000**, *20*, 690–697. [CrossRef] [PubMed]
79. Currier, N.L.; Miller, S.C. *Echinacea purpurea* and melatonin augment natural-killer cells in leukemic mice and prolong life span. *J. Altern. Complement. Med.* **2001**, *7*, 241–251. [CrossRef] [PubMed]
80. Hobbs, C. *The Echinacea Handbook*; Eclectic Medical Publications: Portland, OR, USA, 1989.
81. Islam, J.; Carter, R. Use of Echinacea in upper respiratory tract infection. *South Med. J.* **2005**, *98*, 311–319. [CrossRef] [PubMed]
82. Jukić, H.; Habeš, S.; Aldžić, A.; Durgo, K.; Kosalec, I. Antioxidant and prooxidant activities of phenolic compounds of the extracts of *Echinacea purpurea* (L.). *Bull. Chem. Technol. Bosnia Herzeg.* **2015**, *44*, 43–52.
83. Lee, M.; Lin, W.; Yu, B.; Lee, T. Antioxidant capacity of phytochemicals and their potential effects on oxidative status in animals—A review. *Asian-Australas. J. Anim. Sci.* **2017**, *30*, 299–308. [CrossRef]
84. Yamada, K.; Hung, P.; Park, T.K.; Park, P.J.; Lim, B.O. A comparison of the immunostimulatory effects of the medicinal herbs Echinacea, Ashwagandha and Brahmi. *J. Ethnopharmacol.* **2011**, *137*, 231–235. [CrossRef]
85. Tan, B.K.; Vanitha, J. Immunomodulatory and antimicrobial effects of some traditional Chinese medicinal herbs: A review. *Curr. Med. Chem.* **2004**, *11*, 1423–1430. [CrossRef]
86. Sabouri, Z.; Barzegar, M.; Sahari, M.; Naghdi Badi, H. Antioxidant and antimicrobial potential of *Echinacea purpurea* extract and its effect on extension of cake shelf life. *J. Med. Plants* **2012**, *3*, 28–40.
87. Pellati, F.; Benvenuti, S.; Magro, L.; Melegari, M.; Soragni, F. Analysis of phenolic compounds and radical scavenging activity of *Echinacea* spp. *J. Pharm. Biomed. Anal.* **2004**, *35*, 289–301. [CrossRef]
88. Pellati, F.; Benvenuti, S.; Melegari, M.; Lasseigne, T. Variability in the composition of anti-oxidant compounds in Echinacea species by HPLC. *Phytochem. Anal.* **2005**, *16*, 77–85. [CrossRef]
89. Hudson, J.B. Applications of the phytomedicine *Echinacea purpurea* (Purple Coneflower) in infectious diseases. *BioMed Res. Int.* **2012**, *2012*, 769896.
90. Cruz, I.; Cheetham, J.J.; Arnason, J.T.; Yack, J.E.; Smith, M.L. Alkamides from Echinacea disrupt the fungal cell wall-membrane complex. *Phytomedicine* **2014**, *21*, 435–442. [CrossRef]
91. Birt, D.F.; Widrlechner, M.P.; LaLone, C.A.; Wu, L.; Bae, J.; Solco, A.K.; Price, J.P. Echinacea in infection. *Am. J. Clin. Nutr.* **2008**, *87*, 488S–492S. [CrossRef] [PubMed]
92. Sullivan, A.M.; Laba, J.G.; Moore, J.A.; Lee, T.D. Echinacea-induced macrophage activation. *Immunopharmacol. Immunotoxicol.* **2008**, *30*, 553–574. [CrossRef] [PubMed]
93. Tierra, M. Echinacea: An effective alternative to antibiotics. *J. Herb. Pharmacother.* **2008**, *7*, 79–89. [CrossRef]
94. Bałan, B.J.; Sokolnicka, I.; SkopińSka-różEwSka, E.; Skopiński, P. The modulatory influence of some Echinacea-based remedies on antibody production and cellular immunity in mice. *Central Eur. J. Immu.* **2016**, *41*, 12–18. [CrossRef]
95. Classen, B. Characterization of an arabinogalactan-protein from suspension culture of *Echinacea purpurea*. *Plant Cell Tissue Organ Cult.* **2007**, *88*, 267–275. [CrossRef]
96. Balciunaite, G.; Juodsnukyte, J.; Savickas, A.; Ragazinskiene, O.; Siatkute, L.; Zvirblyte, G.; Savickiene, N. Fractionation and evaluation of proteins in roots of *Echinacea purpurea* (L.) Moench. *Acta Pharm.* **2015**, *65*, 473–479. [CrossRef]
97. Bossy, A.; Blaschek, W.; Classen, B. Characterization and immunolocalization of arabinogalactan-proteins in roots of *Echinacea Purpurea*. *Planta Medica* **2009**, *75*, 1526–1533. [CrossRef]

98. Gallo, M.; Ferracane, R.; Naviglio, D. Antioxidant addition to prevent lipid and protein oxidation in chicken meat mixed with supercritical extracts of *Echinacea angustifolia*. *J. Supercrit. Fluids* **2012**, *72*, 198–204. [CrossRef]
99. Lim, H.S.; Sohn, E.; Kim, Y.J.; Kim, B.Y.; Kim, J.H.; Jeong, S.J. Ethanol Extract of *Elaeagnus glabra f. oxyphylla* Branches Alleviates the Inflammatory Response Through Suppression of Cyclin D3/Cyclin-Dependent Kinase 11p58 Coupled to Lipopolysaccharide-Activated BV-2 Microglia. *Nat. Prod. Commun.* **2022**, *17*. [CrossRef]
100. Haron, M.H.; Tyler, H.L.; Pugh, N.D.; Moraes, R.M.; Maddox, V.L.; Jackson, C.R.; Pasco, D.S. Activities and prevalence of Proteobacteria members colonizing *Echinacea purpurea* fully account for macrophage activation exhibited by extracts of this botanical. *Planta Medica* **2016**, *82*, 1258–1265. [CrossRef] [PubMed]
101. Maggini, V.; Miceli, E.; Fagorzi, C.; Maida, I.; Fondi, M.; Perrin, E.; Fani, R. Antagonism and antibiotic resistance drive a species-specific plant microbiota differentiation in *Echinacea* spp. *FEMS Microbiol. Ecol.* **2018**, *94*, fiy118. [CrossRef] [PubMed]
102. Vaou, N.; Stavropoulou, E.; Voidarou, C.; Tsigalou, C.; Bezirtzoglou, E. Towards advances in medicinal plant antimicrobial activity: A review study on challenges and future perspectives. *Microorganisms* **2021**, *9*, 2041. [CrossRef] [PubMed]
103. Mir-Rashed, N.; Cruz, I.; Jessulat, M.; Dumontier, M.; Chesnais, C.; Juliana, N.G.; Smith, M.L. Disruption of the fungal cell wall by antifungal Echinacea extracts. *Med. Mycol.* **2010**, *48*, 949–958. [CrossRef]
104. Spelman, K. The extraction, stability, metabolism, and bioactivity of the alkylamides in *Echinacea* spp. *Microbiology* **2009**, *3*, 534–540.
105. Luettig, B.; Steinmüller, C.; Gifford, G.E.; Wagner, H.; Lohmann-Matthes, M.L. Macrophage activation by the polysaccharide arabinogalactan isolated from plant cell cultures of *Echinacea purpurea*. *JNCI J. Natl. Cancer Inst.* **1989**, *81*, 669–675. [CrossRef]
106. Chicca, A.; Pellati, F.; Adinolfi, B.; Matthias, A.; Massarelli, I.; Benvenuti, S.; Nieri, P. Cytotoxic activity of polyacetylenes and polyenes isolated from roots of *Echinacea pallida*. *Br. J. Pharmacol.* **2008**, *153*, 879–885. [CrossRef]
107. Sestáková, H.; Turek, B. Effect of Echinacea on cells involved in disease defense. In *Echinacea*; CRC Press: Boca Raton, FL, USA, 2004; pp. 179–184.
108. Kindscher, K. (Ed.) *Echinacea: Herbal Medicine with a Wild History*; Springer: Cham, Switzerland, 2016.
109. Qu, L.; Chen, Y.; Wang, X.; Scalzo, R.; Davis, J.M. Patterns of variation in alkamides and cichoric acid in roots and aboveground parts of *Echinacea purpurea* (L.) Moench. *HortScience* **2005**, *40*, 1239. [CrossRef]
110. Senchina, D.S.; Martin, A.E.; Buss, J.E.; Kohut, M.L. Effects of Echinacea extracts on macrophage antiviral activities. *Phytother. Res.* **2010**, *24*, 810–816. [CrossRef] [PubMed]
111. Vimalanathan, S.; Kang, L.; Amiguet, V.T.; Livesey, J.; Arnason, J.T.; Hudson, J. *Echinacea purpurea*. aerial parts contain multiple antiviral compounds. *Pharm. Biol.* **2005**, *43*, 740–745. [CrossRef]
112. Wu, L.; Bae, J.; Kraus, G.; Wurtele, E.S. Diacetylenic isobutylamides of Echinacea: Synthesis and natural distribution. *Phytochemistry* **2004**, *65*, 2477–2484. [CrossRef] [PubMed]
113. Signer, J.; Jonsdottir, H.R.; Albrich, W.C.; Strasser, M.; Züst, R.; Ryter, S.; Engler, O.B. In vitro virucidal activity of Echinaforce®, an *Echinacea purpurea* preparation, against coronaviruses, including common cold coronavirus 229E and SARS-CoV-2. *Virol. J.* **2020**, *17*, 1–11. [CrossRef] [PubMed]
114. Mistrikova, I.; Vaverkova, S. Echinacea—Chemical composition, immunostimulatory activities and uses. *Thaiszia J. Bot.* **2006**, *16*, 11–26.
115. Farahani, M. Inhibition of HSV-1 multiplication by five species of medicinal plants. *J. Microbiol. Biotechnol. Food Sci.* **2013**, *3*, 69–71.
116. De Oliveira, J.R.; Antunes, B.S.; do Nascimento, G.O.; Kawall, J.C.D.S.; Oliveira, J.V.B.; Silva, K.G.D.S.; Oliveira, C.R. Antiviral activity of medicinal plant-derived products against SARS-CoV-2. *Exp. Biol. Med.* **2022**, *247*, 1797–1809. [CrossRef]
117. Percaccio, E.; De Angelis, M.; Acquaviva, A.; Nicotra, G.; Ferrante, C.; Mazzanti, G.; Di Sotto, A. ECHOPvir: A Mixture of Echinacea and hop extracts endowed with cytoprotective, immunomodulatory and antiviral properties. *Nutrients* **2023**, *15*, 4380. [CrossRef] [PubMed]
118. Awang, D.V. Immune stimulants and antiviral botanicals: Echinacea and ginseng. Perspectives on new crops and new uses. *ASHS Press Alex.* **1999**, *5*, 450–456.
119. Bergner, P. Antiviral botanicals in herbal medicine. *Med. Herbal.* **2005**, *14*, 1–12.
120. Bruni, R.; Brighenti, V.; Caesar, L.K.; Bertelli, D.; Cech, N.B.; Pellati, F. Analytical methods for the study of bioactive compounds from medicinally used Echinacea species. *J. Pharm. Biomed. Anal.* **2018**, *160*, 443–477. [CrossRef]
121. Aucoin, M.; Cooley, K.; Saunders, P.R.; Carè, J.; Anheyer, D.; Medina, D.N.; Garber, A. The effect of Echinacea spp. on the prevention or treatment of COVID-19 and other respiratory tract infections in humans: A rapid review. *Adv. Int. Med.* **2020**, *7*, 203. [CrossRef] [PubMed]
122. Novika, R.G.; Wahidah, N.J.; Yunus, A.; Sumarno, L.; Ilyas, M.F. Clinical effect of *Echinacea purpurea* as an antiviral and its effect on reproductive hormones. *J. Pharm. Pharmacogn. Res.* **2024**, *12*, 255–263. [CrossRef]
123. Sun, Y.; Li, C.; Liu, Z.; Zeng, W.; Ahmad, M.J.; Zhang, M.; He, Q. Chinese herbal extracts with antiviral activity: Evaluation, mechanisms, and potential for preventing PRV, PEDV and PRRSV infections. *Anim. Dis.* **2023**, *3*, 35. [CrossRef]
124. Turner, R.B.; Bauer, R.; Woelkart, K.; Hulsey, T.C.; Gangemi, J.D. An evaluation of *Echinacea angustifolia* in experimental rhinovirus infections. *N. Engl. J. Med.* **2005**, *353*, 341–348. [CrossRef]
125. Gakhar, A. Anti-viral phyto medicine: A review. *J. Pharmacogn. Phytochem.* **2021**, *10*, 2002–2004. [CrossRef]
126. Kindscher, K. Ethnobotany of purple coneflower (*Echinacea angustifolia*, Asteraceae) and other *Echinacea* species. *Econ. Bot.* **1989**, *43*, 498–507. [CrossRef]

127. Naithani, R.; Mehta, R.G.; Shukla, D.; Chandersekera, S.N.; Moriarty, R.M. Antiviral activity of phytochemicals: A current perspective. In *Dietary Components and Immune Function*; Humana Press: Totowa, NJ, USA, 2010; pp. 421–468.
128. Lelešius, R.; Karpovaitė, A.; Mickienė, R.; Drevinskas, T.; Tiso, N.; Ragažinskienė, O.; Šalomskas, A. In vitro antiviral activity of fifteen plant extracts against avian infectious bronchitis virus. *BMC Vet. Res.* **2019**, *15*, 1–10. [CrossRef]
129. Vimalanathan, S.; Shehata, M.; Sadasivam, K.; Delbue, S.; Dolci, M.; Pariani, E.; D'Alessandro, S.; Pleschka, S. Broad antiviral effects of *Echinacea purpurea* against SARS-CoV-2 variants of concern and potential mechanism of action. *Microorganisms* **2022**, *10*, 2145. [CrossRef]
130. LaLone, C.A.; Hammer, K.D.; Wu, L.; Bae, J.; Leyva, N.; Liu, Y.; Birt, D.F. Echinacea species and alkamides inhibit prostaglandin E2 production in RAW264. 7 mouse macrophage cells. *J. Agric. Food Chem.* **2007**, *55*, 7314–7322. [CrossRef]
131. Foster, S. Herbal Remedies: Echinacea: The Cold and Flu Remedy. *Alter Compl Therapies.* **1995**, *1*, 254–257. [CrossRef]
132. Ogal, M.; Johnston, S.L.; Klein, P.; Schoop, R. Echinacea reduces antibiotic usage in children through respiratory tract infection prevention: A randomized, blinded, controlled clinical trial. *Eur. J. Med. Res.* **2021**, *26*, 1–9. [CrossRef] [PubMed]
133. Ghio, S.; Brincat, J.P.; Cetin, Y.; Lia, F. Antiviral activity of natural compounds extracted from Mediterranean medicinal plants against SARS-CoV-2. *Acad. Biol.* **2024**, *2*, 41–49. [CrossRef]
134. Nicolussi, S.; Ardjomand-Woelkart, K.; Stange, R.; Gancitano, G.; Klein, P.; Ogal, M. Echinacea as a potential force against coronavirus infections? A mini-review of randomized controlled trials in adults and children. *Microorganisms* **2022**, *10*, 211. [CrossRef]
135. Mohamadi, N.; Sharififar, F.; Rameshk, M.; Khandani, S.K. A Global Perspective on Medicinal Plants and Phytochemicals with Antiviral Potentials in the Respiratory System. *Anti-Infect. Agents* **2023**, *21*, 56–78. [CrossRef]
136. Hassan, S.T.; Masarčíková, R.; Berchová, K. Bioactive natural products with anti-herpes simplex virus properties. *J. Pharm. Pharmacol.* **2015**, *67*, 1325–1336. [CrossRef]
137. Wagner, L.; Cramer, H.; Klose, P.; Lauche, R.; Gass, F.; Dobos, G.; Langhorst, J. Herbal medicine for cough: A systematic review and meta-analysis. *Forsch. Komplementärmedizin/Res. Complement. Med.* **2015**, *22*, 359–368. [CrossRef]
138. Sadeek, A.; Abdallah, E. Medicinal Plants with Antiviral Properties to Tackle Covid-19 Pandemic: A Short-Review. *Antivirals* **2021**, *2*, 122–127.
139. Wu, Y.H.; Chen, Y.; Zhuang, A.Q.; Chen, S.M. *Natural Phenolic Acids and Their Derivatives against Human Viral Infections*; InTechOpen: Rijeka, Croatia, 2023.
140. Saifulazmi, N.F.; Rohani, E.R.; Harun, S.; Bunawan, H.; Hamezah, H.S.; Nor Muhammad, N.A.; Sarian, M.N. A review with updated perspectives on the antiviral potentials of traditional medicinal plants and their prospects in antiviral therapy. *Life* **2022**, *12*, 1287. [CrossRef]
141. Hudson, J.; Vimalanathan, S.; Kang, L.; Amiguet, V.T.; Livesey, J.; Arnason, J.T. Characterization of antiviral activities in Echinacea. Root preparations. *Pharm. Biol.* **2005**, *43*, 790–796. [CrossRef]
142. Venu, L.N.; Austin, A. Antiviral efficacy of medicinal plants against respiratory viruses: Respiratory Syncytial Virus (RSV) and Coronavirus (CoV)/COVID 19. *J. Pharmacol.* **2020**, *9*, 281–290. [CrossRef]
143. Ghaemi, A.; Soleimanjahi, H.; Farshbaf Moghaddam, M.; Yazdani, N. Evaluation of antiviral activity of aerial part of *Echinacea purpurea* extract against herpes. *Hakim Res. J.* **2007**, *9*, 59–64.
144. Khan, F.; Bamunuarachchi, N.I.; Tabassum, N.; Kim, Y.M. Caffeic acid and its derivatives: Antimicrobial drugs toward microbial pathogens. *J. Agric. Food Chem.* **2021**, *69*, 2979–3004. [CrossRef] [PubMed]
145. Ghaemi, A.; Soleimanjahi, H.; Gill, P.; Arefian, E.; Soudi, S.; Hassan, Z. *Echinacea purpurea* polysaccharide reduces the latency rate in herpes simplex virus type-1 infections. *Intervirology* **2009**, *52*, 29–34. [CrossRef] [PubMed]
146. Hudson, J.; Vimalanathan, S. Echinacea—A source of potent antivirals for respiratory virus infections. *Pharmaceuticals* **2011**, *4*, 1019–1031. [CrossRef]
147. Vimalanathan, S.; Schoop, R.; Suter, A.; Hudson, J. Prevention of influenza virus-induced bacterial superinfection by standardized *Echinacea purpurea*, via regulation of surface receptor expression in human bronchial epithelial cells. *Virus Res.* **2017**, *233*, 51–59. [CrossRef]
148. Meeran, M.N.; Javed, H.; Sharma, C.; Goyal, S.N.; Kumar, S.; Jha, N.K.; Ojha, S. Can Echinacea be a potential candidate to target immunity, inflammation, and infection-The trinity of coronavirus disease 2019. *Heliyon* **2021**, *7*, 65–72.
149. Sharma, M.; Anderson, S.A.; Schoop, R.; Hudson, J.B. Induction of multiple pro-inflammatory cytokines by respiratory viruses and reversal by standardized Echinacea, a potent antiviral herbal extract. *Antivir. Res.* **2009**, *83*, 165–170. [CrossRef]
150. Pleschka, S.; Stein, M.; Schoop, R.; Hudson, J.B. Anti-viral properties and mode of action of standardized *Echinacea purpurea* extract against highly pathogenic avian influenza virus (H5N1, H7N7) and swine-origin H1N1 (S-OIV). *Virol. J.* **2009**, *6*, 1–9. [CrossRef]
151. Farahani, M. Inhibition of HSV-1 multiplication by aqueous extract of *Echinacea purpurea* root. *J. Mashhad Dent. Sch.* **2015**, *39*, 71–80.
152. Stevenson, L.M.; Matthias, A.; Banbury, L.; Penman, K.G.; Bone, K.M.; Leach, D.; Lehmann, R.P. Modulation of macrophage immune responses by Echinacea. *Molecules* **2005**, *10*, 1279–1285. [CrossRef]
153. Kembuan, G.; Lie, W.; Tumimomor, A. Potential usage of immune modulating supplements of the Echinacea genus for COVID-19 infection. Int. J. Med. Rev. *Case Rep* **2020**, *4*, 2020.
154. Di Sotto, A.; Vitalone, A.; Di Giacomo, S. Plant-derived nutraceuticals and immune system modulation: An evidence-based overview. *Vaccines* **2020**, *8*, 468. [CrossRef] [PubMed]

155. Zhai, Z.; Solco, A.; Wu, L.; Wurtele, E.S.; Kohut, M.L.; Murphy, P.A.; Cunnick, J.E. Echinacea increases arginase activity and has anti-inflammatory properties in RAW 264.7 macrophage cells, indicative of alternative macrophage activation. *J. Ethnopharmacol.* **2009**, *122*, 76–85. [CrossRef] [PubMed]
156. Yu, D.; Yuan, Y.; Jiang, L.; Tai, Y.; Yang, X.; Hu, F.; Xie, Z. Anti-inflammatory effects of essential oil in *Echinacea purpurea* L. *Pak. J. Pharm. Sci.* **2013**, *26*, 403–408.
157. Mohammedsaleh, Z.M.; Aljadani, H.M. *Echinacea purpurea* root extract modulates diabetes-induced renal dysfunction in rats through hypoglycemic, antioxidant, and anti-inflammatory activities. *Med. Sci.* **2021**, *25*, 1033–1043.
158. Dobrange, E.; Peshev, D.; Loedolff, B.; Van den Ende, W. Fructans as immunomodulatory and antiviral agents: The case of Echinacea. *Biomolecules* **2019**, *9*, 615. [CrossRef]
159. Bajrai, L.H.; El-Kafrawy, S.A.; Hassan, A.M.; Tolah, A.M.; Alnahas, R.S.; Sohrab, S.S.; Azhar, E.I. In vitro screening of anti-viral and virucidal effects against SARS-CoV-2 by *Hypericum perforatum* and Echinacea. *Sci. Rep.* **2022**, *12*, 21723. [CrossRef]
160. Lim, T.K.; Lim, T.K. *Echinacea purpurea*. Edible Medicinal and Non-Medicinal Plants. *Flowers* **2014**, *7*, 340–371.
161. Melchart, D.; Linde, K.; Worku, F.; Bauer, R.; Wagner, H. Immunomodulation with Echinacea—A systematic review of controlled clinical trials. *Phytomedicine* **1994**, *1*, 245–254. [CrossRef]
162. Oliveira, B.G.D.; Santos, L.F.F.; Costa, M.C.D.; Bastos, R.W.; Carmo, P.H.F.D.; Santos, D.D.A.; César, I.C. Antimicrobial, and immunomodulatory activities of dried extracts of *Echinacea Purpurea*. *Braz. J. Pharm. Sci.* **2022**, *58*, e21026. [CrossRef]
163. Senchina, D.S.; McCann, D.A.; Asp, J.M.; Johnson, J.A.; Cunnick, J.E.; Kaiser, M.S.; Kohut, M.L. Changes in immunomodulatory properties of *Echinacea* spp. root infusions and tinctures stored at 4 C for four days. *Clin. Chim. Acta* **2005**, *355*, 67–82. [CrossRef] [PubMed]
164. Bone, K. Echinacea: Quality, uses, and immunomodulating activity from a phytotherapist's perspective. In *Echinacea*; CRC Press: Boca Raton, FL, USA, 2004; pp. 219–230.
165. Mahmoud, S.H.; Mahmoud, R.M.; Ashoush, I.S.; Attia, M.Y. Immunomodulatory and antioxidant activity of pomegranate juice incorporated with spirulina and echinacea extracts sweetened by stevioside. *J. Agric. Vet. Sci. (Qassim Univ.)* **2015**, *8*, 161–174.
166. Ibrahim, A.; Saleh, R.; Hassan, A.; Amer, M. Immunomodulatory effect of *Echinacea purpurea* and *Curcuma longa* in rabbits. *Mansoura. Vet. Med. J.* **2020**, *22*, 2.
167. Raduner, S.; Majewska, A.; Chen, J.Z.; Xie, X.Q.; Hamon, J.; Faller, B.; Gertsch, J. Alkylamides from Echinacea are a new class of cannabinomimetics: Cannabinoid type 2 receptor-dependent and-independent immunomodulatory effects. *J. Biol. Chem.* **2006**, *281*, 14192–14206. [CrossRef] [PubMed]
168. Park, S.J.; Lee, M.; Kim, D.; Oh, D.H.; Prasad, K.S.; Eun, S.; Lee, J. *Echinacea purpurea* extract enhances natural killer cell activity in vivo by upregulating MHC II and Th1-type CD4+ T cell responses. *J. Med. Food* **2021**, *24*, 1039–1049. [CrossRef] [PubMed]
169. Matthias, A.; Banbury, L.; Stevenson, L.M.; Bone, K.M.; Leach, D.N.; Lehmann, R.P. Alkylamides from Echinacea modulate induced immune responses in macrophages. *Immunol. Investig.* **2007**, *36*, 117–130. [CrossRef]
170. Coeugniet, E.G.; Elek, E. Immunomodulation with Viscum album and *Echinacea purpurea* extracts. *Oncol. Res. Treat.* **1987**, *10*, 27–33. [CrossRef]
171. Aarland, R.C.; Bañuelos-Hernández, A.E.; Fragoso-Serrano, M.; Sierra-Palacios, E.D.C.; Díaz de León-Sánchez, F.; Pérez-Flores, L.J.; Mendoza-Espinoza, J.A. Studies on phytochemical, antioxidant, anti-inflammatory, hypoglycaemic and antiproliferative activities of *Echinacea purpurea* and *Echinacea angustifolia* extracts. *Pharm. Biol.* **2017**, *55*, 649–656. [CrossRef]
172. Dall'Acqua, S.; Perissutti, B.; Grabnar, I.; Farra, R.; Comar, M.; Agostinis, C.; Voinovich, D. Pharmacokinetics and immunomodulatory effect of lipophilic Echinacea extract formulated in softgel capsules. *Eur. J. Pharm. Biopharm.* **2015**, *97*, 8–14. [CrossRef]
173. Classen, B.; Csávás, M.; Borbás, A.; Dingermann, T.; Zündorf, I. Monoclonal antibodies against an arabinogalactan-protein from pressed juice of *Echinacea purpurea*. *Planta Medica* **2004**, *70*, 861–865. [CrossRef]
174. Zorig, A.; Toko, R.; Sukhbold, E.; Takasugi, M.; Arai, H. *Echinacea purpurea* water extracts suppress the release of chemical mediators from mast cells. *Biosci. Biotechnol. Biochem.* **2021**, *85*, 931–940. [CrossRef] [PubMed]
175. Hou, C.C.; Chen, C.H.; Yang, N.S.; Chen, Y.P.; Lo, C.P.; Wang, S.Y.; Shyur, L.F. Comparative metabolomics approach coupled with cell-and gene-based assays for species classification and anti-inflammatory bioactivity validation of Echinacea plants. *J. Nutr. Biochem.* **2010**, *21*, 1045–1059. [CrossRef] [PubMed]
176. Randolph, R.K.; Gellenbeck, K.; Stonebrook, K.; Brovelli, E.; Qian, Y.; Bankaitis-Davis, D.; Cheronis, J. Regulation of human immune gene expression as influenced by a commercial blended Echinacea product: Preliminary studies. *Exp. Biol. Med.* **2003**, *228*, 1051–1056. [CrossRef] [PubMed]
177. Barnes, J.; Anderson, L.A.; Phillipson, J.D. *Herbal Medicines. A Guide for Healthcare Professionals*, updated CDROM of 2nd ed.; Pharmaceutical Press: London, UK, 2004.
178. Binns, S.E.; Hudson, J.; Merali, S.; Arnason, J.T. Antiviral activity of characterized extracts from *Echinacea* spp. (*Heliantheae*: Asteraceae) against Herpes simplex virus (HSV-1). *Planta Med.* **2002**, *68*, 780–783. [CrossRef] [PubMed]
179. Christakis, D.A.; Lehmann, H.P. Can an herbal preparation of echinacea, propolis, and vitamin C reduce respiratory illnesses in children? *Arch. Pediatr. Adolesc. Med.* **2004**, *158*, 222–224.
180. Cohen, H.A.; Varsano, I.; Kahan, E.; Sarrell, M.; Uziel, Y. Effectiveness of an herbal preparation containing Echinacea, propolis, and vitamin C in preventing respiratory tract infections in children. A randomized, double-blind, placebo-controlled, multicenter study. *Arch. Pediatr. Adolesc. Med.* **2004**, *158*, 217–221. [CrossRef]

181. Grimm, W.; Muller, H.H. A randomized controlled trial of the effect of fluid extract of *Echinacea purpurea* on the incidence and severity of colds and respiratory infections. *Am. J. Med.* **1999**, *106*, 138–143. [CrossRef]
182. Lee, A.N.; Werth, V.P. Activation of autoimmunity following use of immunostimulatory herbal supplements. *Arch. Dermatol* **2004**, *140*, 723–727. [CrossRef]
183. Matthias, A.; Penman, K.G.; Addison, R.S.; Dickinson, R.G.; Bone, K.M.; Lehmann, R.P. Bioavailability and pharmacokinetics of alkylamides from Echinacea. *Int. Congr. Nat. Prod. Res. Phoenix Ariz.* **2004**, *57*, p133.
184. Wichtl, M. (Ed.) *Herbal Drugs and Phytopharmaceuticals. A Handbook for Practice on a Scientific Basis*, 3rd ed.; Medpharm Scientific Publishers: Stuttgart, Germany, 2004.
185. Parsons, J.L.; Cameron, S.I.; Harris, C.S.; Smith, M.L. Echinacea biotechnology: Advances, commercialization, and future considerations. *Pharm. Biol.* **2018**, *56*, 485–494. [CrossRef]
186. Catanzaro, M.; Corsini, E.; Rosini, M.; Racchi, M.; Lanni, C. Immunomodulators inspired by nature: A review on curcumin and echinacea. *Molecules* **2018**, *23*, 2778. [CrossRef] [PubMed]
187. Burlou-Nagy, C.; Bănică, F.; Jurca, T.; Vicaș, L.G.; Marian, E.; Muresan, M.E.; Pallag, A. *Echinacea purpurea* (L.) Moench: Biological and pharmacological properties. A review. *Plants* **2022**, *11*, 1244. [CrossRef] [PubMed]
188. Justus, W.; Hossain, M.F. Echinacea, The Immune-Boosting Potential of Nature's Herbal Remedy: A Systematic Review. *Am. J. Nat. Med. Facts* **2024**, *1*, 1–4.
189. Manohar, K.A.; Shahina, N.N.; Sarkar, B.C.; Shukla, G.; Das, S.; Singh, M.; Chakravarty, S. Ethnomedicinal plants: Medicine and nutrition for future generations. In *Bioprospecting of Ethnomedicinal Plant Resources*; Apple Academic Press: Palm Bay, FL, USA, 2025; pp. 11–34.
190. McNeil, B.K.; Renaud, D.L.; Steele, M.A.; Keunen, A.J.; DeVries, T.J. Effects of *Echinacea purpurea* supplementation on markers of immunity, health, intake, and growth of dairy calves. *J. Dairy Sci.* **2023**, *106*, 4949–4965. [CrossRef] [PubMed]
191. Sperber, S.J.; Shah, L.P.; Gilbert, R.D.; Ritchey, T.W.; Monto, A.S. *Echinacea purpurea* for prevention of experimental rhinovirus colds. *Clin. Infect. Dis.* **2004**, *38*, 1367–1371. [CrossRef]

antibiotics

MDPI

Article

Streptomyces rugosispiralis sp. nov., a Novel Actinobacterium Isolated from Peat Swamp Forest Soil That Produces Ansamycin Derivatives and Nocardamines

Trinset Weeraphan [1], Khomsan Supong [2,*], Paranee Sripreechasak [3], Rumpa Jutakanoke [4], Supalerk Kowinthanaphat [1], Somboon Tanasupawat [1], Pattama Pittayakhajonwut [5] and Wongsakorn Phongsopitanun [1,6,*]

1 Department of Biochemistry and Microbiology, Faculty of Pharmaceutical Sciences, Chulalongkorn University, Bangkok 10330, Thailand; trinset.w@chula.ac.th (T.W.); supalerk.k@pharm.chula.ac.th (S.K.); somboon.t@chula.ac.th (S.T.)

2 Department of Applied Science and Biotechnology, Faculty of Agro-Industrial Technology, Rajamangala University of Technology Tawan-ok, Chantaburi 22210, Thailand

3 Office of Educational Affairs, Faculty of Science, Burapha University, Chonburi 20131, Thailand; paranees@go.buu.ac.th

4 Department of Microbiology and Parasitology, Faculty of Medical Science, Naresuan University, Phitsanulok 65000, Thailand; rumpaj@nu.ac.th

5 National Center for Genetic Engineering and Biotechnology (BIOTEC), National Science and Technology Development Agency (NSTDA), Thailand Science Park, Pathum Thani 12120, Thailand; pattamap@biotec.or.th

6 Natural Products and Nanoparticles Research Units (NP2), Chulalongkorn University, Bangkok 10330, Thailand

* Correspondence: khomsan_su@rmutto.ac.th (K.S.); wongsakorn.p@chula.ac.th (W.P.)

Abstract: Actinomycetes, especially the genus *Streptomyces*, are one of the most promising sources of bioactive natural products. In this study, a novel *Streptomyces* strain, RCU-064^T, was isolated from a soil sample collected from a peat swamp forest in Thailand. Strain RCU-064^T showed the highest 16S rRNA gene sequence similarity (99.06%) with *Streptomyces malaysiensis* NBRC 16446^T. Based on a polyphasic approach, strain RCU-064^T represents a novel species of the genus *Streptomyces*, for which the name *Streptomyces rugosispiralis* sp. nov. is proposed. The chemical isolation of the crude ethyl acetate extracts of the strain led to the isolation of six compounds: (**1**) geldanamycin, (**2**) 17-*O*-demethylgeldanamycin, (**3**) reblastatin, (**4**) 17-demethoxyreblastatin, (**5**) nocardamine, and (**6**) dehydroxynocardamine. These compounds were evaluated for their biological activities. All compounds showed no antimicrobial activity against tested microorganisms used in this study. Compounds (**1**)–(**4**) displayed cytotoxic activity against the NCI-H187 cell line, with IC_{50} values ranging from 0.045–4.250 μg/mL. Cytotoxicity against the MCF-7 cell line was found in compounds (**1**) and (**3**) with IC_{50} values of 3.51 and 1.27 μg/mL, respectively. Compounds (**5**) and (**6**) exhibited cytotoxicity only against Vero cells (IC_{50} of 16.57 μg/mL) and NCI-H187 cells (IC_{50} of 13.96 μg/mL), respectively. These results indicate that peat swamp forest soil remains a promising reservoir of novel actinomycetes capable of producing bioactive natural products.

Keywords: actinomycetota; *Streptomyces*; polyphasic taxonomy; natural products; geldanamycin; nocardamines

1. Introduction

Bioactive metabolites are mostly produced from various genera of actinomycetes, including members of *Streptomyces*, *Actinomadura*, *Nonomuraea*, *Micromonospora*, and *Verrucosispora* [1]. *Streptomyces* is the most important and dominant genus within the actinomycete groups. This genus belongs to the family *Streptomycetaceae*, which have a high G+C content in their DNA and form extensively branched substrate and aerial mycelia that later differentiate into spore chains [2]. *Streptomyces* can be differentiated from closely related genera by the presence of *LL*-diaminopimelic acid (*LL*-DAP) in the cell-wall peptidoglycan, but without diagnostic sugars in a whole-cell hydrolysate [3]. Streptomycetes are widely distributed in nature and can be found everywhere, including in terrestrial soils and marine samples [4,5]. In addition, some *Streptomyces* strains are associated with plants, lichens, and insects [6–8]. Streptomycetes are a major source of bioactive metabolites, with more than 70% of known antibiotics being derived from this genus [1]. Streptomycetes have become very useful in the search for bioactive metabolites because they can produce different chemical core-structures, such as macrolides, polyketides, terpenes, and non-ribosomal peptides [9].

Cancer is one of the leading causes of death. According to the Global Cancer Statistic 2020, it was estimated that in 2020 there were 19.3 million new cancer cases and 10.0 million deaths from cancer [10]. *Streptomyces* species are a source of small-molecule anticancer compounds. According to a genome mining study, the genomes of streptomycetes harbor a variable distribution of antitumor biosynthetic gene clusters (BGCs) and so these bacteria are a promising source of molecules for antitumor drug discovery [9]. Examples of anticancer drugs derived from streptomycetes are actinomycin, bleomycin, and doxorubicin [11].

Peat swamp forests are found mainly in Southeast Asia. These ecosystems represent a unique character, distinct from other soil habitats, in terms of their acidic and waterlogged conditions [12]. Peat swap forest soils harbor a large amount soil microbes and have been recognized as a promising source of new actinobacteria. In the past few decades, several novel actinobacteria, including *Dactylosporangium sucinum*, *Streptomyces actinomycinicus*, and *Nocardia rayongensis*, have been isolated from these ecosystems [13–15]. In this present study, we describe a taxonomic study of the new *Streptomyces* strain RCU-064^T based on a polyphasic approach. The bioactive metabolites produced by the strain were elucidated using column chromatography, including Sephadex LH-20 column and high-performance liquid chromatography (HPLC) for purification of the compound, and nuclear magnetic resonance (NMR) and mass spectral analyses for structure determination. The isolated compounds were analyzed for their (i) cytotoxicity against cell lines derived from oral human epidermoid carcinoma (KB), human breast cancer (MCF-7), and human small cell lung cancer (NCI-H187), (ii) anti-malarial activity against the multidrug-resistant *Plasmodium falciparum* K-1, and (iii) anti-bacterial and anti-fungal activities.

2. Results

2.1. Genomic Feature and Phylogeny

The genome of strain RCU-064^T has been deposited at GenBank under the accession number JANIAA000000000, and is 11,017,810 bp in size with a G+C content of 71.3%. The extracted 16S rRNA gene sequence from the genome was 1524 bp.

Strain RCU-064^T showed the highest 16S rRNA gene sequence (accession number: OQ001562) similarity value of 99.06% with *Streptomyces malaysiensis* NBRC 16446^T. The maximum likelihood (ML) phylogeny based on 16S rRNA gene sequences showed that strain RCU-064^T positioned in the same node with *S. malaysiensis* NBRC 16446^T and *S. samsunensis* M1463^T (Figure 1). The core-gene ML phylogeny exhibited that strain RCU-064^T positioned in the node with *S. malaysiensis* NBRC 16446^T, *S. samsunensis* M1463^T, and *S. melanosporafaciens* DSM 40318^T (Figure 2).

The computed ANIb and ANIm values between RCU-067^T and its closely related type strains range from 89.3% to 90.2% and 92.1% to 91.9%, respectively. Furthermore, the dDDH values between strain RCU-064^T and the closely related type strains fall within the range of 43.2% to 43.8% (Table 1). These ANI and dDDH values are lower than the established thresholds of 95–96% for ANI and 70% for dDDH, which are typically employed to distinguish the species [16]. Therefore, it could be concluded that strain RCU-067^T is the novel species of the genus *Streptomyces*.

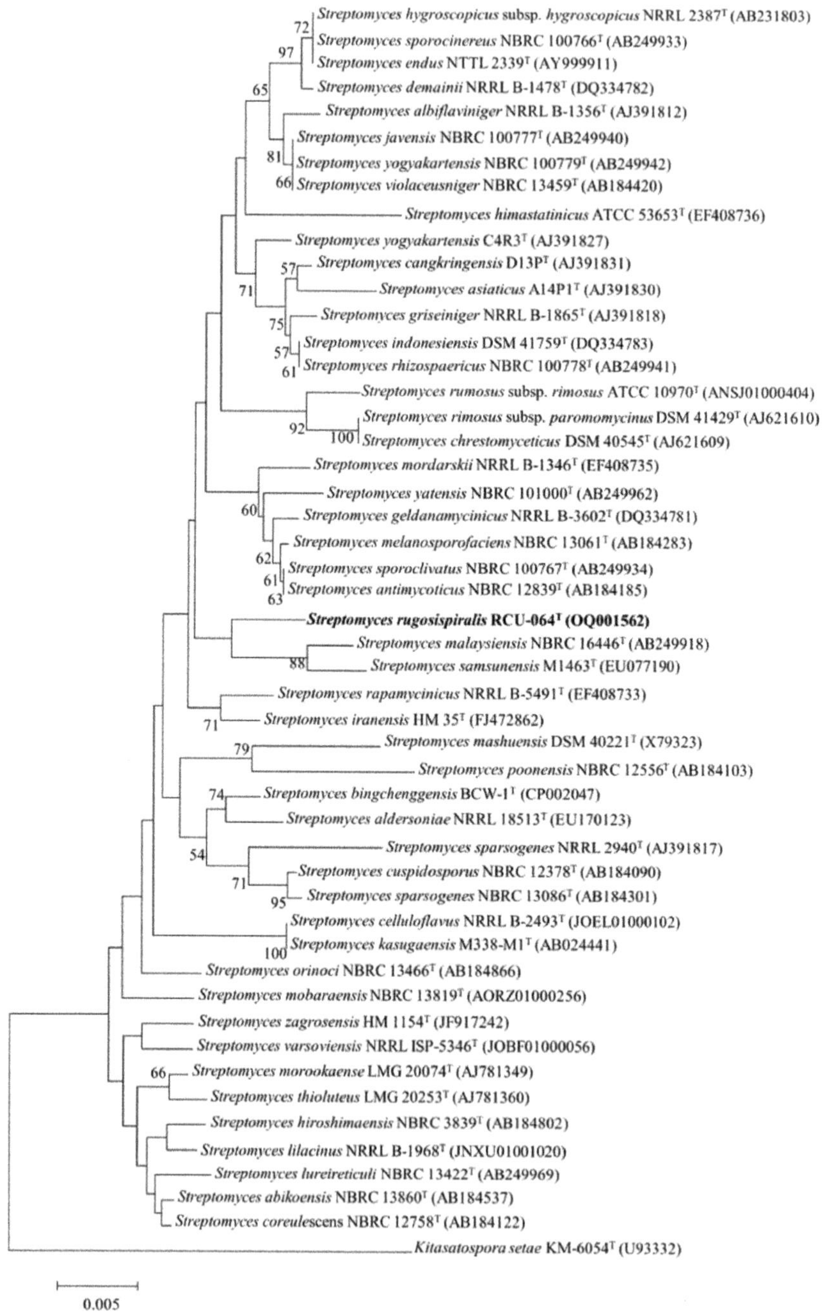

Figure 1. A ML phylogeny based on the 16S rRNA gene sequences of strain RCU-064^T and its closely related *Streptomyces* species. *Kitasatospora setae* KM6054^T was used as an out group. The number at the branch node indicates the bootstrap value (% from 1000 replicates). Only bootstrap values above 50 are shown. Bar, 0.005 substitutions per nucleotides. The bold text shows the position of *Streptomyces rugosispiralis* RCU-064^T in this phylogenetic tree.

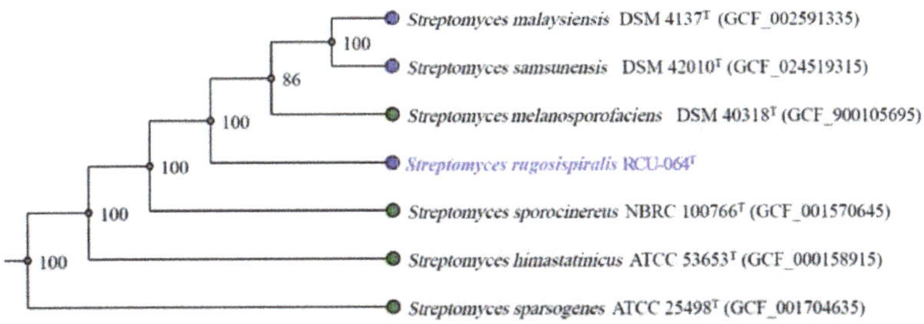

Figure 2. Core-gene ML phylogeny based on the genome of strain RCU-064^T and the closely related *Streptomyces* species. The number on the branch nodes indicate the bootstrap values (% from 1000 replicates). The blue text shows the position of *Streptomyces rugosispiralis* RCU-064^T in this phylogenetic tree.

Table 1. ANIb and ANIm values (%) and the digital DNA-DNA hybridization (dDDH) values between the draft genomes of strain RCU-064^T and its related *Streptomyces* type strains.

Strains	Genome Size (nt)	Accession Number	% GC Content	% dDDH	ANIb	ANIm
RCU-064^T	11017810	GCA_024505145	71.3	-	-	-
S. malaysiensis DSM4137^T	10744231	GCA_002591335	71.1	43.8	90.2	92.1
S. samsunensis DSM 42010^T	11053136	GCF_024519315	70.9	43.5	89.3	92.1
S. melagnosporofaciens DSM 40318^T	10769732	GCA_900105695	71.0	43.2	89.5	91.9

According to the prediction made by the antiSMASH webservice for bacterial BGCs, the genome of strain RCU-064^T contains several BGCs, which encompass non-ribosomal peptide synthases, type 1 polyketide synthases (T1PKS), type 2 polyketide synthases (T2PKS), type 3 polyketide synthases (T3PKS), terpene, siderophore, and aryl polyene as showed in Table 2.

Table 2. The distribution of secondary metabolites biosynthetic gene clusters in the genome of strain RCU-064^T. Only biosynthetic gene clusters with similarity of greater than 50% are shown.

Cluster	Type	Most Similar Known Cluster (Class)	Similarity (%)
1	aryl polyene, ladderane, NRPS, aminocoumarin	Coprisamide C/coprisamide D	95%
2	CDPS	bicyclomycin	100%
3	terpene	pristinol	100
4	NRPS-like, T1PKS	Geldanamycin	69
5	Terpene	2-methylisoborneol	100
6	T1PKS	efomycin K/efomycin L	100
7	T1PKS	ectoine	100
8	NRPS-like	echoside A/echoside B/echosieC/echosideD/echoside E	100
9	T2PKS	spore pigment	83
10	NI-siderophore	Legonoxamine A/desferrioxamine B/legonoxamine B	66
11	Ladderane, aryl polyene	o-dialkylbenzene 1/o-dialkylbenzene 2	61
12	T3PKS, NRPS	feglymycin	84
13	T1PKS	nigericin	63
14	terpene	Hopene	53
15	T1PKS	spirangien O	53

2.2. Chemotaxonomy and Phenotypic Properties of Strain RCU-064^T

The cell wall peptidoglycans of strain RCU-064^T contained LL-DAP and the *N*-acyl type of muramic acid was acetyl. No diagnostic sugars were detected in whole-cell hydrolysates of strain RCU-064^T, with only glucose and ribose being detected. The polar lipids were diphosphatidylglycerol, phosphatidylethanolamine, hydroxy-phosphatidylethanolamine, phosphatidylglycerol, phosphatidylinositol, an unidentified phospholipid, two unidentified glycolipids, and five unidentified lipids. Menaquinones were MK-9(H_2) (10.8%), MK-9(H_4) (24.7%), MK-9(H_6) (54.1%), and MK-9(H_8) (10.4%). The major cellular fatty acids (>4%) were iso-$C_{16:0}$ (21.4%), $C_{16:0}$ (14.4%), anteiso-$C_{15:0}$ (13.0%), iso-$C_{14:0}$ (8.5%), iso-$C_{15:0}$ (8.6%), $C_{17:0}$ cyclo (5.1%), and anteiso-$C_{17:0}$ (4.1%) (Table 3). These chemical composition profiles of strain RCU-064^T exhibited the same pattern as other members of the genus *Streptomyces*.

Table 3. Cellular fatty acid composition of strain RCU-064^T.

Fatty Acid	**RCU-064^T**
Saturated fatty acids	
$C_{14:0}$	2.7
$C_{16:0}$	14.4
$C_{17:0}$ cyclo	5.1
Branched fatty acids	
iso-$C_{14:0}$	8.5
iso-$C_{15:0}$	8.6
anteiso-$C_{15:0}$	13.0
iso-$C_{16:1}$H	3.1
iso-$C_{16:0}$	21.4
iso-$C_{17:0}$	2.3
anteiso-$C_{17:0}$	4.1
Unsaturated fatty acids	
anteiso-$C_{17:1}$ ω9c	2.2
Sum in feature 3 [a]	3.2
Sum in feature 9 [b]	2.5

[a] Summed feature 3 comprised $C_{16:1}$ ω7c and/or $C_{16:1}$ ω6c. [b] Summed feature 8 comprised $C_{16:0}$10-methyl or iso-$C_{17:1}$ ω9c.

Strain RCU-064^T grew well on all tested ISP media. White to grey aerial masses could be observed when grown on ISP2, ISP3, ISP4, ISP5, ISP7, and nutrient agar, but aerial masses were absent on ISP6 (Table 4). The strain did not produce soluble pigment on any agar media used in this study. It produced an extensively branched substrate and aerial mycelia. The mature spore chain was of a spiral type and could be observed on the aerial mycelia (Figure 3A) and the surface of the spores is rugose (Figure 3B). The strain exhibited a positive result for starch hydrolysis but negative results for liquefaction of gelatin, milk peptonization, and nitrate reduction. Growth could be observed at 25–37 °C and at pH 5–9 with an optimum pH of 6–7. No growth was observed at 45 °C. The strain tolerated up to 6% (*w*/*v*) NaCl. The biochemical properties could be used to differentiate strain RCU-064^T from its closely related *Streptomyces* species (Table 5). The details of the biochemical properties and physiology of strain RCU-064^T are summarized in the description of the species.

Table 4. Cultural characteristics of strain RCU-064^T.

Culture Media	**Growth**	**Aerial Masses Color**	**Substrate Mycelia Color**	**Soluble Pigment**
ISP2	Very good	White, light greenish-grey	Dark greenish-yellow	-
ISP3	Very good	White	Dark greenish-yellow	-
ISP4	Good	White, grey	Greyish-yellow	-
ISP5	Good	White	Pale greenish-yellow	-
ISP6	Good	Absent	Greyish-yellow	-
ISP7	Good	White	Greyish-yellow	-
Nutrient agar	Good	White, grey	Greyish-yellow	-

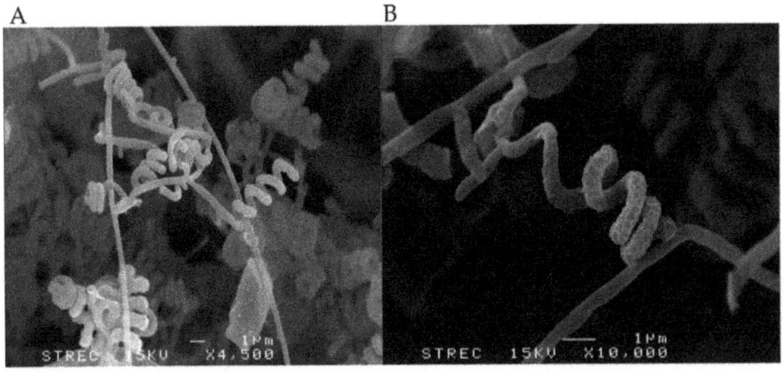

Figure 3. Representative scanning electron micrographs showing the (**A**) spiral spore chains with (**B**) a rugose surface produced by strain RCU-064^T when grown on ISP2 medium for 14 days at 30 °C.

Table 5. Differential characteristics between strain CU-064^T and its closely related *Streptomyces* type strains. * and ** were obtained from [17] and [18], respectively. +, positive; − negative; nd, not determined.

Phenotypic Properties	Strain CU-064^T	*S. malaysiensis* JCM 10672^T	*S. samsunensis* M1463^T *	*S. melanosporofaciens* ISP 5318^T **
Liquefy gelatin	−	+	−	nd
Skim milk peptonization	−	+	nd	nd
Nitrate reduction	−	+	+	nd
NaCl tolerance (% [*w*/*v*])	6%	5%	nd	nd
Carbon utilization of:				
Arabinose	+	+	+	nd
Cellobiose	++	++	+	nd
myo-inositol	+	+	−	+
Salicin	±	+	−	nd
Raffinose	++	+	−	+
Fructose	±	++	+	+
Sucrose	−	−	−	−

2.3. Description of Streptomyces rugosispiralis sp. nov.

Streptomyces rugospiralis (ru.go.si.spi.ra'lis. L. masc. adj. *rugosus*, wrinkled; N.L. masc. adj. *spiralis*, coiled; N.L. masc. adj. *rugosispiralis*, wrinkled and coiled), are Gram-positive, aerobic, mesophilic, filamentous actinomycetes that produce an extensively branched substrate and aerial mycelia. They grow well on ISP2, ISP3, ISP4, ISP5, ISP6, ISP7, and nutrient agar. White to grey aerial masses can be observed when grown on ISP2, ISP3, ISP4, ISP5, ISP7, and nutrient agar, but not on ISP6. The substrate mycelia are dark greenish-yellow to pale greenish-yellow. Type strain does not produce any soluble pigment. Spiral spore chains are produced on the aerial mycelia. The spore surface is rugose. Growth occurs at pH 5–9, with an optimum pH of 6–7, and temperature of 5–37 °C. No growth is observed at 45 °C. Tolerates the presence of NaCl up to 6% (*w*/*v*). Hydrolysis of starch is positive but liquefaction of gelatin, nitrate reduction, and skim milk peptonization are negative. Type strain utilizes arabinose, *myo*-inositol, raffinose, cellobiose, galactose, and rhamnose, and weakly utilizes salicin and fructose, as a sole carbon source but does not utilize ribose and sucrose.

Enzymatic activities for alkaline phosphatase, leucine arylamidase, leucine arylamidase, α-chymotrypsin, acid phosphatase, napthol-AS-BI-phosphohydrolase, and *N*-acetyl-β-glucosaminidase are positive. Weakly positive for esterase (C4), esterase lipase (C8), cystine arylamidase, trypsin, napthol-AS-BI-phosphohydrolase, and α-glucosidase. Type strain shows negative enzyme activities for lipase (C14), α-galactosidase, and α-mannosidase.

Cell wall contains LL-DAP. *N*-acyl type of muramic acid is acetyl. The polar lipids are diphosphatidylglycerol, phosphatidylethanolamine, hydroxy-phosphatidylethanolamine, phosphatidylglycerol, phosphatidylinositol, an unidentified phospholipid, two unidentified glycolipids, and five unidentified lipids. Menaquinones are MK-9(H_2), MK-9(H_4), MK-9(H_6), and MK-9(H_8). The major cellular fatty acids are iso-$C_{16:0}$, $C_{16:0}$, anteiso-$C_{15:0}$, iso-$C_{14:0}$, iso-$C_{15:0}$, $C_{17:0}$ cyclo, and anteiso-$C_{17:0}$. Type strain RCU-064^T (=TBRC 16203^T, = NBRC 115861^T) was isolated from soil collected from Nong Jun Rung peat swamp forest, Rayong province, Thailand. The in silico DNA G+C content of the type strain is 71.3% mol%.

2.4. Isolation and Structure Elucidation of Metabolites

The crude extract of strain RCU-064^T was isolated and enriched by Sephadex-LH20, and HPLC column chromatographic techniques to give six compounds (Figure 4). The chemical structure of compounds (**1**)–(**6**) are shown in Figure 5.

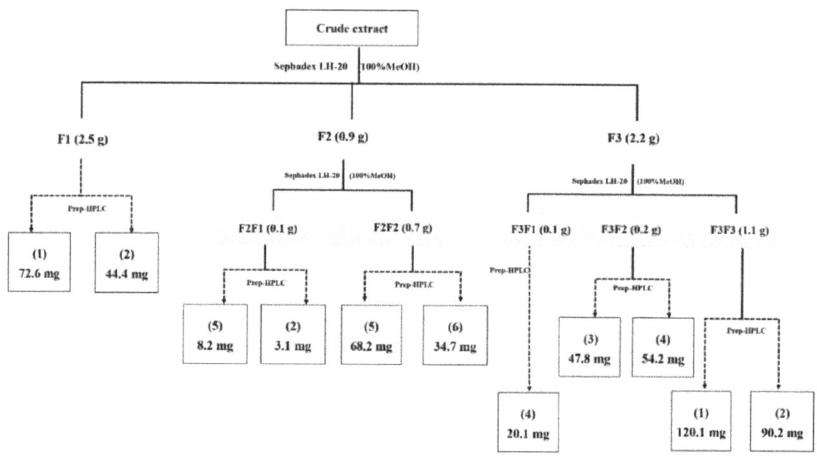

Figure 4. Isolation and purification procedure of compounds from crude EtOAc extract.

- Geldanamycin (**1**): Yellow solid; ^{1}H-NMR (500 MHz, $CDCl_3$) δ: 0.99 (3H, d J = 6.55), 1.00 (3H, d J = 6.40), 1.75 (1H, m), 1.76 (2H, m), 1.79 (3H, s), 2.02 (3H, s), 2.47 (2H, m), 2.77 (1H, m), 3.29 (3H, s), 3.35 (3H, s), 3.39 (1H, m), 4.12 (3H, s), 3.50 (1H, m), 4.31 (1H, d J = 9.22), 5.18 (1H, d J = 4.24), 5.81 (1H, d J = 9.30), 5.86 (1H, m), 6.57 (1H, m), 6.94 (1H, m), 7.41 (1H, s), and 8.7 (1H, s); ^{13}C-NMR (125 MHz, $CDCl_3$) δ: 12.4, 12.5, 12.3, 22.9, 28.0, 32.2, 32.7, 34.7, 56.7, 57.3, 61.7, 72.7, 81.0, 81.3, 81.4, 108.2, 111.8, 126.2, 127.6, 133.1, 133.3, 134.8, 138.1, 140.5, 153.1, 156.0, 157.0, 184.1, and 185.0. HRESIMS m/z 559.2673 $[M-H]^-$ (calcd. for $C_{29}H_{39}N_2O_9$, 559.2661). The ^{1}H-NMR, ^{13}C-NMR and mass spectra of compound (**1**) are shown in Figures S1, S2 and Figure S13, respectively.
- 17-*O*-Demethylgeldanamycin (**2**): Yellow solid; ^{1}H-NMR (400 MHz, $CDCl_3$) δ: 0.94 (3H, d J = 6.93), 1.00 (3H, d J = 5.36), 1.79 (3H, s), 1.76 (2H, m), 1.7–1.8 (1H, m), 2.03 (3H, s), 2.44 (2H, m), 2.79 (1H, m), 3.30 (3H, s), 3.36 (3H, s), 3.37 (1H, m), 3.54 (1H. m), 4.32 (1H, d J = 9.24), 5.17 (1H, s), 5.80 (1H, d J = 9.21), 5.90 (1H, dd J = 10.10), 6.57 (1H, dd J = 11.7), 6.97 (1H, d J = 11.29), 7.41 (1H, s), and 8.96 (1H, s); ^{13}C-NMR (100 MHz, $CDCl_3$) δ: 12.3, 12.4, 12.8, 23.2, 28.1, 32.3, 32.6, 34.5, 56.7, 57.3, 72.9, 81.1, 81.6, 81.8, 108.2, 117.4, 126.1, 127.8, 133.1, 133.4, 134.6, 137.1, 140.6, 153.2, 156.0, 168.1, 183.1, and 184.3; HRESIMS m/z 545.2514 $[M-H]^-$ (calcd. for $C_{28}H_{37}N_2O_9$, 545.2505). The ^{1}H-NMR, ^{13}C-NMR and mass spectra of compound (**2**) are shown in Figures S3, S4 and Figure S14, respectively.
- Reblastatin (**3**): White solid; Partial spectroscopic data from the ^{1}H-NMR (400 MHz, DMSO-d_6) δ: 0.79 (3H, d J = 6.28), 0.90 (3H, d J = 6.53), 1.43 (3H, s), 1.53 (1H, m), 1.67 (3H, s), 1.75 (1H, m), 2.11–2.20 (2H, m), 2.34 (1H, m), 2.36 (2H, m), 2.56 (2H, m), 3.21 (3H, s), 3.33 (3H, s), 3.62 (3H, s), 3.32 (1H, m), 3.28 (1H, m), 3.01 (1H, m), 4.86 (1H, d

J = 7.35), 4.29 (1H, d J = 4.99), 6.29 (1H, s), 5.29 (1H, d J = 9.92), 5.85 (1H, b), 6.86 (1H, s), 9.20 (1H, s), and 9.21 (1H, s); ^{13}C-NMR (100 MHz, DMSO-d_6) δ: 11.6, 12.8, 15.7, 19.9, 23.5, 29.7, 31.0, 33.5, 34.6, 35.7, 56.3, 58.0, 59.7, 73.9, 79.7, 80.5, 81.1, 107.2, 114.5, 129.7, 132.2, 133.3, 133.5, 134.4, 134.5, 142.4, 149.5, 156.0, and 169.9. HRESIMS m/z 571.2987 [M+Na]$^+$ (calcd. for $C_{29}H_{44}N_2NaO_8$, 571.2990). The ^{1}H-NMR, ^{13}C-NMR and mass spectra of compound (**3**) are shown in Figures S5, S6 and Figure S15, respectively.

- 17-Demethoxyreblastatin (**4**): White solid; ^{1}H-NMR (500 MHz, DMSO-d_6) δ: 0.79 (3H, d J = 6.30), 0.89 (3H, d J = 6.43), 1.35 (3H, s), 1.70 (3H, s), 1.78 (1H, b), 2.03–2.15 (2H, m), 2.95 (2H, m), 3.14 (3H, s), 3.28 (3H, s), 4.35 (1H, d J = 4.92), 4.83 (1H, d J = 7.44), 5.20 (1H, d J = 9.44), 5.66 (1H, s), 6.18 (1H, s), 6.24 (1H, s), 6.57 (b), 9.27 (1H, s), and 9.34 (1H, s); ^{13}C-NMR (125 MHz, DMSO-d_6) δ: 12.1, 13.7, 17.3, 19.0, 23.6, 30.0, 30.8, 33.0, 34.5, 43.1, 56.7, 58.8, 73.5, 79.7, 80.9, 81.2, 106.3, 113.2, 128.4, 130.3, 131.0, 132.1, 133.5, 134.4, 140.5, 141.4, 156.6, and 157.8; HRESIMS m/z 541.2900 [M+Na]+ (calcd. for $C_{28}H_{42}N_2NaO_7$, 541.2884). The ^{1}H-NMR, ^{13}C-NMR and mass spectra of compound (**4**) are shown in Figures S7, S8 and Figure S16, respectively.
- Nocardamine (**5**): White solid; ^{1}H-NMR (500 MHz, DMSO-d_6) δ: 1.21 (2H, m), 1.36 (2H, m), 1.46 (2H, m), 2.27 (2H, m), 2.57 (2H, m), 3.00 (2H, m), 3.44 (2H, t), 7.75 (1H, s), and 9.62 (1H, s); ^{13}C-NMR (125 MHz, DMSO-d_6) δ: 23.6, 26.3 27.9, 29.1, 30.4, 38.8, 47.3, 172.0, and 172.5. The ^{1}H-NMR, ^{13}C-NMR and mass spectra of compound (5) are shown in Figures S9, S10 and Figure S17, respectively.
- Dehydroxynocardamine (**6**): White solid. ^{1}H-NMR (400 MHz, DMSO-d_6) δ: 1.21 (2H, m), 1.35 (2H, bs), 1.48 (2H, bs), 2.28 (2H, s), 2.58 (1H, bs), 2.30 (2H, bs), 7.75 (1H, s), and 9.64 (1H, s); ^{13}C-NMR (100 MHz, DMSO-d_6) δ: 23.8, 24.1, 26.5, 28.1, 28.2, 29.2, 29.3, 29.4, 30.7, 31.8, 38.9, 39.0, 47.6, 171.9, 172.0, and 172.2; HRESIMS m/z 607.3429 [M+Na]$^+$ (calcd for $C_{27}H_{48}N_6NaO_8$, 607.3426); HRESIMS at m/z 623.3379 [M+Na]$^+$ (calcd for $C_{27}H_{48}N_6NaO_9$, 623.3375). The ^{1}H-NMR, ^{13}C-NMR and mass spectra of compound (**5**) are shown in Figures S11, S12 and Figure S18, respectively.

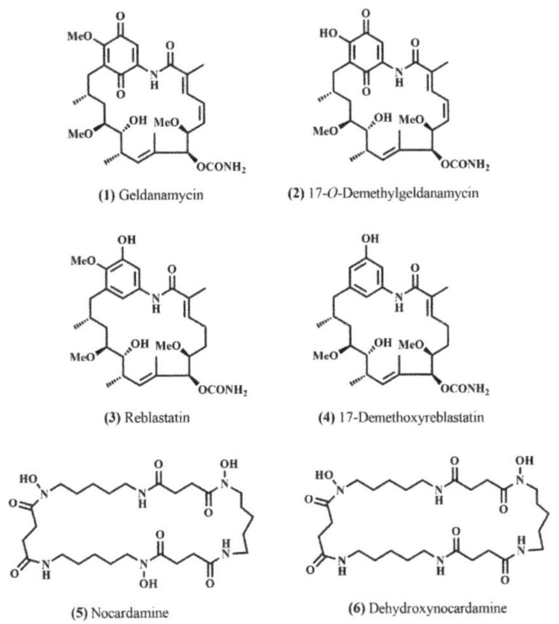

Figure 5. Chemical structure of the isolated compounds (**1**) geldanamycin, (**2**) 17-*O*-demethylgeldanamycin, (**3**) reblastatin, (**4**) 17-deméthoxyreblastatin, (**5**) nocardamine, and (**6**) dehydroxynocardamine.

2.5. Biological Activity of the Isolated Compounds

All compounds were assayed for cytotoxicity against the three human cancer derived cell lines (KB, NCI-H187, and NCF-7) and the untransformed monkey Vero cell line. Compounds (**1**)–(**4**) showed a high cytotoxic activity against NCI-H187 with IC_{50} values ranging from 0.045–4.250 μg/mL. Cytotoxic activity against the MCF-7 cell line was found in compounds (**1**) and (**3**) with IC_{50} values of 3.510 and 1.270 μg/mL, respectively. All compounds showed no antimicrobial activity against *M. tuberculosis* and anti-*P. falciparum* at the final concentration of 50 μg/mL. In addition, the isolated compounds showed no detected inhibitory activity against the bacteria *Acinetobacter baumannii, Escherichia coli* ATCC 25922, and *Mycobacterium tuberculosis* H37Ra; the fungal plant pathogens *Curvularia lunata, Magnaporthe grisea*, and *Alternaria brassicicola*; and the yeast *Candida albicans*. In addition, all compounds had no detected inhibitory activity against the neuraminidase (NA) enzyme. In terms of the biological activities, geldanamycin and its derivatives (**1**)–(**4**) mostly showed a cytotoxic activity, but the nocardamine group (**5**) and (**6**) showed cytotoxicity against only the Vero (IC_{50} of 16.57 μg/mL) and NCI-H187 (IC_{50} of 13.96 μg/mL) cell lines, respectively (Table 6).

Table 6. Biological activity of isolated compound from strain RCU-064^T.

Compound	Anti-*B. cereus* MIC (μg/mL)	Anti-*M. tuberculosis* MIC (μg/mL)	Anti-*P. falciparum* IC_{50} (μg/mL)	Cytotoxicity IC_{50} (μg/mL)			
				Vero	KB	NCI-H187	MCF-7
(1)	inactive	inactive	inactive	0.094	16.72	0.045	3.510
(2)	inactive	inactive	inactive	6.430	inactive	4.250	inactive
(3)	inactive	inactive	inactive	7.750	21.30	0.313	1.270
(4)	inactive	inactive	inactive	13.50	inactive	1.330	inactive
(5)	inactive	inactive	inactive	16.57	inactive	inactive	inactive
(6)	inactive	inactive	inactive	inactive	inactive	13.960	inactive
Vancomycin *	2.00	-	-	-	-	-	-
Rifampicin *	-	0.013	-	-	-	-	-
Ofloxacin *	-	0.391	-	-	-	-	-
Isoniazid *	-	0.047	-	-	-	-	-
Ethambutol *	-	0.938	-	-	-	-	-
Dihydroartemisinine *	-	-	7.02×10^{-4}	-	-	-	-
Mefloquine *	-	-	0.024	-	-	-	-
Ellipticine *	-	-	-	1.580	1.810	1.65	-
Doxorubicin *	-	-	-	-	0.655	0.088	8.07
Tamoxifen *	-	-	-	-	-	-	6.96

* = positive control; -, not determined. Inactive, at the final concentration of 50 μg/mL.

3. Discussion

Based on the results of this polyphasic approach and genomic evidence, it is clear that strain RCU-064^T is a novel species in the genus *Streptomyces*, for which the name *Streptomyces rugosispiralis* sp. nov. is herein proposed. Previous studies have highlighted the presence of novel *Streptomyces* in various ecological niches, including soil environments. For instance, *Streptomyces* have been isolated from diverse soil types worldwide, including agricultural, forest, and grassland soils [19–21]. Although actinomycetes have been isolated from soil for a century, novel species are still being reported from this type of habitat [4], including peat swamp forest soils. In the past decade, several novel species have been isolated from peat swamp forest soils in Thailand. For example, *Actinomadura rayongensis, Amycolatopsis acidicola, Dactylosporangium sucinum, Nocardia rayongensis, Nonomuraea rhodomycinica, Streptoyces actinomycinicus, Streptomyces acididurans*, and *Streptomyces humicola* [13–15,22–25]. These studies underline the adaptability of actinobacteria to different soil conditions and their significant contribution to the microbial diversity in terrestrial ecosystems. In addition, this indicates the unique characteristic of peat land harbors a high diversity of novel actinomycetes.

It is important to note that the physicochemical characteristics of peat swamp forest soil are unique due to its specific habitat. Peat swamp soils are typically characterized by a high organic matter content, acidic pH, waterlogged conditions, and low nutrient availability [26]. These distinct conditions pose challenges for actinomycetes isolation, as certain species may have specific growth requirements or preferential adaptation to different environmental parameters.

In terms of the isolation of actinomycetes, there are a number of essential factors to consider. The selection of suitable isolation techniques is essential for capturing a diverse population. Common techniques include serial dilution, plating on selective media supplemented with particular carbon or nitrogen sources, and altering the pH conditions [27]. These selective methods promote the development and isolation of actinomycetes, such as *Streptomyces*, while inhibiting the growth of competing microorganisms.

Actinomycetes are renowned for their remarkable ability to produce a diverse array of secondary metabolites, many of which possess significant bioactive properties. These bioactive compounds have attracted considerable attention in various fields, including pharmaceutical, agricultural, and industrial applications. Among the numerous secondary metabolites produced by actinomycetes, a key precursor in the biosynthesis of several important classes of compounds is 3-amino-5-hydroxybenzoic acid (AHBA).

Importantly, AHBA serves as a starter unit or building block in the assembly of polyketide or nonribosomal peptide backbones, leading to the formation of diverse bioactive compounds [28]. It can be classified into three distinct structural classes. The predominant class comprises ansamycins, wherein AHBA acts as a starter unit for the synthesis of a polyketide chain, leading to the formation of a macrocyclic lactam. Another class includes the mitomycins, which involve the combination of AHBA with an aminosugar component, resulting in the formation of unique tricyclic structures. Lastly, the saliniketals constitute a third class, characterized by being "degraded ansamycins," although this class has only been observed so far in saliniketal compounds [28].

The ansamycins are a family of polyketides that contain naphthalene/benzene or napthaquinone/benzoquinone rings that are connected at nonadjacent positions by an aliphatic chain. These natural compounds exhibit a variety of biological activities and have clinical applications [29]. Many reports have revealed that they have a wide range of biological activities, including anticancer, antiviral, and antibacterial effects. These compounds are distinguished by the presence of a macrocyclic system that is comprised of an aromatic moiety embedded in an alicycle, which has drawn considerable interest from chemical synthesis and biosynthetic researchers [30].

In this study, two classes of bioactive compounds—ansamycin and cyclic peptides—were isolated from strain RCU-064^T. Geldanamycin (**1**) is the benzoquinone ansamycin, first isolated from the culture broth of *Sreptomyces hygroscopicus* [31]. It exhibited moderate antimicrobial activity against bacteria and fungi with minimum inhibition concentration (MIC) values ranging from 4 to >100 µg/mL. Geldanamycin has been reported to have in vivo anti-parasitic activity against *Syphacia oblevata* but not against *Plasmodium berghei* [31]. However, in this study, the antimicrobial activity against *Bacillus cereus* and *Mycobacterium tuberculosis* of all compounds was negative (MIC > 50 µg/mL). This difference may be attributed to the variation in the tested microorganisms between these studies.

Geldanamycins (**1**) are potent anticancer and antifungal agents, exhibiting their anticancer activity through the inhibition of heat shock protein 90 (Hsp90), a key chaperone protein involved in the stabilization of cancer cell growth and survival [32–34]. By inhibiting the function of Hsp90, geldanamycin (**1**) disrupts multiple signaling pathways involved in cancer progression, leading to cell cycle arrest and apoptosis [35]. Previous work showed that geldanamycin (**1**) inhibited the growth of HPV-18-positive HeLa cells, which are a type of cervical cancer cell line, and also showed antifungal activity against *Setosphaeria turcica* plant pathogens [36].

Geldanamycin (**1**) and its derivatives have been reported to be produced as secondary metabolites in several *Streptomyces* species. In Thailand, *Streptomyces* sp. PC4-3 was isolated from a soil sample collected at Samed Island, Rayong province, Thailand, using starch-casein nitrate agar. The culture broth of *Streptomyces* sp. PC4-3 was extracted with ethyl acetate, concentrated under low pressure to obtain the crude extract, and then subjected to silica gel flash column chromatography and NMR spectroscopic analysis, revealing the active component to be geldanamycin (**1**) [37]. Likewise, the crude extracts of *Streptomyces* sp. BCC71188, which was isolated from a soil sample at Nakhon Si Thammarat Province, Thailand, were subjected to Sephadex LH-20 column chromatography followed by HPLC to yield 19 compounds, including 17-O-demethylgeldanamycin (**2**) [38].

Since geldanamycin (**1**) has demonstrated cytotoxic effects, numerous attempts have been made to identify alternative effective anticancer drugs derived from its molecular structure. These efforts have involved the preparation and biological evaluation of many semi-synthetic derivatives of geldanamycin, often involving modifications at the C-17 position [39,40]. Despite these attempts, an anticancer agent based on the geldanamycin pharmacophore has yet to be approved for clinical use [41]. However, previous research has reported the production of 17-O-demethylgeldanamycin (**2**) by *Streptomyces* DEM20745. This is of particular interest due to its potential as a starting material for the development of new semi-synthetic geldanamycin derivatives for clinical evaluation (41). For example, 17-arylgeldanamycins, synthesized via a triflation/Suzuki coupling approach using synthetic 17-O-demethylgeldanamycin, have been shown to have potent inhibition of Hsp90 [42]. Nevertheless, the limited availability of 17-O-demethygeldanamycin (**2**) has restricted further synthetic work in this area [43]. Therefore, it is of interest that our results revealed the production of 17-O-demethyl-geldanamycin (**2**) as a natural product by *Streptomyces* RCU-064^{T}, which provides future development of a production strain for this potentially valuable compound.

Reblastatin (**3**) and 17-Demethoxyreblastatin (**4**) are phenolic analogues of geldanamycin. Screening for novel compounds with the ability to inhibit phosphorylation of the retinoblastoma protein revealed reblastatin (**3**) [44], isolated as a minor constituent from the cultivation of *Streptomyces hygroscopicus*, which is also known for producing the potent Hsp90 disruptor geldanamycin (**1**) [31,45]. In the original study, reblastatin (**3**) demonstrated significant inhibition of the proliferation of the human histiocytic lymphoma U-937 cell line, with an IC_{50} value of 0.43 μg/mL [44]. Furthermore, it was found to exhibit a potent inhibitory activity in a cell-based oncostatin M signaling assay, with an IC_{50} value of 0.16 μM [46].

17-Demethoxyreblastatin (**4**) is a derivative of reblastatin (**3**), a natural product originally isolated from *Streptomyces* species. It is structurally related to reblastatin (**3**), differing in the presence of a demethoxy group at the C-17 position [45]. This modification alters the chemical properties and potentially affects the biological activities of the compound. Evaluations of its cytotoxic potential have revealed inhibitory effects on cancer cell growth and proliferation, similar to those observed with reblastatin (**3**). However, some research findings indicate that 17-demethoxyreblastatin (**4**) displayed unique biological characteristics when compared to reblastatin (**3**). The specific potency, selectivity, and mechanisms of action may vary between these two compounds due to the structural alteration [47].

Some *Streptomyces* strains have been reported to produce reblastatin (**3**) and 17-demethoxyreblastatin (**4**). The extraction of crude compounds from *Streptomyces hygroscopicus* JCM4427 using ethyl acetate, followed by purifying using octadecyl silica column chromatography and HPLC, revealed the presence of reblastin (**3**) and 17-demethoxyreblastatin (**4**) that exhibited Hsp90 ATPase inhibition activity with IC_{50} values of 0.32 μM and 1.82 μM, respectively, [48]. Despite 17-demethoxyreblastatin (**4**) being a derivative of reblastatin (**3**), there is limited literature available regarding its production from *Streptomyces* species. This scarcity of reports can be attributed to variations in the expression of the BGCs among different *Streptomyces* species [32].

Nocardamine (**5**), also called desferrioxamine, is a cyclic peptide siderophore found in several species of bacteria, including *Nocardia*, *Pseudomonas*, and *Streptomyces* species [49]. Siderophores are compounds synthesized by microorganisms to scavenge and bind iron from the surrounding environment. They act as an iron chelator, facilitating the uptake and utilization of this crucial nutrient by bacteria that require it for their growth and viability. Siderophores exhibit a strong affinity for iron and form stable complexes with the metal, effectively preventing its precipitation or interaction with other molecules present in the environment. Clinically, the nocardamine-type siderophore, Desferol, is used for the treatment of iron intoxication [50–52]. In addition, dehydroxynocardamine (**6**) is a derivative that is structurally related to nocardamine (**5**), with the key difference being the absence of hydroxyl groups in its chemical structure [53].

Nocardamine (**5**) was originally isolated as an antibacterial metabolite from a *Nocardia* strain [52], while nocardamine (**5**) and dehydroxynocardamine (**6**) were isolated from the culture broth of a marine-derived *Streptomyces* isolated from a sponge. Later, both compounds were also reported from soil *Streptomyces* sp. strain TS-2-2 and *Streptomyces* sp. BCC71188 [37,54]. This indicates that the ability to produce nocardamine (**5**) could be found in both terrestrial and marine *Streptomyces* species. In this study, nocardamine (**5**) and dehydroxynocardamine (**6**) were both inactive in the antimicrobial activity test at a concentration of 50 μg/mL, in accord with a previous report [49] that found no antimicrobial activity of both compounds at a final concentration of up to 200 μg/mL. However, in another study, nocardamine (**5**) showed a weak antimicrobial activity against *E. faecium* and *B. subtilis* but no activity against *V. alginolyticus* and *C. albicans* [55]. Moreover, in the same study, nocardamine (**5**) did not inhibit cell proliferation of tumor cell lines, including T-47D, SK-Mel-5, SK-Mel-28, and PRMI-7951, but did inhibit their colony formation [55]. Furthermore, the genetic engineering of *Streptomyces atratus* SCSIO ZH16, a deep-sea-derived *Streptomyces*, by in-frame deletion to activate putative orphan gene clusters, led to the production of new compounds, including nocardamine (**5**) [52].

In the analysis of BGCs, the detection of NRPS-like and T1PKS similar to the previous known BGCs of geldanamycins and the detection of desferrioxamine in the genome of strain RCU-064^T supported that strain RCU-064^T is the producer of geldanamycins (**1**) and nocardamines (**5**). This highlights the remarkable capacity of this genus to function as a potential source for drug production and a rich source of bioactive metabolites. The discovery and production of actinobacterial metabolites has been facilitated by advances in genome sequencing, bioinformatics, and genetic engineering techniques. These approaches have enabled the identification and manipulation of the BGCs responsible for compound synthesis, allowing researchers to optimize system production, enhance yields, and generate novel derivatives with improved properties. Moreover, the exploration of diverse environments, such as soil, marine sediments, and plant-associated microbiomes, has led to the discovery of novel Actinobacterial strains and expanded the diversity of known actinobacterial metabolites.

4. Materials and Methods

4.1. Microorganisms

Soil samples were collected from Nong Jum Rung peat swamp forest, Rayong Province, Thailand, in June 2011. *Streptomyces*, including the new isolate *S. rugosispiralis* sp. nov. (RCU064^T), were isolated following the serial dilution method. Briefly, 1 g of soil sample was added into the basic lauryl sulfate buffer and 10-fold serially diluted to 10^{-4}. Each dilution (0.1 mL) was spread on humic acid vitamin agar supplemented with nalidixic acid (25 mg/L) and cycloheximide (50 mg/L) and incubated at 30 °C for 14 days. After incubation, the colony of strain RCU-064^T was transferred to ISP2 agar and maintained as a working culture. The pure culture was preserved in lyophilized tube for long term preservation. The type strain used for taxonomic comparison was obtained from the Japan Collection of Microorganisms (JCM) and maintained under the same condition used for strain RCU-064^T.

4.2. Phenotypic Study

Morphological observation was performed under light microscopy on the culture grown on ISP2 medium at 30 °C for 14 days. The spore morphology and spore surface were observed using scanning electron microscopy (JSM-5401LV, JEOL, Tokyo, Japan). Cultural characteristics on agar media were determined according to the standard method [56]. The color of aerial mycelia, substrate mycelia, and soluble pigment was determined using the NBS/IBCC colour system [57]. Starch hydrolysis, gelatin liquefaction, skim milk peptonization, and nitrate reduction were determined using the reported methods [58,59]. Carbon utilization was determined following the previously reported method [56]. Enzyme activities were determined using API ZYM (bioMérieux), at 37 °C for 5 h. Growth temperature, pH, and NaCl tolerance were determined on ISP2 medium.

Isomers of diaminopimelic acid, whole-cell sugars, and the presence of mycolic acid were determined using standard thin layer chromatography (TLC) as reported [60,61]. Menaquinones were extracted following [62] and were analyzed using HPLC. *N*-Acyl type of muramic acid was determined as reported [63]. Cellular fatty acids were prepared and analyzed using gas chromatography–mass spectrometry following the MIDI Sherlock Microbial Identification System [64]. Phospholipids were extracted and determined using two-dimensional TLC [65].

4.3. 16S rRNA Gene and Phylogeny

Genomic DNA were obtained from freeze-dried cells following [66] and used for the PCR amplification of 16S rRNA gene as previously reported [67]. The nucleotide sequencing of the PCR products (Macrogen, Seoul, Republic of Korea) was determined using universal primers [68]. BLAST analysis was performed using EzTaxon-e server [69]. The sequence was aligned against the top 48 highest 16S rRNA gene similarity type strains obtained from the GenBank/EMBL/DDBJ database using BioEdit software [70]. The ML phylogenetic trees were constructed using MEGA version 7.0 [71] and the topologies of the resultant trees were evaluated using bootstrap resampling with 1000 replications.

4.4. Genome and Bioinformatics

The genomic DNA of strains RCU-064^T was extracted from the cells grown in ISP2 broth for 5 days using a DNA extraction kit (PureLink, Invitrogen, Thermo Fisher Scientific, Waltham, MA, USA). The QIAGEN FX kit was used for preparing the DNA library. Quality and quantity of the indexed libraries were analyzed using Agilent 2100 Bioanlyzer and Denovix fluorometer and pooled in an equimolar quantity. Cluster generation and paired-end 2 × 150 nucleotide read sequencing were performed on Illumina HiSeq X ten sequencer. FASTQC (Babraham Bioinformatics) was used for checking the quality of the raw read. Trim Galore was used to eliminate the low quality read and adaptors. PATRIC web service was used to assemble and annotate the genome [72]. The assembled genome of strain RCU-064^T was deposited at DDBJ/ENA/GenBank under accession number JANIAA000000000. Prediction of the BCGs in the genome was analyzed using anti-SMASH version 5.0 [73]. Average nucleotide identity (ANI) values were determined using JSpecies web service [74]. Digital DNA-DNA hybridization (dDDH) value was calculated using the Genome-to-Genome Distance Calculator (GGDC 2.1) [75]. The phylogenomic tree was constructed using AutoMLST [76].

4.5. Fermentation and Isolation of Secondary Metabolites

The culture plates of strain RCU-064^T were used for the stock culture, which were grown on ISP2 agar medium at 30 °C for 4 days. The stock culture was inoculated into 250-mL Erlenmeyer flasks containing 150 mL of ISP2 broth (seed medium). The seed culture of strain RCU-064^T was cultivated on a rotary shaker (200 rpm) at 30 °C for 4 days. Then, the seed culture (20 flasks) was transferred into 80 × 1-L Erlenmeyer flasks, each containing 250 mL of ISP 2 broth and cultivated at 30 °C on a rotary shaker (200 rpm) for 14 days. After that, the culture was extracted three times with an equal volume of ethyl acetate, then the pooled extracts were dried over Na_2SO_4 and then evaporated to dryness to yield the crude extract (5.8 g). The crude extract was fractionated through a Sephadex LH-20 column to give three fractions (F1–F3).

Fraction F1 (2.5 g) was enriched using preparative HPLC, eluting with a linear gradient system of 30–95% acetonitrile (CAN) in water (over 40 min at a flow rate of 15 mL/min, to furnish compounds (**1**) (72.6 mg) and (**2**) (44.4 mg).

Fraction F2 (0.8 g) was re-separated by Sephadex LH-20 column chromatography to give two sub-fractions (F2F1 and F2F2). Sub-fractions F2F1 (0.1 g) and F2F2 (0.7 g) were each fractionated by preparative HPLC, eluting with a linear gradient system of 30–95% ACN in H_2O over 40 min at a flow rate of 15 mL/min, to give compounds (**5**) (8.2 mg) and (**2**) (3.1 mg) from F2F1 and compounds (**5**) (68.2 mg) and (**6**) (34.7 mg) from F2F2.

The final major fraction, F3 (2.2 g) was fractionated by Sephadex LH-20 column chromatography to give three sub-fractions (F3F1, F3F2, and F3F3). Each of these sub-fractions were fractioned as per subfractions F2 above to give compound (**4**) (20.1 mg) from F3F1 (0.1 g), compounds (**3**) (47.8 mg) and (**4**) (54.2 mg) from F3F2 (0.2 g), and compounds (**1**) (120.1 mg) and (**2**) (90.2 mg) from F3F3 (1.1 mg). The isolation and enrichment procedure of these compounds is summarized in Figure 4.

4.6. Characterization and Identification of Secondary Metabolites

The NMR spectra were recorded on Bruker Avance 500 MHz and Bruker Avance III 400 MHz NMR spectrometers using acetone-d_6 as an internal standard, while HRESIMS data were obtained from a Bruker MicOTOF spectrometer. Column chromatography was performed on a Sephadex LH-20 column using 100% methanol as the eluent. HPLC was performed on a Dionex-Ultimate 3000 series equipped with a binary pump, an autosampler, and diode array detector. Semi-preparative HPLC was performed on a Sunfire C18 column from Waters (5 µm, diam. 19 mm × 150 mm). Preparative HPLC was performed on a Sunfire C18 column from Waters (10 µm, diam. 19 mm × 250 mm).

4.7. Biological Activity

Antibacterial activity was tested using the resazurin microplate assay (REMA) [77]. The MIC represents the lowest concentration that inhibited growth of the tested bacteria. Vancomycin was used as a positive control. The green fluorescent protein microplate assay (GFPMA) was used for evaluation of cytotoxicity against Vero cells (African green monkey kidney fibroblasts, ATCC CCL-81) and antituberculosis activity against *Mycobacterium tuberculosis* strain H37Ra [78]. Ellipticine and amphotericin B were used as the positive controls for cytotoxicity against Vero cells and anti-phytopathogenic activity, respectively. For antituberculosis, isoniazid, ofloxacin, rifampicin, streptomycin, and ethambutol were used as the positive controls. Antimalarial assay against *Plasmodium falciparum* (K-1, multi-drug resistant strain) was performed using the microculture radioisotope technique [79]. The IC_{50} value represents the concentration that caused a 50% reduction in parasite growth. Dihydroartemisinin and mefloquine were used as the positive controls. Cytotoxicity against KB (oral human epidermoid carcinoma, ATCC CCL-17), MCF-7 (human breast cancer, ATCC HTC-22), and NCI-H187 (human small-cell lung cancer, ATCC CRL-5804) cell lines were evaluated using the resazurin microplate assay (REMA) as previously described [80]. Ellipticine and doxorubicin were used as the positive controls for anti-KB, with tamoxifen and doxorubicin as the positive controls for anti-MCF-7 and doxorubicin was used as the positive control for anti-NCI-H187. The NA inhibition assay was determined using the MUNANA-based enzyme inhibition assay [81].

Supplementary Materials: The following supporting information can be downloaded at: https://www.mdpi.com/article/10.3390/antibiotics12091467/s1, Spectroscopic data of compounds (**1**)–(**6**), including ^{1}H- and ^{13}C-NMR spectra, and mass spectra (see Figures S1–S18). Figure S1. ^{1}H NMR spectrum ($CDCl_3$) of compound (**1**); Figure S2. ^{13}C NMR spectrum ($CDCl_3$) of compound (**1**); Figure S3. ^{1}H NMR spectrum ($CDCl_3$) of compound (**2**); Figure S4. ^{13}C NMR spectrum ($CDCl_3$) of compound (**2**); Figure S5. ^{1}H NMR spectrum (DMSO-d_6) of compound (**3**); Figure S6. ^{13}C NMR spectrum (DMSO-d_6) of compound (**3**); Figure S7. ^{1}H NMR spectrum (DMSO-d_6) of compound (**4**); Figure S8. ^{13}C NMR spectrum (DMSO-d_6) of compound (**4**); Figure S9. ^{1}H NMR spectrum (DMSO-d_6) of compound (**5**); Figure S10. ^{13}C NMR spectrum (DMSO-d_6) of compound (**5**); Figure S11. ^{1}H

NMR spectrum ($CDCl_3$) of compound (**6**); Figure S12. ^{13}C NMR spectrum ($CDCl_3$) of compound (**6**); Figure S13. MS spectrum of compound (**1**); Figure S14. MS spectrum of compound (**2**); Figure S15. MS spectrum of compound (**3**); Figure S16. MS spectrum of compound (**4**); Figure S17. MS spectrum of compound (**5**); Figure S18. MS spectrum of compound (**6**).

Author Contributions: Conceptualization, W.P. and K.S.; methodology, T.W., P.S., K.S. and R.J.; software, T.W., W.P., K.S., R.J. and S.K.; formal analysis, W.P., K.S. and P.P.; investigation, T.W., P.S. and R.J.; resources, W.P., K.S. and P.P.; data curation, W.P., K.S. and P.P.; writing—original draft preparation, T.W., W.P. and K.S.; writing—review and editing, S.T., P.P. and S.K.; supervision, S.T. and P.P.; project administration, W.P. and S.T.; funding acquisition, W.P. and S.T. All authors have read and agreed to the published version of the manuscript.

Funding: This research was supported by the Chulalongkorn University grant to the Natural Products and Nanoparticles Research Unit (GRU 6306433004-1). We also thank the faculty of Pharmaceutical Sciences for the financial support.

Institutional Review Board Statement: Not applicable.

Informed Consent Statement: Not applicable.

Data Availability Statement: The GenBank accession number of the 16S rRNA gene sequences and draft genome of strain RCU-064^T are OQ001562 and JANIAA000000000, respectively.

Acknowledgments: We would like to thank the Natural Products and Nanoparticles Research Unit (NP2) of Chulalongkorn University and the National Center for Genetic Engineering and Biotechnology (BIOTEC) at the National Science and Technology Development Agency (NSTDA) for collaborative support. We thank Pharmaceutical Research Instrument Center, Faculty of Pharmaceutical Sciences, Chulalongkorn University for the scientific instruments. We thank the Rayong Botanical Garden for soil sample collection. Furthermore, this research is supported by Ratchadapisek Somphot Fund for Postdoctoral Fellowship (T.W.), Chulalongkorn University. We thank Aharon Oren for the etymology of the type strain.

Conflicts of Interest: The authors declare no conflict of interest.

Sample Availability: The type strain RCU-064^T is deposited at the culture collections of the Thailand Bioresource Research Center (TBRC) and Biological Resource Center, NITE (NBRC), Japan. Samples of compounds **1–6** are available from KS and PP.

References

1. Bérdy, J. Bioactive Microbial Metabolites. *J. Antibiot.* **2005**, *58*, 1–26. [CrossRef] [PubMed]
2. Barka, E.A.; Vatsa, P.; Sanchez, L.; Gaveau-Vaillant, N.; Jacquard, C.; Meier-Kolthoff, J.P.; Klenk, H.-P.; Clément, C.; Ouhdouch, Y.; van Wezel, G.P. Taxonomy, Physiology, and Natural Products of Actinobacteria. *Microbiol. Mol. Biol. Rev.* **2016**, *80*, 1–43. [CrossRef] [PubMed]
3. Harunari, E.; Hamada, M.; Shibata, C.; Tamura, T.; Komaki, H.; Imada, C.; Igarashi, Y. *Streptomyces hyaluromycini* sp. nov., isolated from a tunicate (*Molgula manhattensis*). *J. Antibiot.* **2016**, *69*, 159–163. [CrossRef] [PubMed]
4. Thawai, C. *Pseudonocardia soli* sp. nov., isolated from mountain soil. *Int. J. Syst. Evol. Microbiol.* **2018**, *68*, 1307–1312. [CrossRef]
5. Buangrab, K.; Sutthacheep, M.; Yeemin, T.; Harunari, E.; Igarashi, Y.; Sripreechasak, P.; Kanchanasin, P.; Tanasupawat, S.; Phongsopitanun, W. *Streptomyces corallincola* and *Kineosporia corallincola* sp. nov., two new coral-derived marine actinobacteria. *Int. J. Syst. Evol. Microbiol.* **2022**, *72*, 005249. [CrossRef]
6. Niemhom, N.; Chutrakul, C.; Suriyachadkun, C.; Thawai, C. *Nonomuraea stahlianthi* sp. nov., an endophytic actinomycete isolated from the stem of *Stahlianthus campanulatus*. *Int. J. Syst. Evol. Microbiol.* **2017**, *67*, 2879–2884. [CrossRef]
7. Somphong, A.; Poengsungnoen, V.; Buaruang, K.; Suriyachadkun, C.; Sripreechasak, P.; Tanasupawat, S.; Phongsopitanun, W. Diversity of the culturable lichen-derived actinobacteria and the taxonomy of *Streptomyces parmotrematis* sp. nov. *Antonie Leeuwenhoek* **2022**, *115*, 911–920. [CrossRef]
8. Bai, L.; Liu, C.; Guo, L.; Piao, C.; Li, Z.; Li, J.; Jia, F.; Wang, X.; Xiang, W. *Streptomyces formicae* sp. nov., a novel actinomycete isolated from the head of *Camponotus japonicus* Mayr. *Antonie Leeuwenhoek* **2016**, *109*, 253–261. [CrossRef]
9. Belknap, K.C.; Park, C.J.; Barth, B.M.; Andam, C.P. Genome mining of biosynthetic and chemotherapeutic gene clusters in *Streptomyces* bacteria. *Sci. Rep.* **2020**, *10*, 2003. [CrossRef]
10. Sung, H.; Ferlay, J.; Siegel, R.L.; Laversanne, M.; Soerjomataram, I.; Jemal, A.; Bray, F. Global Cancer Statistics 2020: GLOBOCAN Estimates of Incidence and Mortality Worldwide for 36 Cancers in 185 Countries. *CA Cancer J. Clin.* **2021**, *71*, 209–249. [CrossRef]
11. Law, J.W.-F.; Law, L.N.-S.; Letchumanan, V.; Tan, L.T.-H.; Wong, S.H.; Chan, K.-G.; Ab Mutalib, N.-S.; Lee, L.-H. Anticancer Drug Discovery from Microbial Sources: The Unique Mangrove Streptomycetes. *Molecules* **2020**, *25*, 5365. [CrossRef] [PubMed]

12. Graham, L.; Giesen, W.; Page, S. A common-sense approach to tropical peat swamp forest restoration in Southeast Asia: Common-sense approach to peat forest restoration. *Restor. Ecol.* **2016**, *25*, 312–321. [CrossRef]
13. Tanasupawat, S.; Phongsopitanun, W.; Suwanborirux, K.; Ohkuma, M.; Kudo, T. *Streptomyces actinomycinicus* sp. nov., isolated from soil of a peat swamp forest. *Int. J. Syst. Evol. Microbiol.* **2016**, *66*, 290–295. [CrossRef]
14. Phongsopitanun, W.; Kudo, T.; Ohkuma, M.; Suwanborirux, K.; Tanasupawat, S. *Dactylosporangium sucinum* sp. nov., isolated from Thai peat swamp forest soil. *J. Antibiot.* **2015**, *68*, 379–384. [CrossRef] [PubMed]
15. Tanasupawat, S.; Phongsopitanun, W.; Suwanborirux, K.; Ohkuma, M.; Kudo, T. *Nocardia rayongensis* sp. nov., isolated from Thai peat swamp forest soil. *Int. J. Syst. Evol. Microbiol.* **2016**, *66*, 1950–1955. [CrossRef] [PubMed]
16. Chun, J.; Oren, A.; Ventosa, A.; Christensen, H.; Arahal, D.R.; da Costa, M.S.; Rooney, A.P.; Yi, H.; Xu, X.-W.; De Meyer, S.; et al. Proposed minimal standards for the use of genome data for the taxonomy of prokaryotes. *Int. J. Syst. Evol. Microbiol.* **2018**, *68*, 461–466. [CrossRef] [PubMed]
17. Sazak, A.; Şahin, N.; Güven, K.; Işık, K.; Goodfellow, M. *Streptomyces samsunensis* sp. nov., a member of the *Streptomyces violaceusniger* clade isolated from the rhizosphere of *Robinia pseudoacacia*. *Int. J. Syst. Evol. Microbiol.* **2011**, *61 Pt 6*, 1309–1314. [CrossRef]
18. al-Tai, A.; Kim, B.; Kim, S.B.; Manfio, G.P.; Goodfellow, M. *Streptomyces malaysiensis* sp. nov., a new streptomycete species with rugose, ornamented spores. *Int. J. Syst. Bacteriol.* **1999**, *49 Pt 4*, 1395–1402. [CrossRef]
19. Cheng, J.; Yang, S.H.; Palaniyandi, S.A.; Han, J.S.; Yoon, T.-M.; Kim, T.-J.; Suh, J.-W. Azalomycin F Complex Is an Antifungal Substance Produced by *Streptomyces malaysiensis* MJM1968 Isolated from Agricultural Soil. *J. Korean Soc. Appl. Biol. Chem.* **2010**, *53*, 545–5522. [CrossRef]
20. Bontemps, C.; Toussaint, M.; Revol, P.-V.; Hotel, L.; Jeanbille, M.; Uroz, S.; Turpault, M.-P.; Blaudez, D.; Leblond, P. Taxonomic and functional diversity of *Streptomyces* in a forest soil. *FEMS Microbiol. Lett.* **2013**, *342*, 157–167. [CrossRef]
21. Quinn, G.A.; Abdelhameed, A.M.; Alharbi, N.K.; Cobice, D.; Adu, S.A.; Swain, M.T.; Castro, H.C.; Facey, P.D.; Bakshi, H.A.; Tambuwala, M.M.; et al. The Isolation of a Novel *Streptomyces* sp. CJ13 from a Traditional Irish Folk Medicine Alkaline Grassland Soil that Inhibits Multiresistant Pathogens and Yeasts. *Appl. Sci.* **2020**, *11*, 173. [CrossRef]
22. Teo, W.F.A.; Srisuk, N.; Duangmal, K. *Amycolatopsis acidicola* sp. nov., isolated from peat swamp forest soil. *Int. J. Syst. Evol. Microbiol.* **2020**, *70*, 1547–1554. [CrossRef] [PubMed]
23. Sripreechasak, P.; Phongsopitanun, W.; Supong, K.; Pittayakhajonwut, P.; Kudo, T.; Ohkuma, M.; Tanasupawat, S. *Nonomuraea rhodomycinica* sp. nov., isolated from peat swamp forest soil in Thailand. *Int. J. Syst. Evol. Microbiol.* **2017**, *67*, 1683–1687. [CrossRef] [PubMed]
24. Chantavorakit, T.; Klaysubun, C.; Duangmal, K. *Streptomyces acididurans* sp. nov., isolated from peat swamp forest soil. *Int. J. Syst. Evol. Microbiol.* **2021**, *71*, 004849. [CrossRef]
25. Klaysubun, C.; Srisuk, N.; Duangmal, K. *Streptomyces humicola* sp. nov., a novel actinobacterium isolated from peat swamp forest soil in Thailand. *Int. J. Syst. Evol. Microbiol.* **2022**, *72*, 005665. [CrossRef]
26. Heller, C.; Ellerbrock, R.H.; Roßkopf, N.; Klingenfuß, C.; Zeitz, J. Soil organic matter characterization of temperate peatland soil with FTIR-spectroscopy: Effects of mire type and drainage intensity. *Eur. J. Soil Sci.* **2015**, *66*, 847–858. [CrossRef]
27. Goodfellow, M. Selective Isolation of Actinobacteria. In *Manual of Industrial Microbiology and Biotechnology*; John Wiley & Sons, Inc.: Hoboken, NJ, USA, 2010; pp. 13–27. [CrossRef]
28. Kang, Q.; Shen, Y.; Bai, L. Biosynthesis of 3,5-AHBA-derived natural products. *Nat. Prod. Rep.* **2012**, *29*, 243–263. [CrossRef]
29. Hill, A.M.; Staunton, J. 1.10—Type I Modular PKS. In *Comprehensive Natural Products II*; Liu, H.-W., Mander, L., Eds.; Elsevier: Oxford, UK, 2010; pp. 385–452.
30. Song, Y.-N.; Zhang, W.-J.; Bi, S.-F.; Jiao, R.-H.; Tan, R.-X.; Ge, H.-M. New ansamycin analogues from the mutant strain of *Streptomyces seoulensis*. *J. Antibiot.* **2015**, *68*, 757–759. [CrossRef]
31. DeBoer, C.; Meulman, P.A.; Wnuk, R.J.; Peterson, D.H. Geldanamycin, a new antibiotic. *J. Antibiot. (Tokyo)* **1970**, *23*, 442–447. [CrossRef]
32. Martín, J.F.; Ramos, A.; Liras, P. Regulation of Geldanamycin Biosynthesis by Cluster-Situated Transcription Factors and the Master Regulator PhoP. *Antibiotics* **2019**, *8*, 87. [CrossRef]
33. Fukuyo, Y.; Hunt, C.R.; Horikoshi, N. Geldanamycin and its anti-cancer activities. *Cancer Lett.* **2010**, *290*, 24–35. [CrossRef] [PubMed]
34. Ochel, H.-J.; Eichhorn, K.; Gademann, G. Geldanamycin: The prototype of a class of antitumor drugs targeting the heat shock protein 90 family of molecular chaperones. *Cell Stress Chaperones* **2001**, *6*, 105–112. [CrossRef] [PubMed]
35. Karkoulis, P.K.; Stravopodis, D.J.; Konstantakou, E.G.; E Voutsinas, G. Targeted inhibition of heat shock protein 90 disrupts multiple oncogenic signaling pathways, thus inducing cell cycle arrest and programmed cell death in human urinary bladder cancer cell lines. *Cancer Cell Int.* **2013**, *13*, 11. [CrossRef]
36. Lin, H.-N.; Wang, K.-L.; Wu, Z.-H.; Tian, R.-M.; Liu, G.-Z.; Xu, Y. Biological and Chemical Diversity of Bacteria Associated with a Marine Flatworm. *Mar. Drugs* **2017**, *15*, 281. [CrossRef] [PubMed]
37. Anansiriwattana, W.; Tanasupawat, S.; Amnuoypol, S.; Suwanborirux, K. Identification and antimicrobial activities of actinomycetes from soils in Samed island, and gedanamycin from strain PC4-3. *Thai. J. Pharm. Sci.* **2006**, *30*, 49–56.

38. Supong, K.; Sripreechasak, P.; Tanasupawat, S.; Danwisetkanjana, K.; Rachtawee, P.; Pittayakhajonwut, P. Investigation on antimicrobial agents of the terrestrial *Streptomyces* sp. BCC71188. *Appl. Microbiol. Biotechnol.* **2017**, *101*, 533–543. [CrossRef] [PubMed]
39. Franke, J.; Eichner, S.; Zeilinger, C.; Kirschning, A. Targeting heat-shock-protein 90 (Hsp90) by natural products: Geldanamycin, a show case in cancer therapy. *Nat. Prod. Rep.* **2013**, *30*, 1299–1323. [CrossRef]
40. Kitson, R.R.A.; Moody, C.J. Learning from Nature: Advances in Geldanamycin- and Radicicol-Based Inhibitors of Hsp90. *J. Org. Chem.* **2013**, *78*, 5117–5141. [CrossRef]
41. Baksh, A.; Kepplinger, B.; Isah, H.A.; Probert, M.R.; Clegg, W.; Wills, C.; Goodfellow, M.; Errington, J.; Allenby, N.; Hall, M.J. Production of 17-O-demethyl-geldanamycin, a cytotoxic ansamycin polyketide, by *Streptomyces hygroscopicus* DEM20745. *Nat. Prod. Res.* **2017**, *31*, 1895–1900. [CrossRef]
42. Le Brazidec, J.-Y.; Kamal, A.; Busch, D.; Thao, L.; Zhang, L.; Timony, G.; Grecko, R.; Trent, K.; Lough, R.; Salazar, T.; et al. Synthesis and biological evaluation of a new class of geldanamycin derivatives as potent inhibitors of Hsp90. *J. Med. Chem.* **2004**, *47*, 3865–3873. [CrossRef]
43. Tadtong, S.; Meksuriyen, D.; Tanasupawat, S.; Isobe, M.; Suwanborirux, K. Geldanamycin derivatives and neuroprotective effect on cultured P19-derived neurons. *Bioorganic Med. Chem. Lett.* **2007**, *17*, 2939–2943. [CrossRef] [PubMed]
44. Takatsu, T.; Ohtsuki, M.; Muramatsu, A.; Enokita, R.; Kurakata, S.-I. Reblastatin, a novel benzenoid ansamycin-type cell cycle inhibitor. *J. Antibiot.* **2000**, *53*, 1310–1312. [CrossRef] [PubMed]
45. Wrona, I.E.; Gabarda, A.E.; Evano, G.; Panek, J.S. Total synthesis of reblastatin. *J. Am. Chem. Soc.* **2005**, *127*, 15026–15027. [CrossRef] [PubMed]
46. Stead, P.; Latif, S.; Blackaby, A.P.; Sidebottom, P.J.; Deakin, A.; Taylor, N.L.; Life, P.; Spaull, J.; Burrell, F.; Jones, R.; et al. Discovery of Novel Ansamycins Possessing Potent Inhibitory Activity in a Cell-based Oncostatin M Signalling Assay. *J. Antibiot.* **2000**, *53*, 657–663. [CrossRef] [PubMed]
47. Choi, J.; Kim, B.-Y.; Son, Y.; Lee, D.; Hong, Y.-S.; Kim, M.S.; Kim, K. Reblastatins Inhibit Phenotypic Changes of Monocytes/Macrophages in a Milieu Rich in 27-Hydroxycholesterol. *Immune Netw.* **2020**, *20*, e17. [CrossRef]
48. Wu, C.Z.; Jang, J.H.; Ahn, J.S.; Hong, Y.S. New geldanamycin analogs from *Streptomyces hygroscopicus*. *J. Microbiol. Biotechnol.* **2012**, *22*, 1478–1481. [CrossRef]
49. Lee, H.-S.; Shin, H.J.; Jang, K.H.; Kim, T.S.; Oh, K.-B.; Shin, J. Cyclic Peptides of the Nocardamine Class from a Marine-Derived Bacterium of the Genus *Streptomyces*. *J. Nat. Prod.* **2005**, *68*, 623–625. [CrossRef]
50. Saha, R.; Saha, N.; Donofrio, R.S.; Bestervelt, L.L. Microbial siderophores: A mini review. *J. Basic Microbiol.* **2013**, *53*, 303–317. [CrossRef]
51. Wang, W.; Qiu, Z.; Tan, H.; Cao, L. Siderophore production by actinobacteria. *BioMetals* **2014**, *27*, 623–631. [CrossRef]
52. Li, Y.; Zhang, C.; Liu, C.; Ju, J.; Ma, J. Genome Sequencing of *Streptomyces atratus* SCSIOZH16 and Activation Production of Nocardamine via Metabolic Engineering. *Front. Microbiol.* **2018**, *9*, 1269. [CrossRef]
53. Information NCfB. PubChem Compound Summary for CID 11606728, Dehydroxynocardamine 2023. Available online: https://pubchem.ncbi.nlm.nih.gov/compound/Dehydroxynocardamine (accessed on 25 June 2023).
54. A Shaaban, K.; Singh, S.; I Elshahawi, S.; Wang, X.; Ponomareva, L.V.; Sunkara, M.; Copley, G.C.; Hower, J.C.; Morris, A.J.; Kharel, M.K.; et al. Venturicidin C, a new 20-membered macrolide produced by *Streptomyces* sp. TS-2-2. *J. Antibiot.* **2014**, *67*, 223–230. [CrossRef] [PubMed]
55. Kalinovskaya, N.I.; Romanenko, L.A.; Irisawa, T.; Ermakova, S.P.; Kalinovsky, A.I. Marine isolate *Citricoccus* sp. KMM 3890 as a source of a cyclic siderophore nocardamine with antitumor activity. *Microbiol. Res.* **2011**, *166*, 654–661. [CrossRef] [PubMed]
56. Shirling, E.B.; Gottlieb, D. Methods for characterization of Streptomyces species. *Int. J. Syst. Evol. Microbiol.* **1966**, *16*, 313–340. [CrossRef]
57. Kelly, K.L.; Judd, D.B.; Inter-Society Color Council; United States National Bureau of Standards. *ISCC-NBS Color-Name Charts Illustrated with Centroid Colors*; U.S. National Bureau of Standards: Washington, DC, USA, 1965.
58. Arai, T. *Culture Media for Actinomycetes*; The Society for Actinomycetes Japan: Tokyo, Japan, 1975.
59. Williams, S.T.; Cross, T. Chapter XI Actinomycetes. In *Methods in Microbiology*; Booth, C., Ed.; Academic Press: Cambridge, MA, USA, 1971; pp. 295–334.
60. Staneck, J.L.; Roberts, G.D. Simplified approach to identification of aerobic actinomycetes by thin-layer chromatography. *Appl. Microbiol.* **1974**, *28*, 226–231. [CrossRef] [PubMed]
61. Tomiyasu, I. Mycolic Acid Composition and Thermally Adaptative Changes in *Nocardia asteroides*. *J. Bacteriol.* **1982**, *151*, 828–837. [CrossRef]
62. Collins, M.D.; Pirouz, T.; Goodfellow, M.; Minnikin, D.E. Distribution of Menaquinones in Actinomycetes and Corynebacteria. *J. Gen. Microbiol.* **1977**, *100*, 221–230. [CrossRef] [PubMed]
63. Uchida, K.; Aida, K. An improved method for the glycolate test for simple identification of the acyl type of bacterial cell walls. *J. Gen. Appl. Microbiol.* **1984**, *30*, 131–134. [CrossRef]
64. Sasser, M. Identification of bacteria by gas chromatography of cellular fatty acids. *USFCC Newsl.* **1990**, *20*, 1–6.
65. Minnikin, D.; O'Donnell, A.; Goodfellow, M.; Alderson, G.; Athalye, M.; Schaal, A.; Parlett, J. An integrated procedure for the extraction of bacterial isoprenoid quinones and polar lipids. *J. Microbiol. Methods* **1984**, *2*, 233–241. [CrossRef]
66. Raeder, U.; Broda, P. Rapid preparation of DNA from filamentous fungi. *Lett. Appl. Microbiol.* **1985**, *1*, 17–20. [CrossRef]

67. Phuengjayaem, S.; Phinkian, N.; Tanasupawat, S.; Teeradakorn, S. Diversity and succinic acid production of lactic acid bacteria isolated from animals, soils and tree barks. *Res. J. Microbiol.* **2017**, *12*, 177–186. [CrossRef]
68. Lane, D.J. 16S/23S rRNA Sequencing. In *Nucleic Acid Techniques in Bacterial Systematic*; Stackebrandt, E., Goodfellow, M., Eds.; John Wiley and Sons: New York, NY, USA, 1991; pp. 115–175.
69. Kim, O.-S.; Cho, Y.-J.; Lee, K.; Yoon, S.-H.; Kim, M.; Na, H.; Park, S.-C.; Jeon, Y.S.; Lee, J.-H.; Yi, H.; et al. Introducing EzTaxon-e: A prokaryotic 16S rRNA gene sequence database with phylotypes that represent uncultured species. *Int. J. Syst. Evol. Microbiol.* **2012**, *62 Pt 3*, 716–721. [CrossRef] [PubMed]
70. Hall, T.A. BioEdit: A user-friendly biological sequence alignment editor and analysis program for Windows 95/98/NT. *Nucleic Acids Symp Ser.* **1999**, *41*, 95–98.
71. Kumar, S.; Stecher, G.; Tamura, K. MEGA7: Molecular Evolutionary Genetics Analysis Version 7.0 for Bigger Datasets. *Mol. Biol. Evol.* **2016**, *33*, 1870–1874. [CrossRef] [PubMed]
72. Davis, J.J.; Wattam, A.R.; Aziz, R.K.; Brettin, T.; Butler, R.; Butler, R.M.; Chlenski, P.; Conrad, N.; Dickerman, A.; Dietrich, E.M.; et al. The PATRIC Bioinformatics Resource Center: Expanding data and analysis capabilities. *Nucleic Acids Res.* **2019**, *48*, D606–D612. [CrossRef] [PubMed]
73. Blin, K.; Shaw, S.; E Augustijn, H.; Reitz, Z.L.; Biermann, F.; Alanjary, M.; Fetter, A.; Terlouw, B.R.; Metcalf, W.W.; Helfrich, E.J.N.; et al. antiSMASH 7.0: New and improved predictions for detection, regulation, chemical structures and visualisation. *Nucleic Acids Res.* **2023**, *51*, W46–W50. [CrossRef]
74. Richter, M.; Rosselló-Móra, R.; Oliver Glöckner, F.; Peplies, J. JSpeciesWS: A web server for prokaryotic species circumscription based on pairwise genome comparison. *Bioinformatics* **2016**, *32*, 929–931. [CrossRef]
75. Meier-Kolthoff, J.P.; Auch, A.F.; Klenk, H.-P.; Göker, M. Genome sequence-based species delimitation with confidence intervals and improved distance functions. *BMC Bioinform.* **2013**, *14*, 60. [CrossRef]
76. Alanjary, M.; Steinke, K.; Ziemert, N. AutoMLST: An automated web server for generating multi-locus species trees highlighting natural product potential. *Nucleic Acids Res.* **2019**, *47*, W276–W282. [CrossRef]
77. Sarker, S.D.; Nahar, L.; Kumarasamy, Y. Microtitre plate-based antibacterial assay incorporating resazurin as an indicator of cell growth, and its application in the in vitro antibacterial screening of phytochemicals. *Methods* **2007**, *42*, 321–324. [CrossRef]
78. Changsen, C.; Franzblau, S.G.; Palittapongarnpim, P. Improved Green Fluorescent Protein Reporter Gene-Based Microplate Screening for Antituberculosis Compounds by Utilizing an Acetamidase Promoter. *Antimicrob. Agents Chemother.* **2003**, *47*, 3682–3687. [CrossRef] [PubMed]
79. Desjardins, R.E.; Canfield, C.J.; Haynes, J.D.; Chulay, J.D. Quantitative assessment of antimalarial activity in vitro by a semiautomated microdilution technique. *Antimicrob. Agents Chemother.* **1979**, *16*, 710–718. [CrossRef]
80. O'Brien, J.; Wilson, I.; Orton, T.; Pognan, F. Investigation of the Alamar Blue (resazurin) fluorescent dye for the assessment of mammalian cell cytotoxicity. *Eur. J. Biochem.* **2000**, *267*, 5421–5426. [CrossRef] [PubMed]
81. Leang, S.K.; Hurt, A.C. Fluorescence-based Neuraminidase Inhibition Assay to Assess the Susceptibility of Influenza Viruses to the Neuraminidase Inhibitor Class of Antivirals. *J. Vis. Exp.* **2017**, e55570. [CrossRef]

antibiotics

MDPI

Article

The Direction of the Antibacterial Effect of Rutin Hydrate and Amikacin

Maria Miklasińska-Majdanik [1,*], Małgorzata Kępa [1], Tomasz J. Wąsik [2], Karolina Zapletal-Pudełko [1], Magdalena Klim [1] and Robert D. Wojtyczka [1]

1 Department of Microbiology and Virology, Faculty of Pharmaceutical Sciences in Sosnowiec, Medical University of Silesia in Katowice, Jagiellońska 4, 41-200 Sosnowiec, Poland; mkepa@sum.edu.pl (M.K.); karolinazapletal@yahoo.com (K.Z.-P.); magdalena.klim@sum.edu.pl (M.K.); rwojtyczka@sum.edu.pl (R.D.W.)

2 Department of Medical Microbiology, Faculty of Medical Sciences in Katowice, Medical University of Silesia in Katowice, Medyków 18, 40-752 Katowice, Poland; twasik@sum.edu.pl

* Correspondence: mmiklasinska@sum.edu.pl; Tel.: +48-32-364-1621

Abstract: The aim of the presented study was to examine the in vitro antimicrobial activity of rutin hydrate (RH) alone and in combination with amikacin against 12 reference strains of Gram-positive and Gram-negative bacteria. The antibacterial activity assay was evaluated in the concentration range of 2–2048 µg/mL. A serial microdilution method was used to determine the minimal inhibitory concentration (MIC) of the examined compound against reference strains. RH showed varying potential against the tested strains with MICs ranging from 128 to 1024 µg/mL. In order to examine the combinatory profile of RH and amikacin, the fractional inhibitory concentrations (FICs) were determined. The RH–amikacin combination was more active against Gram-negative bacteria where four synergism and two additive interactions were noted. For four out of six Gram-positive isolates, an indifferent effect of RH and amikacin was demonstrated, and for two strains, the tested combination had an additive effect. The results of this study showed that RH possesses antimicrobial potential in vitro towards the tested reference isolates. Moreover, it shows a promising combined effect with amikacin against Gram-negative bacteria.

Keywords: rutin hydrate; amikacin; fractional inhibitory concentration

1. Introduction

Antimicrobial Resistance (AMR) is a significant global problem with serious public health risks. The treatment options and ability to control infections are gradually being exhausted, and the duration of infection and hospitalization has increased, all of which have led to an increase in mortality [1]. Due to the ever-growing problem of antibiotic resistance, scientists should focus their attention on finding alternatives to antibiotics as soon as possible. Searching for and testing new chemical compounds showing bacteriostatic or bactericidal activity will increase our chances of therapeutic success in infections caused by antibiotic-resistant bacteria [2,3].

Many previous studies have shown that compounds of natural origin have antibacterial activity alone and in combination with selected antibiotics [4–8]. So far, in our research, we have focused on the antibacterial effect of phenolic acids and flavanols against staphylococcal strains. In this research, we studied the antimicrobial properties of rutin hydrate, which is a representative of glycoside flavonoids, against reference strains of Gram-positive and Gram-negative bacteria. Rutin is composed of aglycone and sugar residue (Figure 1). The aglycone part is composed of quercetin linked with an O-glycosidic bond with rutinose, which is a disaccharide [9,10]. Rutinoside was first isolated from the common rue herb (*Ruta graveolens* L.), from which the name of the organic chemical compound is derived. Some examples of the sources of rutin are Japanese pagoda tree flowers (*Styphnolobium japonicum*), buckwheat herb (*Fagopyrum esculentum*), and eucalyptus leaves (*Eucalyptus* spp.), among many others. Rutin is also commonly found in vegetables and fruits, mainly citrus fruits, and plant-based drinks [9]. Pure rutin takes the form of a yellow powder with a structure of fine crystals. Due to its lipophilic nature, rutoside is soluble in organic solvents, but very poorly soluble in water. To obtain a better assimilable form of rutin, various methods of raw material preparation are used, e.g., with hydration, hydrates are obtained, from which it is easier to prepare the desired solutions of rutin [10].

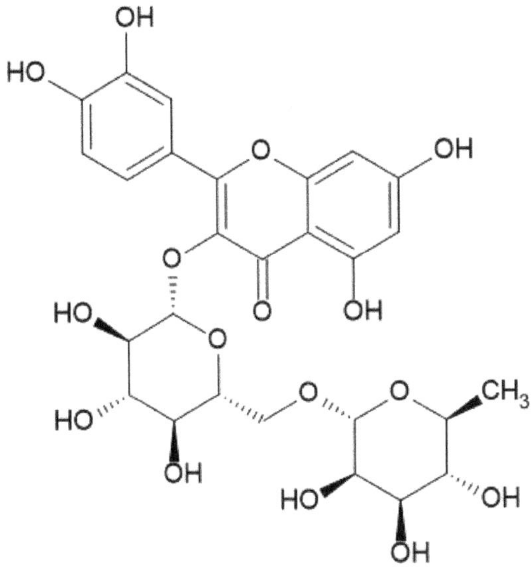

Figure 1. Chemical structure of rutin.

The structure of rutin determines its biological activity, which, in turn, influences its pharmacological properties. The main advantage of rutin is its antioxidant properties. Due to the presence of free hydroxyl groups, rutin has the ability to neutralize reactive oxygen species. By reducing free oxygen radicals, rutin protects the cells of the human body because it limits the formation of damage-causing mutations in the genetic material. In addition, quercetin-3-O-rutoside as an antioxidant prevents the peroxidation of phospholipids that form the cell membrane and consequently reduces the damage caused by free radicals. In this way, rutinoside directly contributes to the protection of cells against apoptosis caused by DNA damage or cell lysis as a result of cell membrane instability [11,12].

In addition, it has been proven that rutin exerts an antiatherogenic effect because it inhibits the oxidation of low-density lipoproteins and consequently reduces the formation of atherosclerotic plaques, which, in turn, have a protective effect on the cardiovascular system. Moreover, rutin slows down the oxidation of vitamin C, which means that ascorbic acid in the presence of rutin has a prolonged antioxidant effect. This property has been used in medical preparations and dietary supplements. Vitamin C, in addition to its important role as a free radical scavenger, is also a cofactor in proline and lysyl hydroxylases, which catalyze the hydroxylation of proline and lysine, respectively. Hydroxyproline and hydroxylysine are the main amino acids of collagen, which is an important structural element of blood vessels because it gives them durability and elasticity. In addition, rutin inhibits the activity of hyaluronidase, which is responsible for the digestion of collagen, and also reduces the activity of metalloproteinases responsible for the degradation of the extracellular matrix. All these properties contribute to the improvement of blood vessel conditions due to an increase in their elasticity and at the same time a reduction in their fragility and permeability [9].

The antibacterial properties of rutin have also been proven, which may find practical applications in the era of antibiotic resistance. Previous scientific research has demonstrated the antimicrobial activity of rutin against both Gram-positive and Gram-negative bacterial strains [13–17].

The antibiotic tested in this study was amikacin, which is used in the treatment of many nosocomial infections caused by Gram-negative bacteria, e.g., urinary tract infections or infections associated with the vascular line. In addition, it acts against some Gram-positive bacteria, e.g., methicillin-resistant *Staphylococcus aureus* (MRSA) [18]. Figure 2 shows the structural formula of amikacin.

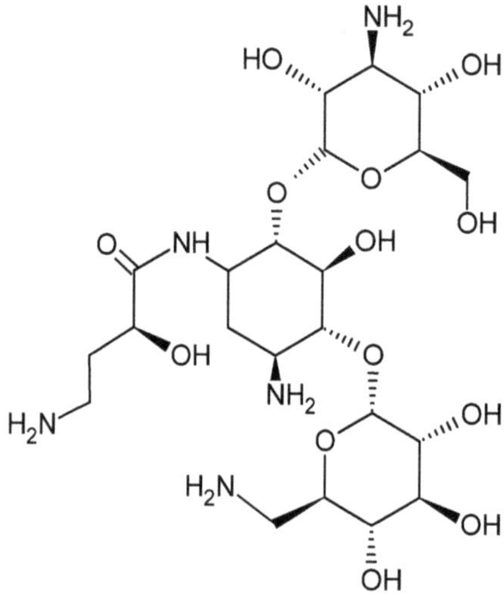

Figure 2. Chemical structure of amikacin.

2. Results

Amikacin turned out to be the most active against the strains *Staphylococcus epidermidis* ATCC 12228 and *Staphylococcus aureus* ATCC 25923, the growths of which were inhibited at concentrations of 0.5 and 1 μg/mL, respectively. In turn, a concentration of 2 μg/mL inhibited the growth of the following strains: *Bacillus subtilis* PMC 2021 and *Enterobacter clocae* ATCC 13047, and a concentration of 4 μg/mL was active against the isolates of *Enterococcus faecalis* ATCC 29212 and *Staphylococcus epidermidis* ATCC 35984. An MIC value of 8 μg/mL proved to work against *Escherichia coli* ATCC 25922 and *Proteus mirabilis* ATCC 7002. An amikacin concentration of 16 μg/mL was found to be active against *Pseudomonas aeruginosa* ATCC 27853. The highest concentration inhibiting the growth of microorganisms (64 μg/mL) was recorded for the following strains: *Staphylococcus aureus* ATCC 43300, *Klebsiella pneumoniae* ATCC 27736, and *Acinetobacter baumannii* ATCC 19606 (Table 1). In summary, the median MIC values obtained for amikacin were 3 μg/mL for Gram-positive bacteria and 12 μg/mL for Gram-negative bacteria. The standard deviation was 25.23 and 29 μg/mL for Gram-positive and Gram-negative strains, respectively. The lower and upper quartiles were 1 and 4 μg/mL for Gram-positive strains and 8 and 64 μg/mL for Gram-negative strains. A statistical analysis showed no differences in the obtained MIC values of amikacin ($p = 0.105$) between Gram-positive and Gram-negative bacteria (Table 2).

Table 1. The MIC values of RH, amikacin alone, and amikacin in combination with RH towards examined strains, along with the obtained FIC index values and their interpretations.

Strain	Gram	MIC of Rutin Hydrate [µg/mL]	MIC of Amikacin [µg/mL]	MIC of Amikacin with Rutin Hydrate [µg/mL]	FIC Index	Interaction
Staphylococcus aureus ATCC 25923	Positive	512	1	0.0625	0.563	additive
Staphylococcus aureus ATCC 43300	Positive	512	64	1	1.016	indifference
Staphylococcus epidermidis ATCC 12228	Positive	512	0.5	0.25	0.656	additive
Staphylococcus epidermidis ATCC 35984	Positive	128	4	4	1.013	indifference
Enterococcus faecalis ATCC 29212	Positive	256	4	0.125	1.031	indifference
Bacillus subtilis PMC 2021	Positive	256	2	0.0625	2.031	indifference
Escherichia coli ATCC 25922	Negative	512	8	0.125	0.078	synergism
Klebsiella pneumoniae ATCC 27736	Negative	256	64	4	0.188	synergism
Proteus mirabilis ATCC 7002	Negative	256	8	2	0.75	additive
Enterobacter clocae ATCC 13047	Negative	128	2	0.5	0.5	synergism
Pseudomonas aeruginosa ATCC 27853	Negative	1024	16	0.5	0.094	synergism
Acinetobacter baumannii ATCC 19606	Negative	1024	64	2	0.532	additive

Table 2. Descriptive and non-parametric statistics for the MIC values of rutin hydrate, amikacin alone, and amikacin with the addition of rutin hydrate for Gram-negative and Gram-positive strains.

	MIC of Rutin Hydrate [μg/mL]		MIC of Amikacin [μg/mL]		MIC of Amikacin with Rutin Hydrate [μg/mL]	
	Gram-Positive Strains	**Gram-Negative Strains**	**Gram-Positive Strains**	**Gram-Negative Strains**	**Gram-Positive Strains**	**Gram-Negative Strains**
Median	384	384	3	12	0.19	1.25
Standard deviation	170.13	400.02	25.23	29	0.38	1.46
Lower quartile	256	256	1	8	0.06	0.5
Upper quartile	512	1024	4	64	0.62	2
Mann–Whitney U test	$p = 0.676$		$p = 0.105$		$p = 0.226$	

Rutin hydrate showed antibacterial activity against all the tested strains. The MIC values of RH for Gram-positive strains ranged from 128 to 512 μg/mL with a median of 384 μg/mL, lower quartile of 256 μg/mL, upper quartile of 512 μg/mL, and standard deviation of 170.13 μg/mL. On the other hand, for the Gram-negative bacteria, the median, lower quartile, upper quartile, and standard deviation were 384, 256, 1024, and 400.02 μg/mL, respectively (Table 2). A statistical analysis showed no differences in the obtained MIC values of rutin hydrate ($p = 0.676$) between Gram-positive and Gram-negative bacteria (Table 2). The lowest MIC value of rutin hydrate amounting to 128 μg/mL was recorded for the *Staphylococcus epidermidis* ATCC 35984 and *Enterobacter clocae* ATCC 13047 strains. The highest MIC value (1024 μg/mL) was observed for two strains: *Pseudomonas aeruginosa* ATCC 27853 and *Acinetobacter baumannii* ATCC 19606. An MIC of 256 μg/mL was noted for four strains: *Klebsiella pneumoniae* ATCC 27736, *Proteus mirabilis* ATCC 7002, *Bacillus subtilis* PCM 2021, and *Enterococcus faecalis* ATCC 29212. The MIC was 512 μg/mL for the remaining four isolates: *Staphylococcus aureus* ATCC 25923, *Staphylococcus aureus* ATCC 43300, *Staphylococcus epidermidis* ATCC 12228, and *Escherichia coli* ATCC 25922 (Table 1).

The final stage of the research was the determination of the FIC index values. The results of the checkerboard assay for the reference strains are presented in Figure 3. Moreover, based on the checkerboard, the MIC values were determined for RH in combination with amikacin and for amikacin in combination with RH. The MIC values of amikacin with RH for Gram-positive strains ranged from 0.0625 to 1 μg/mL with a median of 0.19 μg/mL, lower quartile of 0.06 μg/mL, upper quartile 0.62 of μg/mL, and standard deviation of 0.38 μg/mL. For Gram-negative bacteria, the descriptive statistics above were 1.25, 0.5, 2, and 1.46 μg/mL, respectively (Table 2). The amikacin–RH combination turned out to be more active against Gram-negative strains, where in four cases, a synergistic effect was found, and in two, it was additive. In the group of Gram-positive bacteria, two additive interactions were noted, and for the remaining strains, the effect of combining the compounds was indifferent. No antagonistic effect was noted for any of the tested strains. The results of all the above assays are summarized in Table 1. There were no statistically significant differences in the amikacin MIC, and the MIC decreased after the addition of RH between Gram-positive and Gram-negative strains ($p = 0.226$ and $p = 0.870$, respectively). However, to more precisely investigate differences in the action of the "rutin hydrate—amikacin" combination on Gram-positive vs. Gram-negative bacteria, a larger study group should be used. The descriptive and non-parametric statistics for the MICs of amikacin alone and with rutin hydrate for Gram-negative and Gram-positive strains are presented in Table 2.

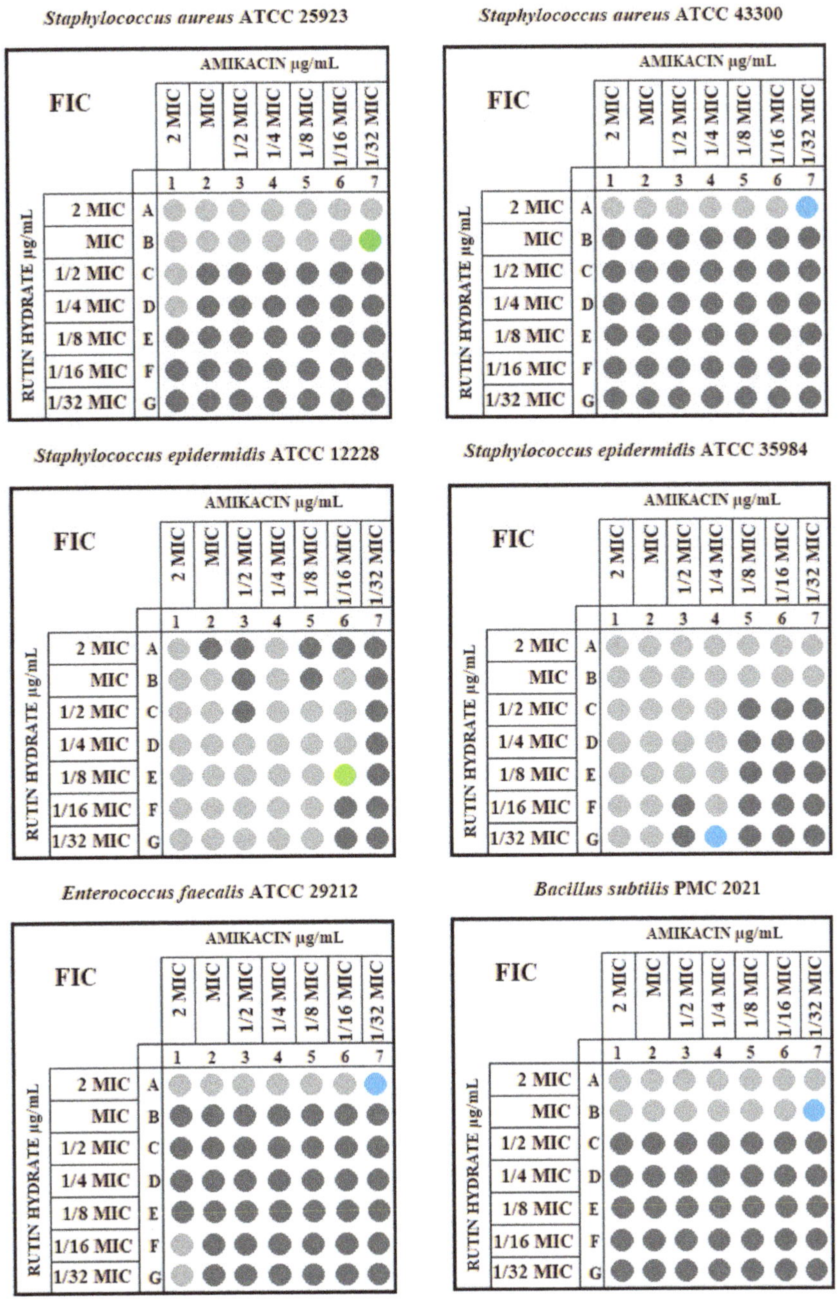

Figure 3. *Cont.*

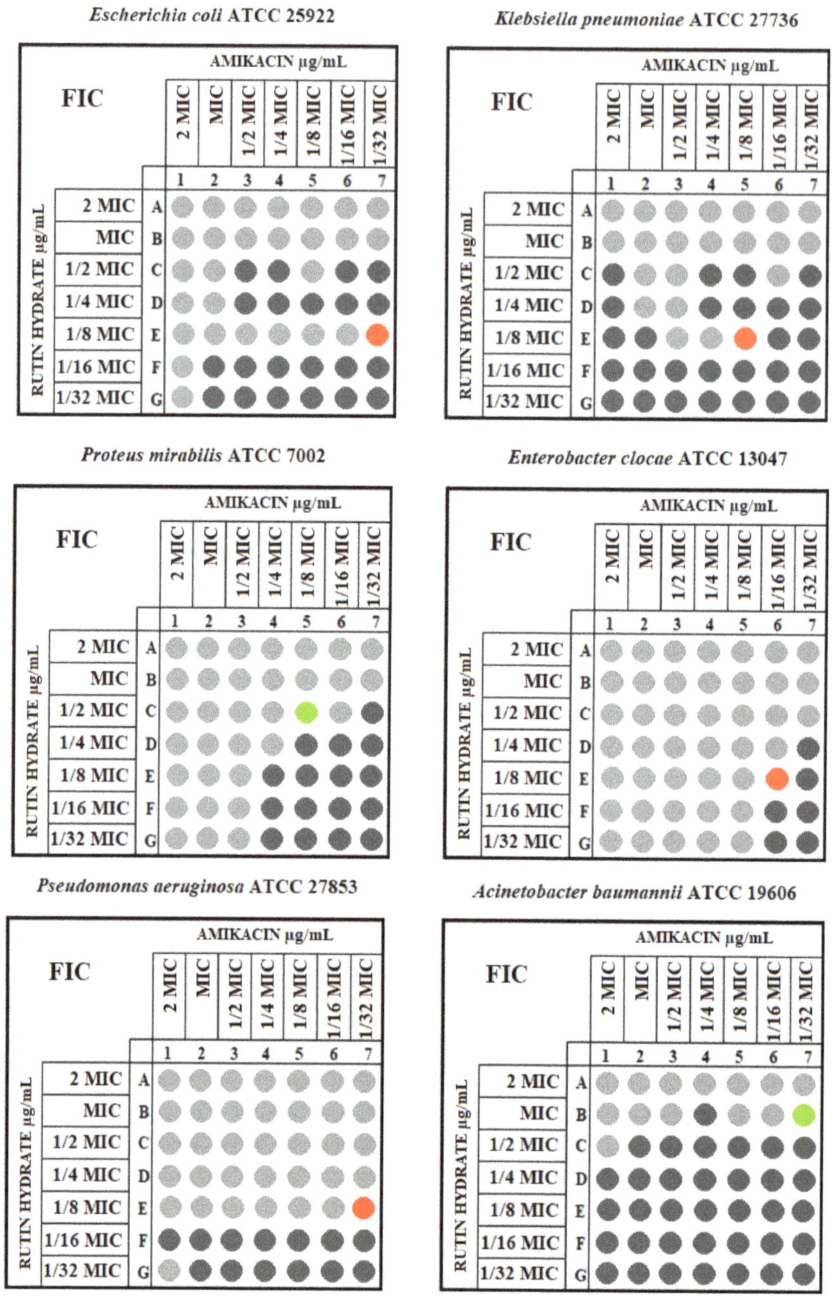

Figure 3. The checkerboard assay for Gram-positive and Gram-negative tested strains. The dark gray shows more than 50% bacterial growth in a well, while the light gray represents less than 50% bacterial growth in a well compared with the growth control. Only light gray wells were used to determine the FIX index. The FIC index for each strain is marked with a color. The blue shows an indifferent, the green an additive, and the red a synergistic interaction. The FIC index was marked on the growth inhibition border and represents the point where a synergistic/additive or indifferent effect was the most visible.

3. Discussion

The need to launch a new antibacterial drug in the era of antibiotic resistance has prompted scientists around the world to return to natural medicine methods and analyze the potential antibacterial mechanisms of action of plant-derived compounds. The antimicrobial potential of polyphenols, especially rutin, has been confirmed in in vitro studies on bacterial cultures [14–17,19–27]. In our study, amikacin, in small concentrations ranging from 0.5 to 16 μg/mL, was active against both Gram-positive and Gram-negative reference strains. Amikacin in its highest concentration (64 μg/mL) inhibited the growth of the following strains: *Staphylococcus aureus* ATCC 43300, *Klebsiella pneumoniae* ATCC 27736, and *Acinetobacter baumannii* ATCC 19606. Due to the resistance of amikacin to most aminoglycoside-modifying enzymes, it is used in the treatment of infections of strains resistant to other aminoglycosides. This antibiotic is the one most frequently applied to semi-synthetic aminoglycoside. However, strains resistant to amikacin have developed over the years. The first acetyltransferases that inactivated amikacin were reported for *P. aeruginosa*. Adenyltransferase, in turn, was found in *K. pneumoniae*, *E. coli*, *Serratia marcescens*, and *Proteus vulgaris*, and phosphotransferases were isolated from *E. coli*. Amikacin is no exception among other antibiotics, and bacteria develop resistance to it as well [28]. The introduction of natural compounds such as rutin hydrate into treatment may increase the potential of amikacin by improving its pharmacokinetic and pharmacodynamic properties, which could lead to a reduction in the doses, and thus reduce side effects associated with its use. This advantage of rutin hydrate as an antibacterial agent may consequently contribute to inhibiting the spread of resistance among bacteria. To the best of our knowledge, studies on the direction of interactions between RH and amikacin have not yet been conducted, but the antibacterial properties of rutin have been studied, and the results of these works are discussed below.

Jhanji et al. in 2021 examined the antimicrobial potential of rutin on four selected reference strains in comparison with commonly used antibiotics, which were streptomycin, ciprofloxacin, and amoxicillin. They observed that the growth of *B. subtilis* in the presence of rutin at a concentration of 256 μg/mL was inhibited at a rate of about 75%. The growth inhibition of *P. aeruginosa* at a concentration of 1024 μg/mL was approximately 90%. In turn, in cultures of *E. coli* and *S. aureus*, a rutin concentration of 512 μg/mL inhibited bacterial growth by approximately 70%. Research conducted by Jhanji et al. showed that the rutin solutions used by them in the concentrations defined in this study as the MIC values inhibited the growth of the indicated bacterial strains in the range of 70–90% [15]. Additionally, Jhanji et al. showed a synergistic effect of the combination "rutin-berberine-streptomycin" against *B. subtilis* (FIC index = 0.25), "rutin-berberine-ciprofloxacin" against *P. aeruginosa* (FIC index = 0.25), and "rutin-berberine-amoxicillin" against *S. aureus* (FIC index = 0.125).

In addition, Jhanji et al., in research conducted in 2020, considered a mechanism of antimicrobial activity in rutin [16]. Researchers have suggested that rutin may inhibit the action of *efflux pumps* and interfere with biofilm formation. Both mechanisms have been confirmed in in silico and in vitro studies on bacterial cultures. Interestingly, in our study, RH turned out to be more active against the reference strain *S. epidermidis* ATCC 35984 (128 μg/mL), which has the ability to form a biofilm, than against the biofilm (-) strain *S. epidermidis* ATCC 12228 (512 μg/mL). Our next studies will focus on assessing the ability to form biofilm under the influence of rutin hydrate.

Wang et al., in their study, focused on the analysis of the antimicrobial potential of rutin against the *K. pneumoniae* ATCC 700603 and *E. coli* ATCC 25922 reference strains. The MIC value of rutin against the *E. coli* strain was 512 μg/mL, which was the same as in this study. In turn, the MIC value for *K. pneumoniae* was 1024 μg/mL, which was four times higher than the concentration of 256 μg/mL obtained in our study against *K. pneumoniae* ATCC 27736. The difference in the obtained MIC values is probably due to the fact that *K. pneumoniae* ATCC 700603, unlike *K. pneumoniae* ATCC 27736, produces extended-spectrum beta-lactamases [17].

In addition, Wang et al., like Jhanji et al., studied the inhibition of biofilm formation in *K. pneumoniae* strains under the influence of rutin. Their research showed that rutin had a strong ability to inhibit biofilm formation in weak, moderate, and strong biofilm-producing strains. The ability to inhibit biofilm formation was confirmed by analyzing the expression profile of 15 genes involved in biofilm formation. A significant reduction in the expression of several genes from this group was observed, which correlated with a reduction in the accumulation of *K. pneumoniae* biomass. A significant inhibition of biofilm formation was observed at rutin concentrations of 512 and 256 μg/mL [17].

The confirmation of the antimicrobial potential of rutin opens many research paths that will be aimed at analyzing the change in the antibacterial properties of rutin in the presence of other polyphenols with a similar effect, as well as antibiotics and various forms of rutin preparation, e.g., in the form of nanoparticles, biomaterials coated with rutin, etc. The validity of searching for compounds against which rutin exhibits synergy and/or potentiates antibacterial activity has been confirmed by research conducted in 2015 by Amin et al. These scientists decided to determine the effect of rutin, morin, and quercetin (in various combinations) with 12 selected antibiotics on 100 clinical MRSA strains and the *S. aureus* ATCC 43300 reference strain. It was found that the tested compounds in combination with antibiotics enhanced the antibacterial effect against the examined staphylococcal strains. The relationship between flavonoids and antibiotics was additive in most cases, but synergism was also observed in a few cases. Moreover, Amin et al. examined potassium release to determine the effect of antibiotic–flavonoid combinations on the cytoplasmic membrane for the tested staphylococci. They proved that flavonoids alone or in combination damage the bacterial cell membrane [24]. The use of a mixture of rutin with other flavonoids may allow for its use in much lower concentrations than the MIC values determined in this study.

The results obtained and presented in this paper confirm the logic and effectiveness of using rutin hydrate as an agent combating antibiotic-resistant bacterial strains. This potential is conditioned by specific mechanisms of action, the study of which is the second step in confirming the usefulness of rutin in bacterial infections. Numerous studies have indicated that rutin, as a polyphenol, modifies the permeability of bacterial cell membranes and changes the stiffness of the cell wall, which leads to the loss of its integrity [25]. In addition, it has been suggested that rutin could alter intracellular functioning by binding hydroxyl residues to important bacterial enzymes [26]. Moreover, it was reported that rutin has the ability to inhibit β-lactamases and biofilm formation [27].

The research results discussed above, as well as the results presented in this paper, indicate the antimicrobial potential of rutin. In addition, they prove that this compound increases the antibacterial potential of antibiotics. Due to the anti-biofilm activity of rutin indicated by several researchers, it seems important to further study this compound in this respect. Moreover, it is necessary to examine the combination "rutin hydrate-amikacin" on clinical strains of Gram-negative bacteria with different resistance mechanisms.

4. Materials and Methods

4.1. Materials

All reference strains of bacteria came from the ATCC culture bank (American Collection of Cell Cultures, Manassas, VA,, USA), except the strain *Bacillus subtilis* PCM 2021, which was obtained from the Polish Collection of Microorganisms (Wroclaw, Poland). The tests were carried out on twelve selected strains of Gram-positive and Gram-negative bacteria: *Staphylococcus aureus* ATCC 25923, *Staphylococcus aureus* ATCC 43300, *Staphylococcus epidermidis* ATCC 12228, *Staphylococcus epidermidis* ATCC 35984, *Enterococcus faecalis* ATCC 29212, *Bacillus subtilis* PCM 2021, *Escherichia coli* ATCC 25922, *Klebsiella pneumoniae* ATCC 27736, *Proteus mirabilis* ATCC 7002, *Enterobacter cloacae* ATCC 13047, *Pseudomonas aeruginosa* ATCC 27853, and *Acinetobacter baumannii* ATCC 19606. Rutin hydrate was obtained from Sigma Chemical Co. (St. Louis, MO, USA).

4.2. Determination of the MIC Values of the Tested Bacterial Strains

In order to determine the lowest bacterial-growth-inhibiting concentrations for rutin hydrate and amikacin, the serial microdilution method was used with sterile, 96-well titer plates (FL Medical, Torreglia, Italy) with a final volume of 200 µL [29,30].

An amount of 100 µL of TSB medium (BTL) was aliquoted into all wells of the titer plates. The next step was to prepare serial dilutions of the tested compounds (from 1024 to 1 µg/mL). Tested compounds were not introduced into the 12th column of the titration plate, which was a growth control. Next, one hundred microliters of mid-logarithmic-phase bacterial cultures (5×10^5 CFU/mL) in TSB was added to each well (rows B–G). Row H wells were used to control the sterility of the medium. In addition, in row A of each plate, a suspension of TSB medium and the tested compound at various concentrations was prepared, which allowed the subsequent measurement of background extinction. Each examined strain was measured in triplicate. The next stage of the study was the incubation of the titer plates at 37 °C for 24 h. After incubation, the optical density of the culture was measured at 595 nm. Absorbance results for individual strains were read using a Multiskan EX reader (Thermo Electron Corp., Vantoa, Finland) [31,32]. MICs were defined as the lowest RH concentrations that completely inhibited bacterial growth [33]. The MIC results obtained in this stage of the research were used to design the "chessboard" and determine the FIC values in the next stage.

4.3. Determination of the FIC Values for the Tested Strains

The sensitivity of the tested reference isolates to the combination of amikacin with RH was assessed by determining the fractionated inhibitory concentration (FIC) value for each strain. The checkerboard microdilution method with modifications [34,35] was used to determine the total susceptibility effect of the tested strains. First, the solutions of the antibiotic and RH were prepared, corresponding to 8 MIC values (according to the MIC values obtained in the first stage of the study). A series of 1/8 MIC dilutions were then produced. An amount of 95 µL of double-concentrated Mueller–Hinton (BLT) medium was added to each well of the titration plate. Then, 50 µL of RH and the appropriate concentration of amikacin were pipetted. Finally, 5 µL of a 0.5 McFarland bacterial suspension was added. The final volume of each well was 200 µL. Therefore, the solutions corresponding to the concentrations of 8 MICs, 4 MICs, 2 MICs, 1 MIC, 1/2 MIC, 1/4 MIC, and 1/8 MIC were prepared for amikacin and RH to account for the dilution of 50 µL of these substances in 200 µL of the solution and were obtained as follows: 2 MICs, 1 MIC, 1/2 MIC, 1/4 MIC, 1/8 MIC, 1/16 MIC, and 1/32 MIC in each of the wells. At the last column and row, respectively, instead of RH and amikacin, 50 µL of medium was added. The scheme of the "chessboard" plate is shown in Figure 4.

The plates prepared in this way were incubated in an aerobic incubator at 37 °C for 24 h. The absorbances at 595 nm were then read. Next, the percentage increase in individual wells relative to the growth control was calculated. Only wells that represented less than 50% bacterial growth compared with the growth control were considered for FIC index determination.

The MICs for rutin hydrate and amikacin for each strain were then recalculated. At the end, the FICs (fractional inhibitory concentrations) were calculated, i.e., the fractional inhibitory concentration for RH and amikacin and their sum for each well. The following formula was used:

$$\text{FIC index} = \text{FICA} + \text{FICB} = (\text{MICA} + \text{B})/\ \text{MICA} + (\text{MICB} + \text{A})/\text{MICB},$$

where:

MICA + B—MIC of the antibiotic in the presence of a polyphenolic compound;
MICB + A—MIC of a polyphenolic compound in the presence of an antibiotic;
MICA—MIC of the antibiotic itself;
MICB—MIC of the polyphenolic compound itself.

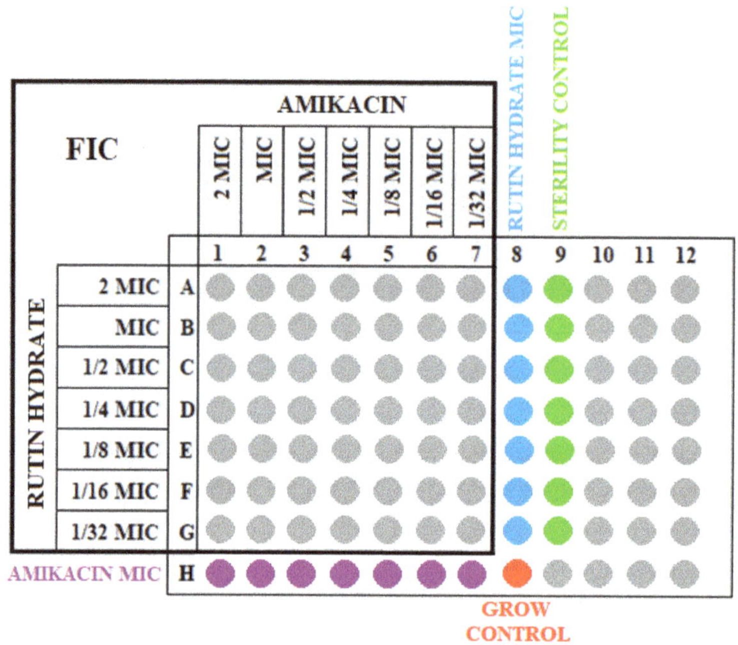

Figure 4. Scheme of the checkerboard method with the simultaneous indication of the FICs and MICs.

Next, on the growth inhibition border, the FIC index was established for each strain. The FIC index was the point where synergistic/additive or indifferent effects were the most visible.

Based on the FIC index value for each strain, the relationship between rutin hydrate and amikacin was assessed according to the following scale:

FIC $\leq$ 0.5—synergism;
0.5 < FIC $\leq$ 1—additive action;
1 < FIC $\leq$ 4—indifference;
FIC > 4—antagonism [35].

4.4. Statistical Analysis

In order to check whether there were differences in the obtained MICs of RH or amikacin values between Gram-positive and Gram-negative bacteria, the Mann–Whitney U test was used for two independent samples. The same test determined whether there were statistically significant differences in the amikacin MICs, and the MICs decreased after the addition of RH between Gram-positive and Gram-negative bacterial strains. Statistical calculations were made in the Statistica 13.0 program. The level of statistical significance was $p < 0.05$.

5. Conclusions

The results of the presented study demonstrate that rutin hydrate possesses antibacterial properties against the tested reference strains, and this effect is similar for both Gram-positive and Gram-negative bacteria. The combination of "amikacin–RH" was effective against Gram-negative bacteria, where in four cases, a synergistic effect was found, and in two, it was additive. On the other hand, two additive interactions and four indifferent effects were noted for Gram-positive bacteria. The in vitro synergistic interaction of RH and amikacin suggests that this effect could also be observed in vivo. Future studies should focus on the mechanism of action of RH on bacterial cells.

Author Contributions: Conceptualization: M.M.-M., M.K. (Małgorzata Kępa) and T.J.W.; methodology: M.M.-M., M.K. (Małgorzata Kępa) and K.Z.-P.; validation: T.J.W., M.M.-M., M.K. (Małgorzata Kępa) and R.D.W.; formal analysis: T.J.W., M.M.-M. and M.K. (Małgorzata Kępa); investigation: M.M.-M., K.Z.-P. and M.K. (Magdalena Klim); data curation: M.M.-M., M.K. (Małgorzata Kępa) and K.Z.-P.; writing—original draft preparation: M.M.-M., M.K. (Małgorzata Kępa) and T.J.W.; writing—review and editing: R.D.W. and T.J.W.; supervision: R.D.W. and T.J.W.; funding acquisition: M.M.-M. and T.J.W. All authors have read and agreed to the published version of the manuscript.

Funding: This research was funded by the Medical University of Silesia in Katowice, Poland, grant numbers PCN-2-018/N/1/I and PCN-2-075/K/2/I.

Institutional Review Board Statement: Not applicable.

Informed Consent Statement: Not applicable.

Data Availability Statement: Not applicable.

Conflicts of Interest: The authors declare no conflict of interest.

References

1. Gupta, R.; Sharma, S. Role of Alternatives to Antibiotics in Mitigating the Antimicrobial Resistance Crisis. *Indian J. Med. Res.* **2022**, *156*, 464–477. [PubMed]
2. Allen, H.K.; Trachsel, J.; Looft, T.; Casey, T.A. Finding Alternatives to Antibiotics. *Ann. N. Y. Acad. Sci.* **2014**, *1323*, 91–100. [CrossRef] [PubMed]
3. Frieri, M.; Kumar, K.; Boutin, A. Antibiotic Resistance. *J. Infect. Public Health* **2017**, *10*, 369–378. [CrossRef] [PubMed]
4. Qu, S.; Dai, C.; Shen, Z.; Tang, Q.; Wang, H.; Zhai, B.; Zhao, L.; Hao, Z. Mechanism of Synergy Between Tetracycline and Quercetin Against Antibiotic Resistant *Escherichia coli*. *Front. Microbiol.* **2019**, *10*, 2536. [CrossRef] [PubMed]
5. Shi, M.; Bai, Y.; Qiu, Y.; Zhang, X.; Zeng, Z.; Chen, L.; Cheng, F.; Zhang, J. Mechanism of Synergy between Piceatannol and Ciprofloxacin against Staphylococcus Aureus. *Int. J. Mol. Sci.* **2022**, *23*, 15341. [CrossRef]
6. Aonofriesei, F. Effect of Methylpyrazoles and Coumarin Association on the Growth of Gram-Negative Bacteria. *Arch. Microbiol.* **2022**, *204*, 160. [CrossRef]
7. El Atki, Y.; Aouam, I.; El Kamari, F.; Taroq, A.; Nayme, K.; Timinouni, M.; Lyoussi, B.; Abdellaoui, A. Antibacterial Activity of Cinnamon Essential Oils and Their Synergistic Potential with Antibiotics. *J. Adv. Pharm. Technol. Res.* **2019**, *10*, 63–67. [CrossRef]
8. Pal, A.; Tripathi, A. Demonstration of Bactericidal and Synergistic Activity of Quercetin with Meropenem among Pathogenic Carbapenem Resistant Escherichia Coli and Klebsiella Pneumoniae. *Microb. Pathog.* **2020**, *143*, 104120. [CrossRef]
9. Samaszko-Fiertek, J.; Roguszczak, P.; Dmochowska, B.; Ślusarz, R.; Madaj, J. Rutin—Structure and Properities. *Wiadomości Chem.* **2016**, *70*, 439–441. Available online: http://yadda.icm.edu.pl/baztech/element/bwmeta1.element.baztech-433ed886-5b08-41bd-a785-41e097496418 (accessed on 23 August 2023).
10. Rotimi, D.E.; Elebiyo, T.C.; Ojo, O.A. Therapeutic Potential of Rutin in Male Infertility: A Mini Review. *J. Integr. Med.* **2023**, *21*, 130–135. [CrossRef]
11. Chua, L.S. A review on plant-based rutin extraction methods and its pharmacological activities. *J. Ethnopharmacol.* **2013**, *150*, 805–817. [CrossRef] [PubMed]
12. Negahdari, R.; Bohlouli, S.; Sharifi, S.; Dizaj, S.M.; Saadat, Y.R.; Khezri, K.; Jafari, S.; Ahmadian, E.; Jahandizi, N.G.; Raeesi, S. Therapeutic Benefits of Rutin and Its Nanoformulations. *Phyther. Res.* **2021**, *35*, 1719–1738. [CrossRef] [PubMed]
13. Ganeshpurkar, A.; Saluja, A.K. The Pharmacological Potential of Rutin. *Saudi Pharm. J.* **2017**, *25*, 149–164. [CrossRef] [PubMed]
14. Rodríguez-Valdovinos, K.Y.; Salgado-Garciglia, R.; Vázquez-Sánchez, M.; Álvarez-Bernal, D.; Oregel-Zamudio, E.; Ceja-Torres, L.F.; Medina-Medrano, J.R. Quantitative Analysis of Rutin by HPTLC and In Vitro Antioxidant and Antibacterial Activities of Phenolic-Rich Extracts from *Verbesina sphaerocephala*. *Plants* **2021**, *10*, 475. [CrossRef]
15. Jhanji, R.; Singh, A.; Kumar, A. Antibacterial Potential of Selected Phytomolecules: An Experimental Study. *Microbiol. Immunol.* **2021**, *65*, 325–332. [CrossRef]
16. Jhanji, R.; Bhati, V.; Singh, A.; Kumar, A. Phytomolecules against Bacterial Biofilm and Efflux Pump: An In Silico and In Vitro Study. *J. Biomol. Struct. Dyn.* **2020**, *38*, 5500–5512. [CrossRef]
17. Wang, Z.; Ding, Z.; Li, Z.; Ding, Y.; Jiang, F.; Liu, J. Antioxidant and Antibacterial Study of 10 Flavonoids Revealed Rutin as a Potential Antibiofilm Agent in Klebsiella Pneumoniae Strains Isolated from Hospitalized Patients. *Microb. Pathog.* **2021**, *159*, 105121. [CrossRef]
18. Hryniewicz, W.; Żukowska, A. *Rekomendacje Diagnostyki, Terapii i Profilaktyki Antybiotykowej Zakażeń w Szpitalu—2020: Materiał Przeznaczony dla Komitetów Terapeutycznych i Zespołów ds. Antybiotykoterapii Polskich Szpitali, Wydanie Drugie*; Narodowy Instytut Leków: Warszawa, Poland, 2020.
19. Cushnie, T.P.T.; Lamb, A.J. Antimicrobial Activity of Flavonoids. *Int. J. Antimicrob. Agents* **2005**, *26*, 343–356. [CrossRef]
20. Xia, X.; Song, X.; Li, Y.; Hou, W.; Lv, H.; Li, F.; Li, Y.; Liu, J.; Li, X. Antibacterial and Anti-Inflammatory ZIF-8@Rutin Nanocomposite as an Efficient Agent for Accelerating Infected Wound Healing. *Front. Bioeng. Biotechnol.* **2022**, *10*, 1026743. [CrossRef]

21. Arima, H.; Ashida, H.; Danno, G. Rutin-Enhanced Antibacterial Activities of Flavonoids against Bacillus Cereus and Salmonella Enteritidis. *Biosci. Biotechnol. Biochem.* **2002**, *66*, 1009–1014. [CrossRef]
22. Motallebi, M.; Khorsandi, K.; Sepahy, A.A.; Chamani, E.; Hosseinzadeh, R. Effect of Rutin as Flavonoid Compound on Photodynamic Inactivation against *P aeruginosa* and *S. aureus*. *Photodiagnosis Photodyn. Ther.* **2020**, *32*, 102074. [CrossRef] [PubMed]
23. Obistioiu, D.; Cocan, I.; Tîrziu, E.; Herman, V.; Negrea, M.; Cucerzan, A.; Neacsu, A.-G.; Cozma, A.L.; Nichita, I.; Hulea, A.; et al. Phytochemical Profile and Microbiological Activity of Some Plants Belonging to the Fabaceae Family. *Antibiotics* **2021**, *10*, 662. [CrossRef] [PubMed]
24. Amin, M.U.; Khurram, M.; Khattak, B.; Khan, J. Antibiotic Additive and Synergistic Action of Rutin, Morin and Quercetin against Methicillin Resistant Staphylococcus Aureus. *BMC Complement. Altern. Med.* **2015**, *15*, 59. [CrossRef]
25. Xu, P.; Xu, X.B.; Khan, A.; Fotina, T.; Wang, S.H. Antibiofilm Activity against Staphylococcus Aureus and Content Analysis of Taraxacum Officinale Phenolic Extract. *Pol. J. Vet. Sci.* **2021**, *24*, 243–251. [PubMed]
26. Bouarab-Chibane, L.; Forquet, V.; Lantéri, P.; Clément, Y.; Léonard-Akkari, L.; Oulahal, N.; Degraeve, P.; Bordes, C. Antibacterial Properties of Polyphenols: Characterization and QSAR (Quantitative Structure–Activity Relationship) Models. *Front. Microbiol.* **2019**, *10*, 829. [CrossRef] [PubMed]
27. Mandal, S.M.; Dias, R.O.; Franco, O.L. Phenolic Compounds in Antimicrobial Therapy. *J. Med. Food.* **2017**, *20*, 1031–1038. [CrossRef]
28. Ramirez, M.S.; Tolmasky, M.E. Amikacin: Uses, Resistance, and Prospects for Inhibition. *Molecules* **2017**, *22*, 2267. [CrossRef]
29. Amsterdam, D. Susceptibility Testing of Antimicrobials in Liquid Media. In *Antibiotics in Laboratory Medicine*, 5th ed.; Loman, V., Ed.; Williams and Wilkins: Philadelphia, PA, USA, 2005; pp. 61–143.
30. European Committee for Antimicrobial Susceptibility Testing (EUCAST) of the European Society of Clinical Microbiology and Infectious Diseases (ESCMID). Determination of Minimum Inhibitory Concentrations (MICs) of Antibacterial Agents by Agar Dilution. *Clin. Microbiol. Infect.* **2000**, *6*, 509–515. [CrossRef]
31. Cudic, M.; Condie, B.A.; Weiner, D.J.; Lysenko, E.S.; Xiang, Z.Q.; Insug, O.; Bulet, P.; Otvos, L. Development of Novel Antibacterial Peptides That Kill Resistant Isolates. *Peptides* **2002**, *23*, 2071–2083. [CrossRef]
32. Devienne, K.F.; Raddi, M.S.G. Screening for Antimicrobial Activity of Natural Products Using a Microplate Photometer. *Braz. J. Microbiol.* **2002**, *33*, 166–168. [CrossRef]
33. European Committee for Antimicrobial Susceptibility Testing (EUCAST) of the European Society of Clinical Microbiology and Infectious Diseases (ESCMID). Determinantion of minimum inhibitory concentrations (MICs) of antibacterial agents by broth dilution. EUCAST discussion document E. dis 5.1. *Clin. Microbiol. Infect.* **2003**, *9*, ix–xv. [CrossRef]
34. Chai, B.; Jiang, W.; Hu, M.; Wu, Y.; Si, H. In Vitro Synergistic Interactions of Protocatechuic Acid and Chlorogenic Acid in Combination with Antibiotics against Animal Pathogens. *Synergy* **2019**, *9*, 100055. [CrossRef]
35. Mazur, P.; Skiba-Kurek, I.; Mrowiec, P.; Karczewska, E.; Drożdż, R. Synergistic ROS-Associated Antimicrobial Activity of Silver Nanoparticles and Gentamicin Against Staphylococcus Epidermidis. *IJN* **2020**, *15*, 3551–3562. [CrossRef] [PubMed]

antibiotics

Article

Biological Characterization of *Cleome felina* L.f. Extracts for Phytochemical, Antimicrobial, and Hepatoprotective Activities in Wister Albino Rats

Heena Yaqub Shaikh [1], Shaik Kalimulla Niazi [2], Asmatanzeem Bepari [3], Mary Anne Wong Cordero [3], Shazima Sheereen [4], Syed Arif Hussain [5], Muthuraj Rudrappa [1], Shashiraj Kariyellappa Nagaraja [1] and Shekappa Ningappa Agadi [1,*]

1 Department of P.G. Studies in Botany, Karnatak University, Dharwad 580003, Karnataka, India; heena.ks@kud.ac.in (H.Y.S.); rmuthuraj@kud.ac.in (M.R.); shashiraj@kud.ac.in (S.K.N.)
2 Department of Preparatory Health Sciences, Riyadh Elm University, Riyadh 12611, Saudi Arabia; kalimullaniazi@gmail.com
3 Department of Basic Health Sciences, College of Medicine, Princess Nourah bint Abdulrahman University, Riyadh 11671, Saudi Arabia; ambepari@pnu.edu.sa (A.B.); macordero@pnu.edu.sa (M.A.W.C.)
4 Department of Pathology, Manipal Academy of Higher Education, Mangalore 576104, Karnataka, India; dr.shazimasheereen@gmail.com
5 Respiratory Care Department, College of Applied Science, Almaarefa University, Diriyah, Riyadh 13713, Saudi Arabia; syhussain@mcst.edu.sa
* Correspondence: snagadi@kud.ac.in

Abstract: The present study aims to explore the phytochemical constitution and biological activities of *Cleome felina* L.f. (Cleomaceae). *C. felina* (leaves, stem, and root) extracts (acetone, methanol, and water) were qualitatively assessed for phytochemical presence. Methanolic leaves extract revealed more positive phyto-compounds among all the extracts; further, methanolic leaves extract was evaluated for FTIR, EDX, GCMS, antimicrobial assay, acute toxicity, and paracetamol-induced hepatoprotective activity in Wister albino rats. FTIR and EDX analysis unveiled important functional groups and elements in the leaves. GCMS analysis of methanolic leaves extract exposed 12 active phyto-compounds: major constituents detected were 1-Butanol, 3-methyl-, formate-48.79%; 1-Decanol, 2-ethyl-13.40%; 1,6-Anhydro-β-d-talopyranose-12.49%; Ethene, 1,2-bis(methylthio)-7.22%; Decane-4.02%; 3-Methylene-7, 11-dimethyl-1-dodecene-3.085%; Amlexanox-2.50%; 1,2,3,4-Cyclopentanetetrol, (1α,2β,3β,4α)-2.07%; L-Cysteine S-sulfate-1.84%; n-Hexadecanoic acid-1.70%; and Flucarbazone-1.55%. The antimicrobial assay showed a moderate zone of inhibition against *S. aureus*, *B. cereus*, *E. coli*, *P. aeruginosa*, *C. albicans*, and *C. glabrata* at 100 μL/mL concentration. Additionally, acute toxicity revealed no behavioral sign of the toxic effect. The significant results were obtained for methanolic leaves extract (low-50 and high-100 mg/kg b.wt. dose) for hepatoprotective activity, where it dramatically reduced serum blood biochemical markers (AST, ALT, ALP, Total bilirubin, and cholesterol) and exhibited elevated hepatic antioxidant enzymes (SOD, CAT, and GSH) concentration with lipid peroxidation retardation. To conclude, *C. felina* methanolic leaves extract ameliorated important phytochemical compounds and showed significant antimicrobial and hepatoprotective efficacy; therefore, utilization of *C. felina* leaves suggested in pharmacological applications, and in numerous cosmetics, herbicides, and food industries, would be a great scope for future hepatoprotective drug designing.

Keywords: *Cleome felina*; phyochemicals; GCMS; antimicrobial; acute toxicity; hepatoprotective

1. Introduction

Plants are essential for human beings in their daily life; they play a vital role as primary and secondary metabolites by providing food as energy, fiber, shelter, phytonutrients, and beneficial health-promoting pharmaceutical applications. In accordance with the World Health Organization (WHO), herbal medicine is utilized as primary health care by about 80% of the global population [1]. The level of primary metabolites determines the nutritional or nutraceutical value of plants, constituting the composition of fat, carbohydrate, protein, fiber, vitamins, and minerals, whereas the level of secondary metabolites determines the medicinal and therapeutic values that have applications in pharmaceutical, food, cosmetics, and fine chemical industries [2]. In the present era, the use of natural plant-based products has increased in the preparation of medicine and nutritional products and in different health sectors, as plants have antibacterial, antifungal, antidiabetic, antioxidant, anti-hyperlipidemic, anti-hypercholesterolemic, analgesic, hepatoprotective, neuroprotective, anticancer, and anti-inflammatory activities [3,4]. Hence, the determination of chemical constituents of herbal plants is essential, which can be achieved by different analytical techniques, such as Fourier-transform infrared spectroscopy (FTIR), energy-dispersive X-ray spectroscopy (EDX), Gas Chromatography–Mass Spectroscopy (GC/MS), etc., which are used to determine functional groups, elemental composition, and identification of the phytochemical compounds in crude extract.

In the past few years, health services have faced problems, as pathogenic bacteria and fungi have adopted new resistance mechanisms to commercial drugs or antimicrobial agents. Hence, it is necessary to find alternate antimicrobial agents that have strong effects towards resistance, along with fewer side effects, which is possible by the discovery of herbal-based antimicrobial agents [5]. Moreover, the use of natural-based products has been recommended by the World Health Organization, but driven attention to their toxicity and safety while using the natural products [6].

On the other hand, synthetic or commercial drugs and xenobiotics act as a toxic agent to most human organs, mainly to the liver, which is one of the largest internal organs and plays a characteristic role in the regulation and synthesis of several metabolic, essential biochemical and physiological processes, which are involved in the fight against infections and the detoxification mechanism of xenobiotics, whereas, at the same time, it is the organ that is readily prone to hepatic injuries by hepatotoxic agents (ethanol, CCl4, thioacetamide, D-galactosamine, environmental toxins, paracetamol) that lead to changes in the physiology and functional mechanism of the liver, as well as later resulting in liver fibrosis and cirrhosis [7,8]. In the present scenario, paracetamol (PC), known as *N*-acetyl-p-aminophenol (acetaminophen), acts as an analgesic and antipyretic drug, and is highly consumed. Moreover, the overdose of PC drug by humans or experimental animals will result in an increase of oxidative stress that induces lipid peroxidation and causes toxicity to hepatic cells [9]. However, various endogenous resistance mechanisms will operate to scavenge ROS to limit undesired cellular damage, but this protection might not be complete; hence, the additional foreign resistance in the form of dietary antioxidants will help to cure excessive cellular damage that was caused by excessive formation of ROS [10,11]. Due to this, researchers are driving their focus to find the substitution herbal treatments with potent antioxidant activities, which exhibit fewer side effects for disease treatments, such as liver diseases [12].

The genus *Cleome* is reported to possess pharmacologically active phytocompounds, which have been isolated, as they perform a vital role in the treatment of several ailments. The various plant parts of the genus *Cleome* have revealed good nutritional and therapeutic value. The most important class of secondary phyto-compounds has been derived from the *Cleome* species, which includes terpenes, sterols, flavonoids, glucosinolates, indole alkaloids, and isothiocyanates, which are distributed in various *Cleome* species [13,14]. *Cleome felina* L.f. is one among the species of the genus *Cleome*, which is a medicinal plant and is endemic to peninsular India [15]. This annual hairy herb is 30–60 cm, with trifoliate leaves, corolla pink, and more than 50 stamens; seedpods with seeds are slightly longer than the pedicel [16]. In epistaxis, the fresh and dry parts of *C. felina* are prescribed, which are pounded in equal quantity and given with milk and sugar. The complete plant is used as an astringent, and the vesicant seeds are given internally as a vermifuge [17]. Further, Wollenweber et al. [18] reported the isolation and characterization of flavonols, namely, 5,3′,4′-triOH-3,6,7,5′-tetraOMe flavone and 5,3′-diOH-3,6,7,4′,5′-pentaOMe-flavone (2), in *C. felina*. To date, several *Cleome* species have been studied for their active phytocompounds and pharmacological applications, but there is a dearth of information on *C. felina*. Hence, the objective of the current study was to screen *C. felina* for phytochemical constituents and to analyze pharmacological applications, such as antimicrobial activity, acute toxicity, and paracetamol-induced hepatoprotective activity, in Wister albino rats. The results of the investigation could provide scientific evidence of *C. felina* for its contribution in the therapeutic field.

2. Results

2.1. The Percentage Yield of Different Solvent Extracts of C. felina

C. felina is a hairy herb with trifoliate leaves (Figure 1). It was collected, and each part was separated; it was then washed and dried. The coarse powder was obtained from the dried part and processed for solvent extraction using organic solvents by Soxhlet apparatus to obtain the extraction yield.

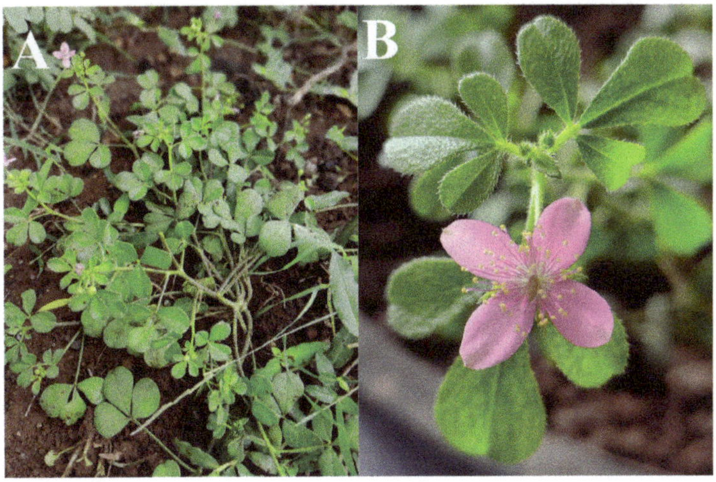

Figure 1. *Cleome felina* plant: (**A**) Plant habitat, (**B**) Plant with flower.

The percentage yield of the acetone, methanol, and water extract of *C. felina* leaves, stem, and root is displayed in Table 1. The leaves extracts of acetone, methanol, and water were 3.65, 17.01, and 13.75 g/100 g, respectively. The estimated amount of acetone, methanol, and water extract of the stem was 1.77, 9.63, and 15.64 g/100 g, respectively, whereas the extracts yield of acetone, methanol, and water for the root account for 1.4, 8.4, and 12.3 g/100 g, respectively.

Table 1. Different solvent extract yields of *C. felina* leaves, stem, and root.

Solvent	Extract Value g/100 g		
	Leaves	**Stem**	**Root**
Acetone	3.65 ± 0.03 [g]	1.77 ± 0.01 [h]	1.4 ± 0.03 [i]
Methanol	17.01 ± 0.33 [a]	9.63 ± 0.01 [e]	8.4 ± 0.03 [f]
Water	13.75 ± 0.01 [c]	15.64 ± 0.02 [b]	12.3 ± 0.03 [d]

Data are mean ± standard error (n = 3). Different letters in superscript indicate significant difference ($p < 0.05$).

2.2. Preliminary Screening of Phytocompounds for Different Solvent Extracts of C. felina

The various parts of *C. felina*, such as leaves, stem, and root, were extracted using organic solvents (acetone, methanol, and water). Each selective plant part with its chosen solvent was qualitatively analyzed for the presence of phytochemical constituents, such as carbohydrates, amino acids, glycosides, cardiac glycoside, phenolic, flavonoids, saponins, terpenoids, anthraquinones glycosides, and quinones, present in it for the screening of better solvent extracts to be used for further research work (Table 2). The phyto-compounds screening of leaves extract was estimated to show the presence of 6 acetone, 12 methanol, and 9 water metabolites. On the other hand, stem extract showed the presence of 10 acetone, 10 methanol, and 8 water phytochemicals, while the study of root extract exhibited the presence of 5 acetone, 9 methanol, and 6 water plant metabolites.

Table 2. Qualitative phytochemical screening of different solvent extracts of *C. felina* leaves, stem, and root.

Test Name	Leaves			Stem			Root		
	A	M	W	A	M	W	A	M	W
Carbohydrates									
Fehling's test	+	+	+	+	+	−	+	−	−
Protein									
Biuret test	−	−	+	−	+	+	+	+	+
Amino acids									
Ninhydrin test	−	+	−	−	+	+	+	+	+
Glycosides									
Salkowski's test	−	+	−	+	−	−	−	+	−
Cardiac glycoside									
Keller–Kiliani test	+	+	−	+	+	+	+	−	−
Phenolics									
Ferric chloride test	+	+	+	−	−	+	−	−	+
Flavonoids									
Alkaline reagent test	+	+	+	+	+	−	−	+	−
Saponins									
Froth Test	−	+	+	+	+	+	−	−	+
Terpenoids									
Salkowski's test	−	+	−	+	−	−	−	+	−
Anthraquinones glycosides									
Borntrager's test	+	+	+	+	+	+	−	−	+
Tannins									
Ferric chloride test	+	+	−	+	−	−	−	−	−
Alkaloids									
Mayer's test	−	+	−	−	+	+	−	+	+
Wagner's test	−	−	+	−	−	−	−	+	−
Betacyanins									
Sodium hydroxide test	−	−	+	+	+	+	−	+	−
Quinones	−	+	+	+	+	−	+	+	−

Note: A = Acetone, M = Methanol, W = Water, "+" = Present, and "−" = Absent.

2.3. *Fourier-Transform Infrared Spectroscopy (FT-IR) and Energy-Dispersive X-ray Spectroscopy (EDX) Analysis*

The IR spectrum for methanolic extract of the *C. felina* leaves was obtained by a NICOLET 67000 FTIR Spectrophotometer (NICOLET, Thermo Fisher Scientific, Waltham, MA, USA), and the transmittance of FT-IR analysis was recorded under the range of the 400–4000 cm^{-1} IR region. Wavenumber (cm^{-1}) intensities for a functional group and compound class were documented as presented in Figure 2 and Table 3. For the absorption spectrum of the methanolic leaves extract, the main peak showed the occurrence of various classes of compounds, such as alcohols, amine salt, conjugated alkenes, sulfonyl chloride, and halo compounds. Major bands were observed at 3383.67 cm^{-1}, 2920.81 cm^{-1}, 2850.61 cm^{-1}, 1384.43 cm^{-1}, 1176.30 cm^{-1}, and 824.86 cm^{-1} due to the vibration of O-H, N-H, S=O, C-O, C-Cl, and C-Br, respectively. Meanwhile, the mineral composition of *C. felina* leaves was analyzed by the energy-dispersive X-ray spectroscopy (EDX) technique with respect to the mass % and is presented in Figure 3 and Table 4. The minerals found in leaves were carbon, oxygen, magnesium, aluminum, silicon, phosphorus, sulfur, chlorine, potassium, and calcium of 36.48, 39.74, 1.80, 0.35, 0.46, 0.58, 1.01, 2.15, 2.31, and 15.13 mass %, respectively.

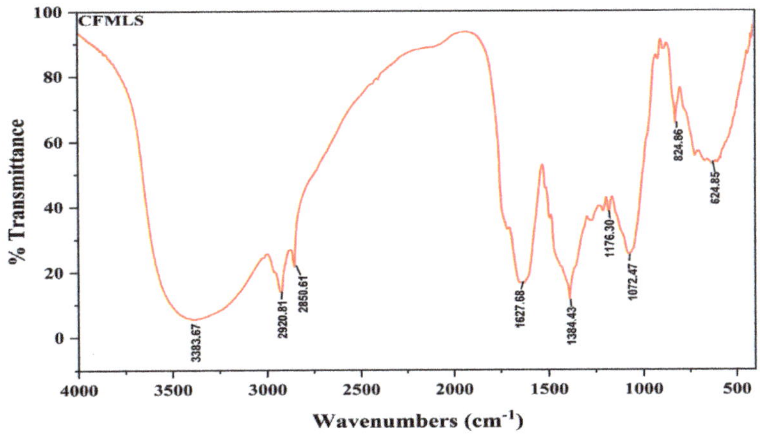

Figure 2. FT-IR chromatogram showing peak values for bioactive functional groups of *C. felina* methanolic leaves extract.

Table 3. FT-IR peak values interpretation for bioactive functional groups of *C. felina* methanolic leaves extract.

Wavenumber (cm^{-1})	Intensities of Functional Group	Functional Group	Compound Class
3383.67	Strong, broad	O-H stretching	Alcohols
2920.81	Strong	N-H stretching	Amine salts
2850.61	Strong	N-H stretching	Amine salts
1627.68	Medium	C=C stretching	Conjugated alkene
1384.43	Strong	S=O stretching	Sulfonyl chloride
1176.30	Strong	C-O stretching	Tertiary alcohol
1072.47	Medium	C-N stretching	Amines
824.86	Strong	C-Cl stretching	Halo compounds
624.85	Strong	C-Br stretching	Halo compounds

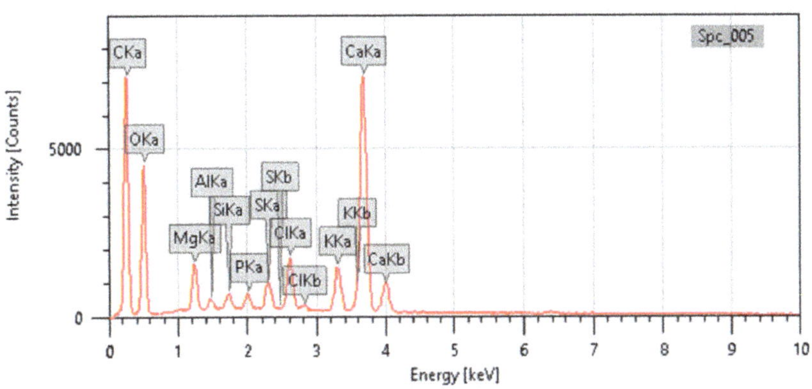

Figure 3. EDX chromatogram of *C. felina* leaves indicating elemental peaks.

Table 4. Element composition of *C. felina* leaves.

Serial No.	Elements	Mass % Leaves
1	C	36.48 ± 0.08
2	O	39.74 ± 0.19
3	Na	ND
4	Mg	1.80 ± 0.02
5	Al	0.35 ± 0.01
6	Si	0.46 ± 0.01
7	P	0.58 ± 0.01
8	S	1.01 ± 0.01
9	Cl	2.15 ± 0.02
10	K	2.031 ± 0.02
11	Ca	15.13 ± 0.06
Total		100.00

Note: ND- Not determined.

2.4. Phytochemical Determination of *C. felina* Methanolic Leaves Extract by Gas Chromatography–Mass Spectrometry (GCMS) Analysis

The methanolic leaves extract of *C. felina* were investigated for volatile phytochemical composition by GCMS analysis and were confirmed by NIST library mass spectrum. In total, 12 different phyto-compounds were identified in the leaves, and methanolic extract are of important applications. The retention time, peak area, area percent, name of the compound, molecular formula, and molecular weight are separately depicted for each identified phyto-compound in Figure 4 and Table 5. The phyto-constituents with high-percent composition were found to be 1-Butanol, 3-methyl-, formate (48.79%); 1-Decanol, 2-ethyl- (13.40%); 1,6-Anhydro-β-d-talopyranose (12.49%); Ethene, 1,2-bis(methylthio)- (7.22%); and Decane (4.02%), while considerable-percent composition of phyto-compounds detected were 3-Methylene-7, 11-dimethyl-1-dodecene (3.085); Amlexanox (2.50%); 1,2,3,4-Cyclopentanetetrol, (1α,2β,3β,4α) (2.07%), L-Cysteine S-sulfate (1.84%); n-Hexadecanoic acid (1.70%); Flucarbazone (1.55%); and 4-Bromo-2, 6-difluorobenzyl alcohol (1.35%). Each identified compound is specific for biological activities and is a specific role of metabolite.

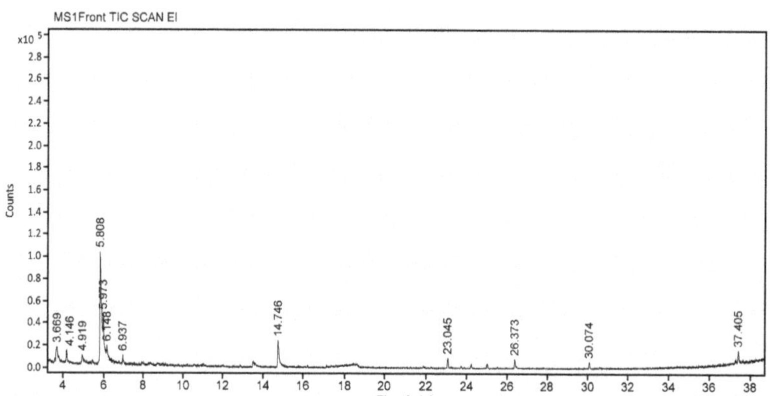

Figure 4. GCMS chromatogram showing peak values for volatile phytochemicals of *C. felina* methanolic leaves extract.

Table 5. Chemical composition of *C. felina* methanolic leaves extract screened by GCMS analysis.

Retention Time	Area	Identified Compound Name	Area (%)	Molecular Formula	Molecular Weight
3.669	76,453.684	Ethene, 1,2-bis(methylthio)-	7.21	$C_4H_8S_2$	120.2 g/mol
4.146	42,618.846	Decane	4.02	$C_{10}H_{22}$	142.28 g/mol
4.919	16,409.742	Flucarbazone	1.55	$C_{12}H_{11}F_3N_4O_6S$	396.30 g/mol
5.808	516,902.062	1-Butanol, 3-methyl-, formate	48.79	$C_6H_{12}O_2$	116.16 g/mol
5.973	141,915.824	1-Decanol, 2-ethyl-	13.40	$C_{12}H_{26}O$	186.33 g/mol
6.148	21,971.905	1,2,3,4-Cyclopentanetetrol, (1α,2β,3β,4α)	2.07	$C_5H_{10}O_4$	134.13 g/mol
6.937	19,474.186	L-Cysteine S-sulfate	1.84	$C_3H_7NO_5S_2$	201.2 g/mol
14.746	132,340.738	1,6-Anhydro-β-d-talopyranose	12.49	$C_6H_{10}O_5$	162.14 g/mol
23.045	32,613.550	3-Methylene-7,11-dimethyl-1-dodecene	3.08	$C_{15}H_{28}$	208.38 g/mol
26.373	17,986.273	n-Hexadecanoic acid	1.70	$C_{16}H_{32}O_2$	256.42 g/mol
30.074	14,265.444	4-Bromo-2,6-difluorobenzyl alcohol	1.35	$C_7H_5BrF_2O$	223.01 g/mol
37.405	26,479.282	Amlexanox	2.50	$C_{16}H_{14}N_2O_4$	298.29 g/mol
Total %			100.00		

2.5. Antimicrobial Activity of *C. felina* Methanolic Leaves Extract

Antimicrobial activity for two positive *Staphylococcus aureus* (*S. aureus*) and *Bacillus cereus* (*B. cereus*) bacteria, two negative *Escherichia coli* (*E. coli*) and *Pseudomonas aeruginosa* (*P. aeruginosa*) bacteria, and two yeast *Candida albicans* (*C. albicans*) and *Candida glabrata* (*C. glabrata*) strains was studied by the agar well diffusion method for *C. felina* methanolic leaves extract at 25, 50, 75, and 100 μL/mL concentrations, depicted in Figure 5 and Table 6, wherein streptomycin and nystatin were used as the positive control and DMSO as the negative control. The observations for the formation of the inhibition zone by methanolic leaves extract were made, which implies that methanolic leaves extract was found to show a potential zone of inhibition against *S. aureus*-12.3 ± 7.84 mm, *B. cereus*-13.67 ± 8.69 mm, *E. coli*-11.33 ± 7.21 mm, *P. aeruginosa*-10.67 ± 6.78 mm, *C. albicans*-14.67 ± 9.33 mm, and *C. glabrata*-12.33 ± 7.84 mm at a 100 μL/mL concentration, which was comparable to the positive control, while the moderate zone of inhibition was observed at a 75 μL/mL concentration against *S. aureus*-8.67 ± 5.51 mm, *B. cereus*-10.67 ± 6.78 mm, *E. coli*-7.67 ± 4.87 mm, *P. aeruginosa*-7.67 ± 4.87 mm, *C. albicans*-11.67 ± 7.42 mm, and *C. glabrata*-7.33 ± 4.66 mm; further, *P. aeruginosa*-5.33 ± 3.39 mm and *C. glabrata*-5.67 ± 3.60 mm were also found to be sensitive at a 50 μL/mL concentration, whereas all selected pathogens showed resistance at a 25 μL/mL concentration, except *C. glabrata*-3.33 ± 2.12 mm.

Table 6. Antimicrobial activity of the *C. felina* methanolic leaves extract against Gram-positive, Gram-negative bacteria, and two yeast strains.

Organisms	Zone of Inhibition in mm					
	Positive Control	CFMLS Extract				Negative Control
	100 μL	25 μL	50 μL	75 μL	100 μL	100 μL
S. aureus	18.33 ± 11.66 [cd]	ND	ND	8.67 ± 5.51 [j]	12.3 ± 7.84 [g]	ND
B. cereus	20.33 ± 12.94 [a]	ND	ND	10.67 ± 6.78 [i]	13.67 ± 8.69 [f]	ND
E. coli	14.33 ± 9.12 [ef]	ND	ND	7.67 ± 4.87 [k]	11.33 ± 7.21 [hi]	ND
P. aeruginosa	18.67 ± 11.87 [bc]	ND	5.33 ± 3.39 [l]	7.67 ± 4.87 [k]	10.67 ± 6.78 [i]	ND
C. albicans	19.33 ± 12.30 [b]	ND	ND	11.67 ± 7.42 [gh]	14.67 ± 9.33 [e]	ND
C. glabrata	17.67 ± 11.24 [d]	3.33 ± 2.12 [m]	5.67 ± 3.60 [l]	7.33 ± 4.66 [k]	12.33 ± 7.84 [g]	ND

Data are mean ± standard error (n = 3). Different letters in superscript indicate significant difference ($p < 0.05$); the same superscript letters indicates no significant difference ($p < 0.05$) between each other, and ND = not determined. CFMLS: *C. felina* methanolic leaves extract.

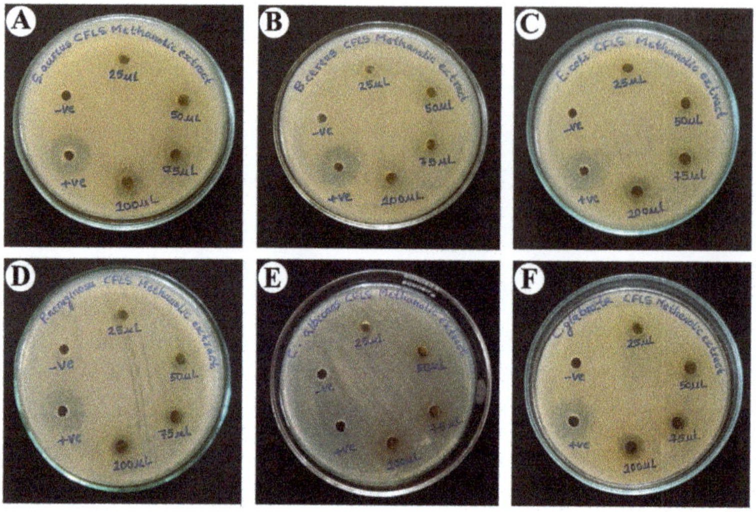

Figure 5. Antimicrobial activity of methanolic leaves extract of *C. felina* showing zone of inhibition at different concentrations against (**A**) *S. aureus*, (**B**) *B. cereus*, (**C**) *E. coli*, (**D**) *P. aeruginosa*, (**E**) *C. albicans*, and (**F**) *C. glabrata*.

2.6. Acute Toxicity of *C. felina* Methanolic Leaves Extract

The acute toxicity for the methanolic leaves extract of *C. felina* was evaluated according to Organization for Economic Co-operation and Development (OECD) guidelines 425 by oral administration of the single-extract dose at concentrations of 84, 80, and 70 mg to the body weight (42, 40, and 35 g, respectively) of Swiss albino mice. The limit dose given per oral administration was 2000 mg/kg b.wt. The dosed animals were under uninterrupted observation for 4 h for gross behavioral and toxicological signs; they were further monitored for the next 14 days. From the results, it was interpreted that no such behavioral and toxicological signs were manifested, which implies that the selected dose of methanolic leaves extract was nontoxic and showed no side effects, as death did not occur in the treated animals.

2.7. Paracetamol-Induced Hepatoprotective Activity by *C. felina* Methanolic Leaves Extract in Wister Albino Rats

2.7.1. Estimation of Serum Blood Biochemical Markers

Early hepatic damage is measured by the estimation of biochemical markers, such as aspartate aminotransferase-AST (Figure 6A), alanine aminotransferase-ALT (Figure 6B), alkaline phosphatase -ALP (Figure 6C), total bilirubin (Figure 6D), and total cholesterol (Figure 6E), present in the serum blood of experimental animals at the end of the practical day, presented in Figure 6A–E and Table 7. The conducted study showed that group 2 rats (control) constituted blood serum AST (857.7 ± 2.67 U/L), ALT (722.9 ± 3.20 U/L), ALP (736.9 ± 0.67 U/L), total bilirubin (1.98 ± 0.00 mg/dL), and total cholesterol (60.50 ± 1.12 mg/dL). In comparison, group 1 (normal) animal models of AST (136.2 ± 0.40 U/L), ALT (76.20 ± 0.48 U/L), ALP (238.1 ± 1.19 U/L), total bilirubin (0.48 ± 0.003 mg/dL), and total cholesterol (35.77 ± 0.38 mg/dL) was detrimental to group 1 animal serum, whereas group 3 (standard) rats' blood serum AST (127.3 ± 0.91 U/L), ALT (70.85 ± 0.85 U/L), ALP (224.0 ± 0.49 U/L), total bilirubin (0.45 ± 0.001 mg/dL), and total cholesterol (33.13 ± 0.13 mg /dl) was minimal. Paracetamol-induced hepatoprotective activity by methanolic leaves extract of *C. felina* of group 4 (low dose-50 mg/kg b.wt.) rats with AST (220.5 ± 0.79 U/L), ALT (47.18 ± 0.82 U/L), ALP (203.1 ± 2.38 U/L), total bilirubin (0.21 ± 0.00 mg /dl), and total cholesterol (38.46 ± 0.67 mg /dl) was significant; similarly, the animals of group 5 (high dose-100 mg/kg b.wt.) in blood serum AST (248.0 ± 5.30 U/L),

ALT (34.48 ± 0.48 U/L), ALP (445.0 ± 1.45 U/L), total bilirubin (0.17 ± 0.002 mg/dL), and total cholesterol (39.03 ± 0.41 mg/dL) were in considerable concentrations.

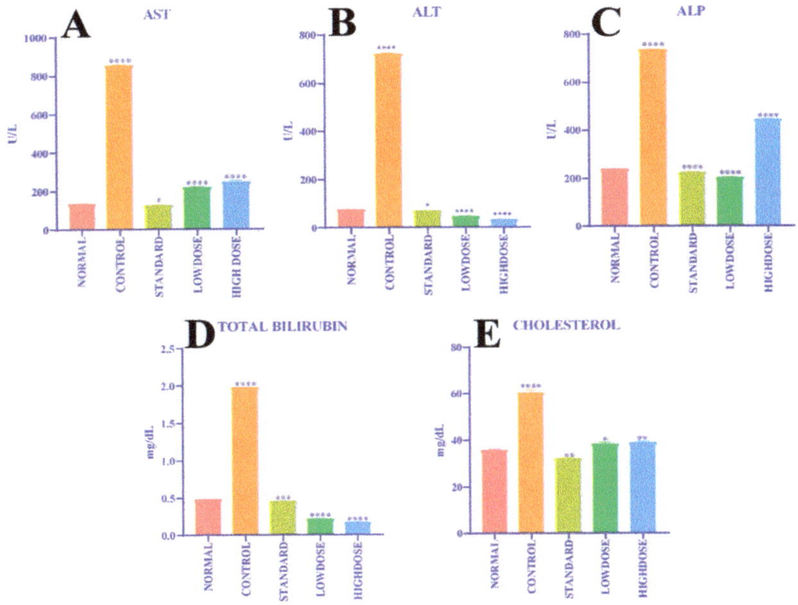

Figure 6. (**A**) Effect of different doses of CFMLS methanolic extract on AST level; (**B**) Effect of different doses of CFMLS methanolic extract on ALT level; (**C**) Effect of different doses of CFMLS extract on ALP level; (**D**) Effect of different doses of CFMLS methanol extract on total bilirubin level; and (**E**) Effect of different doses of CFMLS methanol extract on cholesterol level. All values presented as mean ± SEM, one-way Analysis of Variance (ANOVA), followed by multiple Dunnett's test, * $p < 0.05$, ** $p < 0.01$, *** $p < 0.001$, and **** $p < 0.0001$ compared with normal group. (CFMLS: *C. felina* methanolic leaves extract).

Table 7. The effect of *C. felina* methanolic leaves extract towards serum blood biochemical markers.

Groups	Treatment	AST (U/L)	ALT (U/L)	ALP (U/L)	Total Bilirubin (mg/dL)	Total Cholesterol (mg/dL)
Group-1 Normal	Vehicle	136.2 ± 0.40	76.20 ± 0.48	238.1 ± 1.19	0.48 ± 0.003	35.77 ± 0.38
Group-2 Control	Paracetamol (PC)	857.7 ± 2.65 ****	722.9 ± 3.20 ****	736.9 ± 0.67 ****	1.98 ± 0.00 ****	60.50 ± 1.12 ****
Group-3 Standard	Silymarin	127.3 ± 0.91 *	70.85 ± 0.85 *	224.0 ± 0.49 ****	0.45 ± 0.001 ***	33.13 ± 0.31 **
Group-4 Low dose	PC + CFMLS (50 mg/kg p. o)	220.5 ± 0.79 ****	47.18 ± 0.82 ****	203.1 ± 2.38 ****	0.21 ± 0.00 ****	38.46 ± 0.67 *
Group-5 High dose	PC + CFMLS (100 mg/kg p. o)	248.0 ± 5.30 ****	34.48 ± 0.48 ****	445.0 ± 1.45 ****	0.17 ± 0.002 ****	39.03 ± 0.41 **

All values of table presented as mean ± SEM, one-way Analysis of Variance (ANOVA), followed by multiple Dunnett's test, * $p < 0.05$, ** $p < 0.01$, *** $p < 0.001$, and **** $p < 0.0001$ compared with normal group. (CFMLS: *C. felina* methanolic leaves extract).

2.7.2. Assessment of Liver Antioxidant Potential

The methanolic leaves extract effects on the concentration of antioxidant enzymes, such as glutathione-GSH (Figure 7A), catalase-CAT (Figure 7B), superoxide dismutase (SOD (Figure 7C)), and level of lipid peroxidation-LPO (Figure 7D), in hepatic homogenate of experimental rats were analyzed and are displayed in Figure 7A–D and Table 8. Paracetamol-treated group 2 (control) rats exhibited a decline in the concentration of hepatic GSH (59.93 ± 0.30 n mol/mg of protein), CAT (0.02 ± 0.001 n mol/mg of protein), and SOD (208.9 ± 7.57 n mol/mg of protein) level and an increase in the LPO (465.7 ± 28.54 n mol/mg of protein) process; in relation to this, group

1 (normal) untreated PC animals showed an increased hepatic GSH (100.8 ± 1.53 n mol/mg of protein), CAT (0.10 ± 0.00 n mol/mg of protein), and SOD (337.2 ± 2.47 n mol/mg of protein) level and a decreased LPO (264.0 ± 17.48 n mol/mg of protein) reaction. The estimated amount of hepatic GSH (346.4 ± 6.77 n mol/mg of protein), CAT (0.93 ± 0.04 n mol/mg of protein), SOD (353.9 ± 0.58 n mol/mg of protein) level and LPO (40.00 ± 8.13 n mol/mg of protein) was significant in group 3 (standard) rats treated with silymarin. Methanolic leaves extract effects in group 4 (low dose-50 mg/kg b.wt.) and group 5 (high dose-100 mg/kg b.wt.) experimental rats were determined, where, in group 4 rats, the estimated concentration of hepatic GSH (51.29 ± 1.05 n mol/mg of protein), CAT (0.18 ± 0.003 n mol/mg of protein), and SOD (218.5 ± 0.00 n mol/mg of protein) antioxidant enzymes and LPO (72.65 ± 2.41 n mol/mg of protein) was significant. Meanwhile, group 5 rats' antioxidant enzymes level for hepatic GSH (81.50 ± 3.80 n mol/mg of protein), CAT (0.17 ± 0.1 n mol/mg of protein), and SOD (407.9 ± 6.16 n mol/mg of protein) concentration and LPO (194.0 ± 0.59 n mol/mg of protein) reaction was as mentioned.

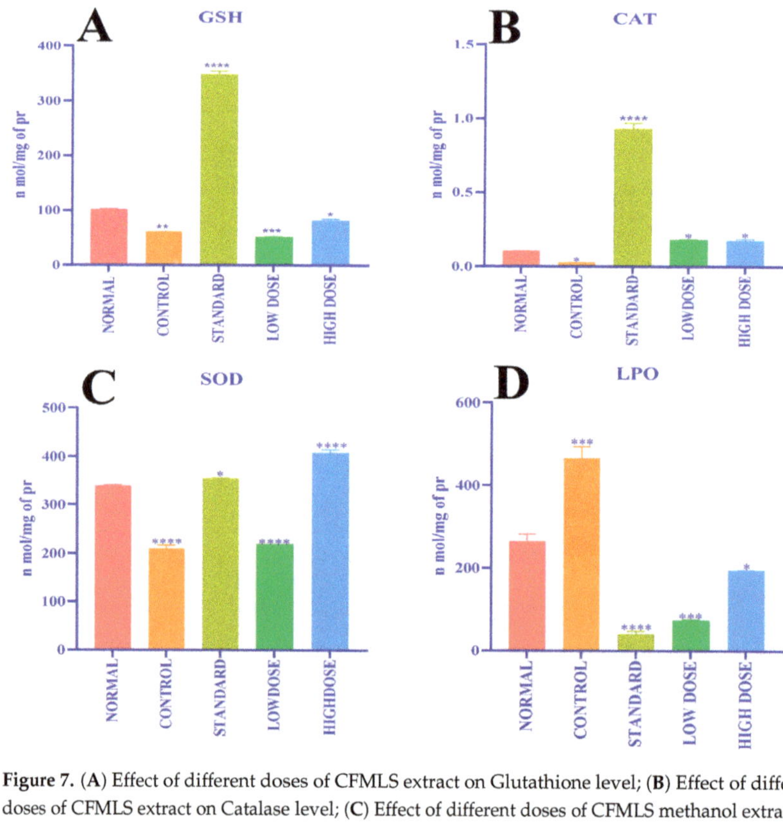

Figure 7. (**A**) Effect of different doses of CFMLS extract on Glutathione level; (**B**) Effect of different doses of CFMLS extract on Catalase level; (**C**) Effect of different doses of CFMLS methanol extract on SOD level; and (**D**) Effect of different doses of CFMLS methanol extract on Lipid peroxidation level. All values presented as mean ± SEM, one-way Analysis of Variance (ANOVA), followed by multiple Dunnett's test, * $p < 0.05$, ** $p < 0.01$, *** $p < 0.001$, and **** $p < 0.0001$ compared with normal group. (CFMLS: *C. felina* methanolic leaves extract).

Table 8. The effect of *C. felina* methanolic leaves extract towards in vivo antioxidant enzymes and lipid peroxidation.

Groups	Treatment	GSH (n mol/mg of Protein)	CAT (n mol/mg of Protein)	SOD (n mol/mg of Protein)	LPO (n mol/mg of Protein)
Group-1 Normal	Vehicle	100.8 ± 1.53	0.10 ± 0.00	337.2 ± 2.47	264.0 ± 17.48
Group-1 Control	Paracetamol (PC)	59.93 ± 0.30 **	0.02 ± 0.001 *	208.9 ± 7.57 ****	465.7 ± 28.54 ***
Group-1 Standard	Silymarin	346.4 ± 6.77 ****	0.93 ± 0.04 ****	353.9 ± 0.58 *	40.00 ± 8.13 ****
Group-1 Low dose	PC + CFMLS (50 mg/kg p.o)	51.29 ± 1.05 ***	0.18 ± 0.003 *	218.5 ± 00 ****	72.65 ± 2.41 ***
Group-1 High dose	PC + CFMLS (100 mg/kg p.o)	81.50 ± 3.80 *	0.17 ± 0.1 *	407.9 ± 6.16 ****	194.0 ± 0.59 *

All values of table presented as mean ± SEM, one-way Analysis of Variance (ANOVA), followed by multiple Dunnett's test, * $p < 0.05$, ** $p < 0.01$, *** $p < 0.001$, and **** $p < 0.0001$ compared with normal group. (CFMLS: *C. felina* methanolic leaves extract).

3. Discussion

Natural plant-based products are rich pockets of minerals and nutrients and have essential phyto-compounds with therapeutic properties. Worldwide, about 25% of prescribed drugs are obtained from plants, where, at present, about 121 active phyto-compounds are in use. The World Health Organization (WHO) has emphasized the basics and essentials of the 252 drugs; while 11% are tremendous of plant origin, polyphenols play a pivotal role in the maintenance of cellular antioxidant status by reducing free radicals, which inactivates inflammatory cytokines and production of chemokines and, as well, minimizes the generation of reactive oxygen species (ROS) and lipid peroxidation [19,20]. The extraction yield varies in accordance with the purity of the crude compound and the polarity of the solvent [21]. The present results of *C. felina* revealed that the leaves methanolic (17.01 g/100 g) extract yield was higher than the other solvent extracts. The high methanolic extract yield represents the occurrence of major polar chemical groups, such as phenols, flavonoids, alkaloids, steroids, glycosides, and other secondary metabolites [21].

Among the other parts of the *C. felina*, the methanolic leaves extract exhibited a maximum number of phytochemical compounds, such as carbohydrates, amino acids, glycosides, cardiac glycoside, phenolic, flavonoids, saponins, terpenoids, anthraquinones glycosides, and quinones. The closest abundance of phyto-constituents was noticed in the leaves (water) and stem (acetone and methanolic) extracts. The presence of bioactive compounds in the different parts of *C. felina* contributes to the therapeutic values of the plants in the treatment of diseases. In contrast to this, previously, several *Cleome* species were studied for the existence of phytochemical compounds in *C. spinosa* leaves and root extracts of cyclohexane, chloroform, ethyl acetate, and methanolic solvents [22]; *C. rutidosperma* leaves to water and ethanolic extracts [23], *C. gynandra* methanolic leaves extract [24], and *C. arabica* whole-plant aqueous-methanol, butanol, and water extracts [25], and it was reported the presence of flavonoids, saponins, terpenoids, anthraquinones, cardiac glycosides, tannins, carbohydrates, amino acids, proteins, polyphenols, reducing sugars, and alkaloids. The early preliminary findings reported by Silva et al. [22] and Alkhatib et al. [25] have determined that among comparative analyses between the different solvent extracts, the methanolic extract exhibited stronger positivity towards active phytochemical constitution than the other selective solvents during their studies.

The FTIR absorption spectrum of *C. felina* methanolic leaves extract revealed strong peaks at 3383.67 cm^{-1}, 2920.81 cm^{-1}, 2850.61 cm^{-1}, 1384.43 cm^{-1}, 1176.30 cm^{-1}, and 824.86 cm^{-1}, respectively, for the occurrence of alcohols, amines, conjugated alkenes, sulfonyl chloride, and halo compounds. The identified functional group contributes to the structural configuration of important compounds that are involved in different pharmacological activities and biosynthesis of functional metabolites. Similarly, Pillai and Nair [26] reported that whole-plant methanolic extract of *C. viscosa* and *C. burmanni* revealed the presence of phenols, alkanes, aldehydes, ketones, amines, amides, alkenes, carboxylic acids, sulfur compounds, alcohols, alkynes, and alkyl halides groups, while reports by Lingegowda et al. [27] on FT-IR analysis of methanolic leaves extract of *C. gynandra* exhibited the functional groups for important classes of compounds, i.e., phenols, amines and amides, carboxyl acid, silicon compounds, ketones, alkyl ketone, alkyl amine, alkanes, the alcohol hydroxyl group, and alkyl halides. Also, EDX analysis of *C. felina* methanolic leaves extract reports the presence of carbon, oxygen, sodium, magnesium, aluminum, silicon, phosphorus, sulfur, chlorine, potassium, and calcium elements. Similarly, Singh et al. [28] reported EDX analysis of *C. viscosa* seeds and confirmed the occurrence of carbon and oxygen, whereas a trace amount of magnesium, aluminum, silicon, sulfur, and calcium was observed. Elemental composition contributes to nutritional value and is proven for specific functions in metabolic activities and therapeutic values.

The current study on GCMS analysis of *C. felina* methanolic leaves extract exhibited 12 different phyto-compounds, in that the compound 1-Butanol,3-methyl-, formate, also known as isoamyl formate, is a short-chain ester possessing an aroma property, whose odor smells like pineapple, pear, and strawberry. Hence, it is utilized for flavoring and to intensify the flavor odor [29]. Earlier, Al-Dalali et al. [30] reported for 1-Butanol, 3-methyl-, formate, which is detected by GCMS analysis from vinegar, the compound 1-Decanol, 2-ethyl, which is alcoholic in nature, and 1,6-Anhydro-β-d-talopyranose is an exopolysaccharide. Ibrahim et al. [31] screened the 3% sulfuric acid leaves extract of *Gmelina arborea* (Verbenaceae family) for phyto-compounds by GCMS, in which 1,6-Anhydro-β-d-talopyranose was one among the other compounds detected, as well as it was reported that this compound acts as a toasted oak wood indicator and is used during wines ageing and distillates. The other compounds detected in *C. felina* methanolic leaves extract were Ethene, 1,2-bis(methylthio)-, Decane, 3-Methylene-7,11-dimethyl-1-dodecene, Amlexanox 1,2,3,4-Cyclopentanetetrol, (1α,2β,3β,4α) (carbohydrates), L-Cysteine S-sulfate, n-Hexadecanoic acid, Flucarbazone, and 4-Bromo-2,6-difluorobenzyl alcohol. The occurrence of Decane in the 80% ethanol extract of the *Cleome amblyocarpa* Barr. and Murb (stem) was reported by Khlifi et al. [32], estimated by GCMS analysis. The Amlexanox (azoxanthone drug) was used for curing mouth aphthous ulcers as a 5% topical oral paste and is the one approved clinically by the US FDA for aphthous ulcers treatment. It also exhibits novel applications in pharmacy [33–36]. L-Cysteine S-sulfate is an organic thiosulfate. It is an important class of L-cysteine molecule, which is S-substituted with a specified sulfur group. It is present as a plant and human metabolite and is involved in post-translation modifications, metabolisms, and pharmaceutical synthesis. In addition, it has detrimental effects on processes of cellular adhesive and tissue dehydration and has a role in the inactivation and clearance of small biomolecules of plasma [37,38]. n-Hexadecanoic acid is a saturated fatty acid. Most of the fatty acids are popular to possess antibacterial and antifungal activities. n-Hexadecanoic acid is highly studied and found to exhibit natural antioxidant, anti-inflammatory, antibacterial, anti-androgenic flavor, hypocholesterolemic nematicide, 5-Alpha reductase inhibitor, pesticide, hemolytic, and potent mosquito larvicide properties [39–41]. Perumal et al. [42] has reported the presence of n-Hexadecanoic acid in the *C. viscose* whole-plant ethyl extract analyzed by GCMS, species of the Cleomaceae family. Flucarbazone, previously called Flucarbazone-sodium, is a sulfonylurea herbicide. This herbicide is used to control dicotyledon weeds, such as Little seed Canarygrass, wild oats, and green foxtail, and reduces bermudagrass clippings grown as a weed during wheat and durum farming. However, it has been registered as an herbicide and growth regulator of turf grasses by U.S registration [43–45].

The evaluation of the antimicrobial assay of methanolic leaves extract has shown a significant inhibition zone against *S. aureus*, *B. cereus*, *E. coli*, *P. aeruginosa*, *C. albicans*, and *C. glabrata* at a 100 μL/mL concentration. Similarly, Weli et al. [46] reported the antimicrobial activity of *Cleome austroarabica* methanolic and different organic solvent extracts against *E. coli*, *H. influenza*, *E. faecalis*, and *S. aureus*, which did not show a zone of inhibition at selected concentrations. Another study conducted by Ghosh et al. [23] for antimicrobial activity of water and 70% ethanolic extract of *C. arabica* leaves against *S. aureus*, *E. coli*, and *V. cholerae*, individually, exhibited a moderate zone of inhibition. Khlifi et al. [32] performed the antimicrobial activity of *C. amblyocarpa* leaves and stem hydroalcoholic extract against four Gram-positive, four Gram-negative, and four yeast microorganisms using agar diffusion and micro-dilution methods. The growth inhibition of the entire tested microorganism at a dose-dependent manner was observed, and *E. coli* was found to be more sensitive among all.

The harmful side effects of the remedial substances were determined within 14 days by administrating the single-dose via oral routes and are carried to determine the median lethal dose (LD_{50}) of specific toxic substances in experimental rats or mice [47]. The results of acute toxicity of *C. felina* methanolic leaves extract were non-toxic at the lethal dose of 2000 mg/kg b.wt. on single oral dose administration in Swiss albino mice. Previously, del Carmen et al. [48] analyzed the acute oral toxicity of dichloromethane ethanol and methanol at 0.5, 1, and 2 g/kg b.wt., hexane, and dichloromethane at 2 g/kg b.wt. extract of *Cleoserrata serrata* (Jacq.) Iltis. (Syn. *Cleome serrata* Jacq.) observed for the gain of body weight and alteration of organs (spleen, liver, kidney). Changes were not noticed in the body weight and organs of experimental rats examined at the microscopic level. Similarly, hydroalcoholic extract of *C. amblyocarpa* leaves and stem showed no mortality rate and no behavioral changes studied for the oral acute toxicity at 0.5, 1, and 3 g/kg b.wt. [32].

The current paracetamol-induced hepatoprotective study revealed that *C. felina* methanolic leaves extract at a low dose of 50 mg/kg b.wt. (group 4) and high dose-100 mg/kg b.wt. (group 5) remarkably deduced the serum blood biochemical markers for AST, ALT, ALP, total bilirubin, and total cholesterol. In the study, it was found that the level of serum blood biomarkers at the low dose-50 mg/kg b.wt. was significant when compared to the high dose-100 mg/kg b.wt. The significant reduction in the serum blood biomarkers by *C. felina* methanolic leaves extract was attributed to the healing ability of hepatic parenchymal tissues and hepatocytes. In contrast to this, Begum and Kiran [49] demonstrated the hepatoprotective activity of whole-plant methanolic extract of *C. chelidonii* induced by paracetamol and ethanol to estimate serum biomolecule markers. The 100, 200, and 400 mg/kg b.wt. doses were found to reduce the serum ALP, SGPT, SGOT, and TBIL levels.

The present study implies the in vivo antioxidant potential of *C. felina* methanolic leaves extract for hepatoprotective activity. The results of the experiment depicted that the methanolic leaves extract at the low dose-50 mg/kg b.wt. (group 4) and high dose-100 mg/kg b.wt. (group 5) ameliorated significant elevation of hepatic antioxidant enzymes with LPO retardation. Results of the conducted study indicate that the antioxidant enzyme estimation of hepatic tissue treated with *C. felina* methanolic leaves extract has exhibited similar results as that of the serum blood biochemical marker estimation, wherein the rats treated with a low extract concentration exhibited stronger effectiveness towards the hepatic oxidation than that of the animals treated with a high extract concentration. The significant elevation of antioxidant enzymes, such as GSH, CAT, and SOD, in rats treated with the methanolic leaves extract is the result restoration of metabolic enzymes that have been reduced due to endogenous oxidative stress induced by paracetamol. In relation to this, Singh et al. [14], in their review article, described the hepatoprotective activity of *C. viscosa* (leaves ethanolic extract, isolated coumarinolignoids from seeds, and seeds), administrated in a dose-dependent manner, and was equally significant to the standard drug Silymarin induced by CCl_4. The reason of hepatoprotective activity might be due to the presence of polyphenols and flavonoids that have strong antioxidant activity reported to be present in *Cleome* species. Hence, from the overview of the present study, hepatoprotective activity exhibited by methanolic leaves extract of *C. felina* might be due to the presence of active phyto-metabolites, such as 1,6-Anhydro-β-d-talopyranose, n-Hexadecanoic acid, L-Cystein S-sulfate, and other examined compounds, detected in methanolic leaves extract of *C. felina* analyzed by GCMS; the conclusion of the results can be drawn that *C. felina* leaves possess a novel hepatoprotective activity, and disputes its richness of phyto-compounds illustrated by functional group, elements, and phyto-compounds identification. Results of the analysis specify the abundance of *C. felina* in bioactive compounds, which could be alternatively used in the pharmacy field for isolation and preparation of eco-friendly drugs and would be a great scope for future hepatoprotective drug designing and an alternate resource as that of Silymarin.

4. Materials and Methods

4.1. Collection and Preparation of Plant Material

Wild *Cleome felina* L.f. plant was collected from the mountains of Darikonur (17.0268155 N, 75.3761952 E) village, Taluk-Jat, District-Sangli, Maharashtra, India. The plant specimens were authenticated and identified by Dr. Manoj M. Lekhak, professor (assistant) of the Department of Botany, Shivaji University, Kolhapur. The research plant herbarium was deposited at the Shivaji University, Kolhapur, labeled with the voucher specimen number HYS-02. The collected *C. felina* plant material (leaves, stem, and root) was washed under running tap water and shade-dried for 30–35 days. Each dried part of the *C. felina* was separately made into powder form using an electric blender and was stored in airtight containers at 4 °C and used for further analysis.

The 20 g powder of leaves, stem, and root was extracted with 250 mL of different solvents (acetone, methanol, and water) in the range of increasing polarity with its specific boiling temperature by a Soxhlet apparatus for 8–10 h. Then, the obtained extracts were filtered and made solvent-free under vacuum pressure. The obtained extracts were used for further analysis.

4.2. The Percentage Yield of Different Solvent Extracts

It was calculated as the total amount of the extract obtained, divided by the total amount of the powder of the plant samples. All the percentage yield of extract was repeated thrice and calculated by the following equation.

$$\text{Yield } (\%) = \frac{\text{weight of extract} - \text{weight of solvent free extract}}{\text{Total weight of powder}} \times 100$$

4.3. Preliminary Screening of Phytocompounds for Different Solvent Extracts of C. felina

4.3.1. Tests for Carbohydrates

Fehling's Test

An equal volume of Fehling's solution (A and B) was mixed and was added drop-wise to each heated extract solution. Brick-red precipitation was observed, which indicates the presence of reducing sugars [50].

4.3.2. Test for Proteins

Biuret Test

A total of 1 mL of NaOH (10%) solution was combined with each extract and heated. To this, a few drops of $CuSO_4$ (0.7%) solution was added, and the presence of proteins was indicated by the formation of a purplish-violet color [51].

4.3.3. Test for Amino Acids

Ninhydrin Test

To each extract (2 mL), 2–5 drops of Ninhydrin solution (2%) was added and incubated for 1–2 min in a boiling water bath. The formation of purple color indicated the presence of amino acids [51].

4.3.4. Test for Glycosides

Salkowski's Test

A total of 1 mL of extract was combined with chloroform (2 mL), followed by treatment with concentrated H_2SO_4, and was then gently shaken. The presence of a steroidal ring was determined by the formation of a reddish-brown color [52].

4.3.5. Test for Cardiac Glycosides

Cardiac Glycoside (Keller–Kiliani Test)

Plant extract (2 mL) was mixed with 5 mL distilled water and was shaken, followed by the addition of 2 mL glacial acetic acid (prepared by the addition of a few drops of ferric chloride). To this, 1 mL H_2SO_4 was added by the sides of the test tube. It was then observed for brown ring formation at the interface that shows the occurrence of cardiac glycosides, and also the formation of a violet ring might be noticed below the brown ring [53].

4.3.6. Test for Phenols

Ferric Chloride Test

Test extracts were diluted in distilled water (3 mL) and reacted with ferric chloride (5% aqueous solution). A deep-blue or black color shows the positivity of phenols [51].

4.3.7. Test for Flavonoids

Alkaline Reagent Test

Plant extracts were combined with 2% of NaOH solution (2 mL), which resulted in a deep-yellow color, which became colorless upon the addition of diluted acid (a few drops). This determines the presence of flavonoids [52].

4.3.8. Test for Saponins

A total of 2 mL of plant extract was added to 10 mL distilled water and then shaken vigorously to obtain stable forth that indicates the presence of Saponins [53].

4.3.9. Test for Terpenoids

Salkowski's Test

Test extract (2 mL) was added to a test tube containing chloroform (2 mL), and they were thoroughly shaken to homogenize them. To this, 2 mL concentrated H_2SO_4 was added by the side of the test tube; the presence of terpenoids was indicated by the formation of a reddish-brown ring at the interface [53].

4.3.10. Anthraquinones Glycosides

Borntrager's Test

The sample extracts were shaken vigorously with a benzene layer and separated. To this, 10% ammonia solution was added in half the taken volume of the benzene layer. In the ammoniacal phase, pink, red, or violet color was observed for the anthraquinones glycosides presence [54].

4.3.11. Test for Tannins

A total of 10 mL of distilled water was mixed with each extract and then filtered. To this, 5% ferric chloride (few drops) was added. The presence of tannins was determined by the formation of black or blue–green coloration or precipitation [53].

4.3.12. Test for Alkaloids

A total of 2 mL of each extract was individually treated with 5 mL of hydrochloric acid (1.5% *v*/*v*) and filtered. The obtained filtrates were reacted with Mayer's reagent (mercuric chloride (1.36 g) and potassium iodide (5 g) prepared in 100 mL distilled water). The presence of alkaloid was determined by the observation of yellow cream precipitation [51].

4.3.13. Test for Betacyanins

Test extracts were reacted with 2 N NaOH and heated at 100 °C for 5 min; the occurrence of yellow color indicates the presence of betacyanins [55].

4.3.14. Test for Quinone's

An equal volume of extract was treated with concentrated H_2SO_4 and observed for the red color indicating the presence of quinone's [51].

4.4. Fourier-Transform Infrared Spectroscopy (FT-IR) and Energy-Dispersive X-ray Spectroscopy (EDX) Analysis

The NICOLET 67000 FTIR spectrophotometer (NICOLET, Thermo Fisher Scientific, Waltham, MA, USA) was used for functional group identification. The obtained methanolic extract of leaves was dried under vacuum pressure for complete removal of moisture, grounded with crystals of potassium bromide, and pressed between guides by applying a vacuum to make the thin discs. Then, the spectrum of the extract was recorded in the transmittance mode between 400 cm^{-1} and 4000 cm^{-1} at a resolution of 4 cm^{-1}. An elemental analysis of leaves powder was carried out to determine the elemental composition. The mass % of elements was determined by generating the spectra of the various micro and macro mineral elements using energy-dispersive X-ray spectroscopy (EDX) (JSM-IT 500LA, Tokyo, Japan) [19].

4.5. Phytochemical Determination of C. felina Methanolic Leaves Extract by Gas Chromatography–Mass Spectrometry (GCMS) Analysis

GCMS analysis of extract was performed using an Agilent 8890 MS gas chromatograph coupled to an Agilent 5977B Mass spectrometer detector, Palo Alto, CA, USA (MSD). Compounds were separated on a fused silica capillary column with a column dimension 30 m × 250 μm × 0.25 μm. The temperature of the injector was 250 °C, and 1 μL of the sample was injected in the split mode with a split ratio of 15:1. Helium (He) was used as a carrier gas, and the flow rate of the gas was 3 mL/min. The temperature program was as follows: initial temperature of 75 °C held for 0.5 min, followed by the ramping up of the temperature at a rate of 5 °C/min up to 300 °C, which was held for 20 min. The temperature of the MSD transfer line was 280 °C. For mass spectra determination, the MSD was operated in electron ionization (EI) mode, with ionization energy of 70 eV, while the mass range scanned was 50 m/z. The temperature of the ion source was 230 °C, and that of the MS quadrupole was 150 °C. The name, molecular weight, and structure of the components of the test materials were ascertained by comparing the mass spectra with the known compounds using an automated library search on the NIST MS Search program (version 2.3 accessed on 13 April 2023).

4.6. Antimicrobial Activity of C. felina Methanolic Leaves Extract

The *C. felina* methanolic leaves extract was analyzed for antimicrobial activity against selected pathogenic organisms by the agar well diffusion method in triplicates, according to the method of Rudrappa et al. [56]. The respective two Gram-positive bacteria: *S. aureus* (MTCC 6908) and *B. cereus* (MTCC 11778); two Gram-negative bacteria: *E. coli* (MTCC 40), *P. aeruginosa* (MTCC 9027); two yeast strains: *C. albicans* (MTCC 227) and *C. glabrata* (MTCC 3019) organisms were analyzed, which were procured from IMTECH, Chandigarh, India. The leaves methanolic (99%) extract of 100 mg/mL was prepared by dissolving in Dimethyl-sulfoxide DMSO (99%). Pathogenic organisms to be screened were cultured with a loopful of inoculation loop in Muller–Hinton broth (Himedia, Pvt Ltd, Mumbai, India), which was then incubated at 37 °C overnight. Pre-cultured pathogenic organisms were swabbed on separate nutrient agar plates in 0.5 McFarland concentrations, and a sterilized cork borer was used to produce 6 mm wells on cultured nutrient plates. For each organism, the respective wells were loaded with 100 μL of positive control (streptomycin for bacteria and nystatin for yeast, 100 μg/mL of each); 100 μL of negative control (DMSO);

and 25, 50, 75, and 100 μL of *C. felina* methanolic leaves extract (100 mg/mL). All cultured plates were incubated at 37 °C for 24 h, and the zone of inhibition was recorded after the incubation period.

4.7. Experiment Animals

The male and female Wister albino rats (200–250 g) were facilitated from a central animal facility present in H.S.K. College of Pharmacy and Research Centre, Bagalkot. The experimental rats were maintained in a controlled environment of room temperature (22–28 °C), followed by relative humidity (65 ± 10%) and a light–dark cycle of 12 h. They were under observation in accordance to the guidelines of the Institutional Animal Ethics Committee (IAEC) and were provided with standard laboratory feed (Amruth, Sangli, Maharashtra, India) and were in continuous access to water as needed. Ethical approval was acquired from the Institutional Animal Ethics Committee (IAEC) of Hangal Shri Kumareshwar College of Pharmacy, Bagalkot-587101, Karnataka, India, with reference number HSKCP/IAEC, Clear/1/2022-23/R&D/ KUD 02.

4.8. Acute Toxicity of C. felina Methanolic Leaves Extract

The acute toxicity of Swiss albino mice was examined in accordance with the Organization for Economic Co-operation and Development (OECD) guidelines 425, by administering a single dose of *C. felina* methanolic leaves extract orally at concentrations of 84, 80, and 70 mg to the body weight (42, 40, and 35 g). The limit dose given per oral administration was 2000 mg/kg. The mice were closely monitored for 4 h for behavioral and toxicological signs. Subsequent observations continued for 14 days. The observations were made for various parameters, such as changes in the skin, fur, eyes, and mucous membranes; special attention was given to tremors, convulsions, salivation, diarrhea, lethargy, sleep, and coma. The determination of screening doses for the selected extract to evaluate their hepatoprotective activity was based on the results obtained from this study.

4.9. Paracetamol-Induced Hepatoprotective Activity by C. felina Methanolic Leaves Extract in Wister Albino Rats

The Wister albino rats were grouped into five sets, each consisting of four animals. In group 1 (Normal), rats were given a normal saline solution (vehicle) at a dosage of 10 mL/kg b.wt.; group 2 (Control) rats were treated with Paracetamol (PC), commonly known as *N*-acetyl-p-aminophenol (acetaminophen). Group 3 (standard) rats received Silymarine 20 mg/kg b.wt. Groups 4 and 5 were administered with *C. felina* methanolic leaves extract at a 50 and 100 mg/kg b.wt. dose, respectively, for 12 days duration via oral administration. All the group rats were sacrificed at the end of the experiment after 24 h of the last dose administration. Serum blood and liver tissue homogenates from all the experimental animals were collected and analyzed for biochemical markers and in vivo antioxidant enzyme activities.

4.9.1. Biochemical Estimation in Blood Serum

After 24 h intervals of the final administration of PC, serum blood samples were obtained from each animal via the tail vein. The collected blood samples were then subjected to centrifugation at 3000 rpm for 10 min in order to separate the serum. The separated serum was utilized for the measurement of aspartate transaminase (AST), alanine transaminase (ALT), alkaline phosphatase (ALP), Total Bilirubin, and Total cholesterol levels by employing the described experiments of Iqbal et al. [57], using standard Biochemical diagnostic kits BIO-LA-TEST (Erbamannheim, Transasia Bio-Medicals Pvt Ltd., Mumbai, India).

Assessment of Aspartate Transaminase or Serum Glutamic Oxaloacetic Transaminase (AST/SGOT)

AST activity was estimated by following the method of Iqbal et al. [57], with minor adjustments. This assay was determined by preparing a fresh working reagent by combining 4 volumes of Reagent 1 with 1 volume of Reagent 2. To establish a baseline, a blank was analyzed using distilled water. For the test samples, 50 μL of serum was mixed with 500 μL of the working reagent at a temperature of 37 °C. The oxidation rate of NADH was measured kinetically by tracking the decrease in absorbance at 340 nm using an Auto analyzer (CPC Stat Fax 3000 Plus, Shimadzu, Kyoto, Japan).

Assessment of Alanine Transaminase or Serum Glutamic Pyruvic Transaminase (ALT/SGTP)

ALT activity was measured by employing the described procedure of Iqbal et al. [57], with a few concentration alterations. A working reagent was prepared by mixing Reagent with Reagent 2 to perform the estimation. The blank was analyzed using distilled water as a reference. For the test sample, 50 μL of serum was mixed with 500 μL of the working reagent at a temperature of 37 °C. The rate of NADH oxidation was determined kinetically by observing the decrease in absorbance at 340 nm using Auto analyzer (CPC Stat Fax 3000 Plus, Shimadzu, Kyoto, Japan).

Assessment of Alkaline Phosphatase (ALP)

ALP activity level was determined using Tietz et al. [58] method, with a few alterations. To determine the level of ALP activities, 20 μL of serum was combined with 1000 μL of ALP reagent. The ALP reagent consisted of Reagent 1. The change in absorbance caused by the formation of the yellow color was measured kinetically at 405 nm using an Auto analyzer (CPC Stat Fax 3000 Plus, Shimadzu, Kyoto, Japan). The magnitude of the absorbance change was directly proportional to the ALP activity present in the sample.

Assessment of Total Bilirubin

The estimation of Total Bilirubin was conducted using the Diazo method developed by Pearlman and Lee [59]. In this method, the working reagent used for this process was a combination of two components. Reagent 1 was the total Bilirubin reagent, and Reagent 2 was the sodium nitrite reagent (sodium nitrite). The analysis was carried out by preparing a blank solution consisting of 500 μL of the working reagent mixed with 25 μL of distilled water. Following this, the test sample is prepared by combining 500 μL of the working reagent with 25 μL of the test serum. The mixture was thoroughly mixed and then incubated for 5 min at 37 °C. The absorbance of the test sample was measured at a wavelength of 546 nm using an Auto analyzer (CPC Stat Fax 3000 Plus, Shimadzu, Kyoto, Japan).

Assessment of Total Cholesterol

Total cholesterol assessment was performed using the conducted experiment of Iqbal et al. [57], with some modifications. The assay was conducted using the PEG-CHOD-PAP (Polyethylene glycol-cholesterol oxidase-peroxidase-4- aminoantipyrine) method as an endpoint assay, incorporating the Lipid Clearing Factor (LCF). The standard was prepared by combining 100 μL of Reagent 1 with 10 μL of Reagent 2, namely, the Cholesterol standard containing cholesterol, preservatives, and stabilizers. To analyze the test sample, 1000 μL of the enzyme reagent is mixed with 10 μL of the sample and incubated at 37 °C for 10 min. The analysis was carried out using the reagent blank, followed by the standard and the test sample. The absorbance of the colored dye was measured at 505 nm using an Auto analyzer (CPC Stat Fax 3000 Plus, Shimadzu, Kyoto, Japan).

4.9.2. In Vivo Antioxidant Estimation of Hepatic Tissues

In vivo antioxidant estimation of hepatic tissues was assessed. First, blood samples were collected from each animal through the tail vein using sterile centrifuge tubes containing heparin. Subsequently, all groups of rats were sacrificed, and their livers were removed. The excised livers were then rinsed with ice-cold normal saline to eliminate any remaining blood constituents. After rinsing, the livers were weighed and homogenized in cold phosphate buffer (0.1 M, pH 7.4). To obtain the post-mitochondrial supernatant (PMS), the tubes containing the liver homogenates were placed in a refrigerated centrifuge (high speed brushless centrifuge, MPW-350R (Shimadzu, Kyoto, Japan) and spun at 10,000 rpm for 10 min at 4 °C. The supernatant obtained from this step was further centrifuged at 17,000 rpm for 1 h at 4 °C. The resulting supernatant was used to evaluate liver function, reduced glutathione (GSH), catalase (CAT), superoxide dismutase (SOD), and lipid peroxidation (LPO).

Assay for Glutathione

Reduced glutathione was examined by the described method of Moron et al. [60], with some modifications. The preparation of reagents involves the following steps. A solution of 0.6 mM 5,5′-dithiobis (2-nitrobenzoic acid) (DTNB) was made by dissolving 0.00238 g of DTNB in 10 mL of methanol. For the phosphate buffer solution (PBS) with a pH 8, 9.4 mL of potassium hydrogen phosphate and 3 mL of potassium di-hydrogen phosphate are combined. Next, 1 mL of tissue homogenate was mixed with 6 mL of PBS at pH 8 and 1 mL of 0.6 mM DTNB. This mixture was then incubated at room temperature for 10 min, after which the absorbance was measured at 412 nm using an analyzer (CPC Stat Fax 3000 Plus, Shimadzu, Kyoto, Japan) against appropriate blank samples. To determine the glutathione content, a standard plot was used under the same experimental conditions.

Assay for Catalase

Catalase activity was assessed by employing the Claiborne method of Zeashan et al. [61], with minor changes. In summary, the assay mixture comprised 50 mM Phosphate Buffered Saline (PBS) at pH 7. To create a solution of 0.7 mM H_2O_2, 0.160 mL of H_2O_2 was combined with 100 mL of PBS. Following this, 1.95 mL of PBS at pH 7, 1 mL of H_2O_2, and 50 units of tissue homogenate were added together. Alterations in absorbance were measured at 240 nm using an auto analyzer (CPC Stat Fax 3000 Plus, Shimadzu, Kyoto, Japan) both at 0 min and 1 min. Catalase activity was determined in units per milligram of protein.

Assay for Superoxide Dismutase

Superoxide dismutase assay was determined using the procedure of Natikar et al. [62]. The sodium carbonate buffer, 0.5 N HCl, and epinephrine solution were prepared during the analysis. To initiate the experiment, combine 0.8 g of sodium carbonate buffer with 0.1 mL of tissue homogenate. Subsequently, the epinephrine solution was put into the quartz cuvettes. Another mixture of 0.8 g of sodium carbonate buffer and 0.1 mL of tissue homogenate was added to a separate cuvette. Absorbance was recorded at 295 nm using auto analyzer (CPC Stat Fax 3000 Plus, Shimadzu, Kyoto, Japan) both at 0 min and 1 min.

Assay for Lipid Peroxidation

The LPO reaction was determined by following the Buege and Aust [63] procedure with a few changes. To estimate the presence of thiobarbituric acid reactive substances (TBARS) in the tissue homogenate, 500 µL of 10% tissue homogenate was combined with 300 µL of 15% trichloroacetic acid (TCA), 300 µL of 0.375% thiobarbituric acid (TBA), and 30 µL of 5 N HCl. This mixture was then incubated at 95 °C for 15 min using a hot water bath. After cooling, the mixture was centrifuged at 2000 rpm, and the absorbance of the resulting supernatant was measured at 535 nm against an appropriate blank.

4.10. Statistical Analysis

All values were expressed as mean ± SEM. Results were analyzed statistically by using One-Way Analysis of Variance (ANOVA), by using Duncan's multiple range test (DMRT) using IBM SPSS Statistics software version 20, followed by multiple Dunnett's test (GraphPad Prism 10). The $p < 0.05$ was considered as significant. The effects of different treated groups were compared with that of normal groups.

5. Conclusions

The results of the current study on *C. felina* reports for the occurrence of remarkable secondary metabolites, such as glycosides, phenolics, flavonoids, saponins, terpenoids, and a few more. The fatal functional groups, like alcohols, amine salt, conjugated alkenes, sulfonyl chloride, halo compounds and major elements, like carbon, oxygen, magnesium, aluminum, silicon, phosphorus, sulfur, chlorine, potassium, and calcium, were revealed by FTIR and EDX spectroscopy analysis. Furthermore, the methanolic leaves extract exhibited the nutritional and pharmacological active phyto-compounds being detected as 1-Butanol, 3-methyl-, formate, 1-Decanol, 2-ethyl, 1,6-Anhydro-β-d-talopyranoseEthene, 1,2-bis(methylthio)-, Decane, 3-Methylene-,11-dimethyl-1-dodecene, AmLexanox, 1,2,3,4-Cyclopentanetetrol, (1α,2β,3β,4α), L-Cysteine S-sulfate, n-Hexadecanoic acid, and Flucarbazone screened by the GCMS technique. Despite phytochemical constitutions, methanolic leaves extract depicted potent antimicrobial, acute oral toxicity, and paracetamol-induced hepatoprotective activity. The exhibition of antimicrobial and hepatoprotective activity might be due to the 1, 6-Anhydro-β-d-talopyranose and n-Hexadecanoic acid, as these compounds were reported for their pharmacological applications. Overall, from the present data of the study, it can be concluded that *C. felina* leaves would be immense bedrock for the isolation of active phytochemicals, can be a future scope for treating microbial and hepatotoxic diseases, and could be utilized in numerous cosmetics, herbicides, and food industries. Future study is required for isolation and analysis of active phyto-components commencements for the antimicrobial and hepatoprotective activity of the *C. felina* leaves.

Author Contributions: Conceptualization, H.Y.S., S.K.N. (Shaik Kalimulla Niazi) and S.N.A.; methodology, H.Y.S. and S.N.A.; software, S.K.N. (Shaik Kalimulla Niazi), A.B. and S.S.; validation, S.N.A., M.R. and S.K.N. (Shashiraj Kariyellappa Nagaraja); formal analysis, H.Y.S.; investigation, H.Y.S.; resources, S.A.H. and S.N.A.; data curation, A.B., S.S., S.A.H. and M.A.W.C.; writing—original draft preparation, H.Y.S. and S.N.A.; writing—review and editing, S.A.H., M.R. and S.K.N. (Shashiraj Kariyellappa Nagaraja); visualization, S.N.A.; supervision, S.N.A.; project administration, H.Y.S., S.N.A. and S.K.N. (Shaik Kalimulla Niazi); funding acquisition, A.B. and M.A.W.C. All authors have read and agreed to the published version of the manuscript.

Funding: This research is funded by Princess Nourah bint Abdulrahman University Researchers Supporting Project number (PNURSP2023R147), Princess Nourah bint Abdulrahman University, Riyadh, Saudi Arabia.

Institutional Review Board Statement: Ethical approval was acquired from the Institutional Animal Ethics Committee (IAEC) of Hangal Shri Kumareshwar College of Pharmacy, Bagalkot-587101, Karnataka, India, with reference number HSKCP/IAEC, Clear/1/2022-23/R&D/ KUD 02.

Informed Consent Statement: Not applicable.

Data Availability Statement: Data are available upon request.

Acknowledgments: The authors gratefully acknowledge the P.G. Department of Studies in Botany, Karnatak University, Dharwad, for providing lab facilities. The authors extend their gratitude to H.S.K. College of Pharmacy and Research Centre, Bagalkot, for its support and provision of lab facilities to complete acute oral toxicity and hepatoprotective activity. The authors are also thankful to the University Scientific Instrumentation Centre (USIC) and Sophisticated Analytical Instrumentation Facility (SAIF), Karnatak University, Dharwad, for its essential instrumentation services.

Conflicts of Interest: The authors declare no conflict of interest.

References

1. El-Saadony, M.T.; Zabermawi, N.M.; Zabermawi, N.M.; Burollus, M.A.; Shafi, M.E.; Alagawany, M.; Yehia, N.; Askar, A.M.; Alsafy, S.A.; Noreldin, A.E.; et al. Nutritional aspects and health benefits of bioactive plant compounds against infectious diseases: A review. *Food. Rev. Int.* **2021**, *39*, 2138–2160. [CrossRef]
2. Shraim, A.M.; Ahmed, T.A.; Rahman, M.M.; Hijji, Y.M. Determination of total flavonoid content by aluminum chloride assay: A critical evaluation. *LWT* **2021**, *150*, 111932. [CrossRef]

3. Memariani, Z.; Farzaei, M.H.; Ali, A.; Momtaz, S. Nutritional and bioactive characterization of unexplored food rich in phytonutrients. In *Phytonutrients in Food*; Woodhead Publishing, Elsevier: Amsterdam, The Netherlands, 2020; pp. 157–175.
4. Radha, K.M.; Puri, S.; Pundir, A.; Bangar, S.P.; Changan, S.; Choudhary, P.; Parameswari, E.; Alhariri, A.; Samota, M.K.; Damale, R.D.; et al. Evaluation of nutritional, phytochemical, and mineral composition of selected medicinal plants for therapeutic uses from cold desert of Western Himalaya. *Plants.* **2021**, *10*, 1429. [CrossRef] [PubMed]
5. Nagaraja, S.K.; Nayaka, S.; Kumar, R.S. Phytochemical analysis, GC-MS profiling, and *in vitro* evaluation of biological applications of different solvent extracts of *Leonotis nepetifolia* (L.) R.Br. flower buds. *Appl. Biochem. Biotechnol.* **2023**, *195*, 1197–1215. [CrossRef] [PubMed]
6. Lawal, B.; Shittu, O.K.; Oibiokpa, F.I.; Mohammed, H.; Umar, S.I.; Haruna, G.M. Antimicrobial evaluation, acute and sub-acute toxicity studies of *Allium sativum*. *J. Acute Dis.* **2016**, *5*, 296–301. [CrossRef]
7. Saidurrahman, M.; Mujahid, M.; Siddiqui, M.A.; Alsuwayt, B.; Rahman, M.A. Evaluation of hepatoprotective activity of ethanolic extract of *Pterocarpus marsupium* Roxb. leaves against paracetamol-induced liver damage via reduction of oxidative stress. *Phytomedici. Plus* **2022**, *2*, 100311. [CrossRef]
8. Henneh, I.T.; Ahlidja, W.; Alake, J.; Kwabil, A.; Ahmed, M.A.; Kyei-Asante, B.; Adinortey, M.B.; Ekor, M.; Armah, F.A. *Ziziphus abyssinica* root bark extract ameliorates paracetamol-induced liver toxicity in rats possibly via the attenuation of oxidative stress. *Toxicol. Rep.* **2022**, *9*, 1929–1937. [CrossRef] [PubMed]
9. Lin, H.H.; Hsu, J.Y.; Tseng, C.Y.; Huang, X.Y.; Tseng, H.C.; Chen, J.H. Hepatoprotective activity of *Nelumbo nucifera* Gaertn. seed pod extract attenuated acetaminophen-induced hepatotoxicity. *Molecules* **2022**, *27*, 4030. [CrossRef]
10. Feki, F.; Mahmoudi, A.; Denev, P.; Feki, I.; Ognyanov, M.; Georgiev, Y.; Choura, S.; Chamkha, M.; Trendafilova, A.; Sayadi, S. A jojoba (*Simmondsia chinensis*) seed cake extract express hepatoprotective activity against paracetamol-induced toxicity in rats. *Biomed. Pharmacother.* **2022**, *153*, 113371. [CrossRef]
11. Sinaga, E.; Fitrayadi, A.; Asrori, A.; Rahayu, S.E.; Suprihatin, S.; Prasasty, V.D. Hepatoprotective effect of *Pandanus odoratissimus* seed extract on paracetamol-induced rats. *Pharm. Biol.* **2021**, *59*, 31–39. [CrossRef]
12. Abd El-Ghffar, E.A.; El-Nashar, H.A.; Eldahshan, O.A.; Singab, A.N.B. GC-MS analysis and hepatoprotective activity of the n-hexane extract of *Acrocarpus fraxinifolius* leaves against paracetamol-induced hepatotoxicity in male albino rats. *Pharm. Biol.* **2017**, *55*, 441–449. [CrossRef] [PubMed]
13. Chand, J.; Panda, S.R.; Jain, S.; Das, A.M.; Kumar, G.J.; Naidu, V.G.M. Phytochemistry and polypharmacology of *Cleome* species: A comprehensive Ethnopharmacological review of the medicinal plants. *J. Ethnopharmacol.* **2022**, *282*, 114600. [CrossRef] [PubMed]
14. Singh, H.; Mishra, A.; Mishra, A.K. The chemistry and pharmacology of *Cleome* genus: A review. *Biomed. Pharmacother.* **2018**, *101*, 37–48. [CrossRef] [PubMed]
15. Hanumantha Rao, V. Endemic and threatened plants of uranium mining area. Na. *Int. Res. J. Environ. Sci.* **2016**, *5*, 40–46.
16. Joseph, M.; Vincent, A.R.; Charles, A. The anticancer activity of ethanolic extract of *Cleome felina* linn. *J. Pharm. Res.* **2014**, *8*, 1223–1225.
17. Manjuparkavi, K.; Jayanthi, G. Micromorphological studies of *Cleome felina* L.f. *Int. J. Curr. Res. Biosci. Plant Biol.* **2019**, *6*, 32–41. [CrossRef]
18. Wollenweber, E.; Valant-Vetschera, K.M.; Roitman, J.N. Chemodiversity studies on exudate flavonoids of Cleomaceae species (Brassicales). *Nat. Prod. Commun.* **2007**, *2*, 997–1002. [CrossRef]
19. Nagaraja, S.K.; Niazi, S.K.; Bepari, A.; Assiri, R.A.; Nayaka, S. *Leonotis nepetifolia* flower bud extract mediated green synthesis of silver nanoparticles, their characterization, and *in vitro* evaluation of biological applications. *Materials.* **2022**, *15*, 8990. [CrossRef]
20. Riaz, S.; Abid, R.; Ali, A. Phenolic compounds and elements of leaves as an aid for the taxonomic delimitation of the genus *Cleome* L. (Cleomaceae) from pakistan. *Int. J. Biol. Biotech.* **2021**, *18*, 307–313.
21. Ghosh, P.; Rahaman, C.H. Pharmacognostic studies and phytochemical screening of aerial and root parts of *Cyanotis tuberosa* (Roxb.) Schult. & Schult. f.-an ethnomedicinal herb. *World J. Pharmaceut. Res.* **2016**, *5*, 1580–1601.
22. Silva, A.P.; Nascimento da Silva, L.C.; Martins da Fonseca, C.S.; De Araujo, J.M.; Correia, M.T.; Cavalcanti, M.D.S.; Lima, V.L. Antimicrobial activity and phytochemical analysis of organic extract from *Cleome spinosa* Jaqc. *Front. Microbiol.* **2016**, *7*, 963. [CrossRef] [PubMed]
23. Ghosh, P.; Biswas, M.; Biswas, S.; Dutta, A.; Hazra, L.; Nag, S.K.; Sil, S.; Chatterjee, S. Phytochemical screening, anti-oxidant and anti-microbial activity of leaves of *Cleome rutidosperma* DC. (Cleomaceae). *J. Pharm. Sci. Res.* **2019**, *11*, 1790–1795.
24. Wakhisi, C.W.; Michael, G.M.; Mwangi, E. Mineral and phytochemical composition of *Cleome gynandra* methanolic extract. *Adv. J. Grad. Res.* **2020**, *8*, 18–26. [CrossRef]
25. Alkhatib, R.Q.; Almasarweh, A.B.; Abdo, N.M.; Mayyas, A.S.; Al-Qudah, M.A.; Abu-Orabi, S.T. Chromatographic analysis (LC-MS and GC-MS), antioxidant activity, antibacterial activity, total phenol, and total flavonoid determination of *Cleome arabica* L. growing in Jordan. *Int. J. Food Prop.* **2022**, *25*, 1920–1933. [CrossRef]
26. Pillai, L.S.; Nair, B.R. Functional group analysis of *Cleome viscosa* L. and C. burmanni W. & A. (Cleomaceae) extract by FT-IR. *J. Pharmacogn. Phytochem.* **2014**, *2*, 120–124.
27. Lingegowda, D.C.; Kumar, J.K.; Prasad, A.D.; Zarei, M.; Gopal, S. FTIR spectroscopic studies on *Cleome gynandra*- Comparative analysis of functional group before and after extraction. *Rom. J. Biophys.* **2012**, *22*, 137–143.
28. Singh, H.; Mishra, A.; Mishra, A.K. Pharmacognostical and physicochemical analysis of *Cleome viscosa* L. seeds. *Pharmacogn. J.* **2017**, *9*, 372–377. [CrossRef]

29. Tang, K.; Tian, X.; Ma, Y.; Sun, Y.; Qi, X.; Miu, C.; Xu, Y. Aroma characteristics of cabernet sauvignon wines from loess plateau in China by QDA®, Napping® and GC–O analysis. *Eur. Food Res. Technol.* **2020**, *246*, 821–832. [CrossRef]
30. Al-Dalali, S.; Zheng, F.; Xu, B.; Abughoush, M.; Li, L.; Sun, B. Processing technologies and flavor analysis of Chinese cereal vinegar: A comprehensive review. *Food Anal. Methods* **2023**, *16*, 1–28. [CrossRef]
31. Ibrahim, H.; Ayilara, S.; Nwanya, K.; Zanna, A.; Adegbola, O.; Nwakuba, D. Exploring *Gmelina arborea* leaves for biofuels and petrochemical and pharmaceutical feed stocks. *Chem. Sci. Int. J.* **2017**, *18*, 1–7. [CrossRef]
32. Khlifi, A.; Chrifa, A.B.; Lamine, J.B.; Thouri, A.; Adouni, K.; Flamini, G.; Oleszek, W.; Achour, L. Gas chromatography-mass spectrometry (GM-MS) analysis and biological activities of the aerial part of *Cleome amblyocarpa* Barr. and Murb. *Environ. Sci. Pollut. Res.* **2020**, *27*, 22670–22679. [CrossRef] [PubMed]
33. Bell, J. Amlexanox for the treatment of recurrent aphthous ulcers. *Clin. Drug Investig.* **2005**, *25*, 555–566. [CrossRef] [PubMed]
34. Bailly, C. The potential value of a mlexanox in the treatment of cancer: Molecular targets and therapeutic perspectives. *Biochem. Pharmacol.* **2022**, *197*, 114–895. [CrossRef] [PubMed]
35. Gonzalez-Hilarion, S.; Beghyn, T.; Jia, J.; Debreuck, N.; Berte, G.; Mamchaoui, K.; Mouly, V.; Gruenert, D.C.; Déprez, B.; Lejeune, F. Rescue of nonsense mutations by amlexanox in human cells. *Orphanet J. Rare Dis.* **2012**, *7*, 58. [CrossRef] [PubMed]
36. Atanasova, V.S.; Jiang, Q.; Prisco, M.; Gruber, C.; PiñónHofbauer, J.; Chen, M.; Has, C.; Bruckner-Tuderman, L.; McGrath, J.A.; Uitto, J.; et al. Amlexanox enhances premature termination codon read-through in COL7A1 and expression of full length type VII collagen: Potential therapy for recessive dystrophic epidermolysis bullosa. *J. Investig. Dermatol.* **2017**, *137*, 1842–1849. [CrossRef] [PubMed]
37. National Center for Biotechnology Information. PubChem Compound Summary, S-Sulfocysteine. CID 115015. Available online: https://pubchem.ncbi.nlm.nih.gov/compound/S-Sulfocysteine (accessed on 22 July 2023).
38. Wang, Q.; Qin, Z.; Hou, G.L.; Yang, Z.; Valiev, M.; Wang, X.B.; Zheng, X.; Cui, Z. Properties of gaseous deprotonated L-Cysteine S-Sulfate Anion [cysS-SO_3]−: Intramolecular H-bond network, electron affinity, chemically active site, and vibrational fingerprints. *Int. J. Mol. Sci.* **2023**, *24*, 1682. [CrossRef] [PubMed]
39. Aparna, V.; Dileep, K.V.; Mandal, P.K.; Karthe, P.; Sadasivan, C.; Haridas, M. Anti-inflammatory property of n-hexadecanoic acid: Structural evidence and kinetic assessment. *Chem. Biol. Drug Des.* **2012**, *80*, 434–439. [CrossRef] [PubMed]
40. Abubakar, M.N.; Majinda, R.R. GC-MS analysis and preliminary antimicrobial activity of *Albizia adianthifolia* (Schumach) and *Pterocarpus angolensis* (DC). *Medicines* **2016**, *3*, 3. [CrossRef] [PubMed]
41. Ganesan, T.; Subban, M.; Christopher Leslee, D.B.; Kuppannan, S.B.; Seedevi, P. Structural characterization of n-hexadecanoic acid from the leaves of *Ipomoea eriocarpa* and its antioxidant and antibacterial activities. *Biomass Convers. Bioref.* **2022**, 1–12. [CrossRef]
42. Perumal, G.; Prabhu, K.; Rao, M.R.K.; Janaki, C.S.; Kalaivannan, J.; Kavimani, M. The GC MS Analysis of ethyl acetate extract of one herbal plant, *Cleome Viscosa. Nat. Volatiles Essent. Oils J.* **2021**, *8*, 4066–4072.
43. McCullough, P.E.; Sidhu, S.S.; Singh, R.; Yu, J. Seashore paspalum growth regulation with flucarbazone-sodium. *Crop Sci.* **2014**, *54*, 1197–1204. [CrossRef]
44. Kamel, A.H.; Amr, A.E.G.E.; Abdalla, N.S.; El-Naggar, M.; Al-Omar, M.A.; Alkahtani, H.M.; Sayed, A.Y. Novel solid-state potentiometric sensors using polyaniline (PANI) as a solid-contact transducer for flucarbazone herbicide assessment. *Polymers* **2019**, *11*, 1796. [CrossRef] [PubMed]
45. Bayat, M.; Zargar, M. Postemergence herbicide combinations for effective Little seed Canarygrass (*Phalaris minor*) control in winter wheat (*Triticumaestivum* L.). *Acta Physiol. Plant.* **2021**, *43*, 150. [CrossRef]
46. Weli, A.M.; Al-Harrasi, A.; Al Baiti, N.H.; Philip, A.; Hossain, A.; Gilani, S.A.; Banioraba, N. Biological and toxicological evaluation of aerial parts extract of locally grown *Cleome austroarabica. J. King Saud. Univ. Sci.* **2020**, *32*, 753–757. [CrossRef]
47. Alelign, T.; Chalchisa, D.; Fekadu, N.; Solomon, D.; Sisay, T.; Debella, A.; Petros, B. Evaluation of acute and sub-acute toxicity of selected traditional antiurolithiatic medicinal plant extract in Wistar albino rats. *Toxicol. Rep.* **2020**, *7*, 1356–1365. [CrossRef] [PubMed]
48. del Carmen Juárez-Vázquez, M.; Zamilpa, A.; León-Díaz, R.; Martínez-Vázquez, M.; López-Torres, A.; Luna-Herrera, J.; Yépez-Mulia, L.; Alarcón-Aguilar, F.; Jiménez-Arellanes, M.A. Phytochemical screening and anti-inflammatory potential of the organic extract from *Cleoserrata serrata* (Jacq.) Iltis. *Pharmacogn. J.* **2021**, *13*, 1225–1241. [CrossRef]
49. Begum, M.M.; Kiran, K.R. Evaluation of methanolic extract of *Cleome chelidonii* for hepatoprotective activity against paracetamol and ethanol induced hepatotoxicity in rats. *Int. J. Pharm. Sci. Rev. Res.* **2016**, *5*, 28–36.
50. Evans, W.C. *Trease and Evans Pharmacognosy*; Elsevier Health Sciences: Edinburgh, UK, 2009.
51. Alotaibi, A.A.; Bepari, A.; Assiri, R.A.; Niazi, S.K.; Nayaka, S.; Rudrappa, M.; Nagaraja, S.K.; Bhat, M.P. *Saussurea lappa* exhibits anti-oncogenic effect in hepatocellular carcinoma, HepG2 cancer cell line by Bcl-2 mediated apoptotic pathway and mitochondrial cytochrome C release. *Curr. Issues Mol. Biol.* **2021**, *43*, 1114–1132. [CrossRef] [PubMed]
52. Yadav, R.N.S.; Agarwala, M. Phytochemical analysis of some medicinal plants. *J. Phytol.* **2011**, *3*, 10–14.
53. Iqbal, E.; Salim, K.A.; Lim, L.B. Phytochemical screening, total phenolics and antioxidant activities of bark and leaf extract of *Goniothalamus velutinus* (Airy Shaw) from Brunei Darussalam. *J. King Saud Univ.-Sci.* **2015**, *27*, 224–232. [CrossRef]
54. Abbhi, V.; Joseph, L.; George, M. Phytochemical analysis of fruit extract of *Myrsine africana. Int. J. Pharm. Pharm. Sci.* **2011**, *3*, 427–430.
55. Harborne, J.B. Photochemical methods. In *A Guide to Modern Techniques of Plant Analysis*; Chapman A and Hall.: London, UK, 1973.

56. Rudrappa, M.; Rudayni, H.A.; Assiri, R.A.; Bepari, A.; Basavarajappa, D.S.; Nagaraja, S.K.; Chakraborty, B.; Swamy, P.S.; Agadi, S.N.; Niazi, S.K.; et al. *Plumeria alba*-mediated green synthesis of silver nanoparticles exhibits antimicrobial effect and anti-oncogenic activity against glioblastoma U118 MG cancer cell line. *Nanomaterials.* **2022**, *12*, 493. [CrossRef] [PubMed]
57. Iqbal, S.S.; Mujahid, M.; Kashif, S.M.; Khalid, M.; BadruddeenArif, M.; Bagga, P.; Akhtar, J.; Rahman, M.A. Protection of hepatotoxicity using *Spondia spinnata* by prevention of ethanol-induced oxidative stress, DNA-damage and altered biochemical markers in Wistar rats. *Integr. Med. Res.* **2016**, *5*, 267–275. [CrossRef] [PubMed]
58. Tietz, N.W.; Burtis, C.; Duncan, P.; Ervin, K.; Petitclerc, C.; Rinker, A.; Shuey, D.; Zygowicz, E. A reference method for measurement of alkaline phosphatase activity in human serum. *Clin. Chem.* **1983**, *29*, 751–761. [CrossRef] [PubMed]
59. Pearlman, F.C.; Lee, R.T. Detection and measurement of total bilirubin in serum, Gram-positive bacteria: *Staphylococcus aureus* (MTCC) and *Bacillus cereus* (MTCC); two Gram-negative bacteria: *Escherichia coli* (MTCC40), *Pseudomonas aeruginosa* (MTCC9027); and two fungal strains: *Candida albicans* (MTCC227) and *Candida glabrata* (MTCC3019) with use of surfactants as solubilizing agents. *Clinchemis* **1974**, *20*, 447–453.
60. Moron, M.S.; Depierre, J.W.; Mannervik, B. Levels of glutathione, glutathione reductase and glutathione S-transferase activities in rat lung and liver. *Biochim. Biophys. Acta* **1979**, *582*, 67–78. [CrossRef]
61. Zeashan, H.; Amresh, G.; Singh, S.; Rao, C.V. Hepatoprotective activity of *Amaranthus spinosus* in experimental animals. *Food Chem. Toxicol.* **2008**, *46*, 3417–3421. [CrossRef]
62. Natikar, N.A.; Mangannavar, C.V.; Shalavadi, M.H.; Kolli, S.S. Hepatoprotective activity of *Curcuma vamana* ethanolic rhizome extract against paracetamol and CCl_4 induced hepatotoxicity in albino rats. *RGUHS J. Pharm. Sci.* **2020**, *10*, 23–32.
63. Buege, J.A.; Aust, S.D. Microsomal lipid peroxidation. In *Methods in Enzymology*; Academic Press: Cambridge, MA, USA, 1978; Volume 52, pp. 302–310.

antibiotics

MDPI

Article

Antibacterial Efficiency of *Tanacetum vulgare* Essential Oil against ESKAPE Pathogens and Synergisms with Antibiotics

Horațiu Roman [1,2,3], Adelina-Gabriela Niculescu [2,4,*], Veronica Lazăr [3] and Mihaela Magdalena Mitache [5]

1 Interdisciplinary School of Doctoral Studies (ISDS), University of Bucharest, 050095 Bucharest, Romania; horatiu.roman@bio.unibuc.ro
2 Research Institute of the University of Bucharest (ICUB), University of Bucharest, 050095 Bucharest, Romania
3 Faculty of Biology, University of Bucharest, 050095 Bucharest, Romania; veronica.lazar@bio.unibuc.ro
4 Department of Science and Engineering of Oxide Materials and Nanomaterials, National University of Science and Technology Politehnica Bucharest, 011061 Bucharest, Romania
5 Department of General Medicine, Titu Maiorescu University, 040441 Bucharest, Romania; magdalena.mitache@prof.utm.ro
* Correspondence: adelina.niculescu@upb.ro

Abstract: Medicinal plants with multiple targets of action have become one of the most promising solutions in the fight against multidrug-resistant (MDR) bacterial infections. *Tanacetum vulgare* (Tansy) is one of the medicinal plants with antibacterial qualities that deserve to be studied. Thus, this research takes a closer look at tansy extract's composition and antibacterial properties, aiming to highlight its potential against clinically relevant bacterial strains. In this respect, the antibacterial test was performed against several drug-resistant pathogenic strains, and we correlated them with the main isolated compounds, demonstrating the therapeutic properties of the extract. The essential oil was extracted via hydrodistillation, and its composition was characterized via gas chromatography. The main isolated compounds known for their antibacterial effects were α-Thujone, β-Thujone, Eucalyptol, Sabinene, Chrysanthenon, Camphor, Linalool oxide acetate, *cis*-Carveol, *trans*-Carveyl acetate, and Germacrene. The evaluation of the antibacterial activity was carried out using the Kirby–Bauer and binary microdilution methods on Gram-positive and Gram-negative MDR strains belonging to the ESKAPE group (i.e., *Enterococcus faecium*, *Staphylococcus aureus*, *Klebsiella pneumoniae*, *Acinetobacter baumannii*, *Pseudomonas aeruginosa*, and *Enterobacter* spp.). Tansy essential oil showed MIC values ranging from 62.5 to 500 μg/mL against the tested strains. Synergistic activity with different classes of antibiotics (penicillins, cephalosporins, carbapenems, monobactams, aminoglycosides, and quinolones) has also been noted. The obtained results demonstrate that tansy essential oil represents a promising lead for developing new antimicrobials active against MDR alone or in combination with antibiotics.

Keywords: natural products; *Tanacetum vulgare*; tansy extract; multidrug resistance; bioactive compounds; antibacterial activity; synergism with antibiotics

1. Introduction

The therapy of infectious diseases is going through a major crisis due to the extent of the phenomenon of antibiotic resistance (AR), which has reached alarming proportions. The World Health Organization (WHO) list (27 February 2017) [1] of priority pathogens for research and development of new antibiotics comprises three priority levels: critical, high, and medium. The critical level includes multidrug-resistant pathogens (MDR—bacteria resistant to three or more classes of antibiotics) ESKAPE, Gram-negative pathogens, *A. baumannii* (carbapenem-resistant), *P. aeruginosa* (carbapenem-resistant), *K. pneumoniae* (resistant to third-generation cephalosporins), and Enterobacter spp. (resistant to third-generation cephalosporins). The high level includes ESKAPE Gram-positive pathogens, *Enterococcus faecium* (vancomycin-resistant), and *S. aureus* (intermediate methicillin-resistant and vancomycin-resistant). These pathogens are often isolated from clinical settings associated with life-threatening nosocomial infections [2].

The design of new (classes of) antibiotics is difficult to achieve. Although efforts are made to stop and reduce the phenomenon, the monitoring studies do not report the positive effects of these policies, as the incidence of multidrug and pandrug-resistant strains is continuously increasing [3]. New antibiotics that entered the market in recent decades are variations of pre-existent antibiotics discovered up to the 1980s [4]. The lack of progress in antibiotic development highlights the need to explore innovative approaches to treating bacterial infections.

The list of plants with curative effects against a wide variety of chronic and infectious diseases has expanded, especially in recent decades. Analytical methods have identified diverse compounds with therapeutic effects, especially against bacterial infectious diseases, in the context of the expansion of the phenomenon of antibiotic resistance [5,6]. In vitro tests have shown that some plant species that are used to treat non-infectious diseases (e.g., *Panax ginseng*, *Achillea* sp., *Cichorium intybus* L., *Cynara cardunculus* L., *Foeniculum vulgare* Mill., which regulate liver functions [7], or plants that regulate the nervous system, such as *Ginkgo biloba* L., *Panax ginseng* C.A. Mayer, *Scutellaria baicalensis* Georgi [8]) also have antibacterial activity [9–14]. More than a quarter of the medicines administered in industrialized countries are obtained directly or indirectly from plants. The antimicrobial action of plant extracts results from their complex chemical composition, the compounds acting synergistically and having multiple action targets. These preparations are generically referred to as "non-antibiotic" antibacterial agents [15] and were proven to be active against a large spectrum of bacterial and fungal strains [16].

The use of essential oils (EOs), resulting from the secondary metabolism of plants, has been known since Neolithic times when they were extracted via pressing. The Egyptians used to extract oils by infusing a plant into a fatty substance. By boiling, the flavor evaporates and is fixed in the fat [17]. The oldest medicine book, "Shennong's Herbal", dating back to 2700 BC, contains instructions for using 365 medicinal plants belonging to Chinese folklore. Hippocrates, the father of modern medicine, documented the medical benefits of fumigation with aromatic oils in treating plague. There are 12 different types of EOs mentioned in the Holy Bible. In 1990, in the book "L'Aromatherapie Exactement", the medical properties of more than 270 EOs are described, representing a start for many studies [18].

The main chemical compounds found in the composition of EOs include terpenes, terpenoids, alkaloids, and phenolic compounds. EOs are obtained from raw vegetable material, steam distillation, or dry distillation. Yields vary greatly depending on plant parts' pre-processing techniques and agronomic factors (climate, soil, oral harvest interval) [19,20]. In general, the increase in drying temperature is proportional to the decrease in the EO content [21]. Thus, drying plants at 30 °C leads to concentration losses of 16%, while drying at higher temperatures of 60 °C leads to 65% losses [22]. Therefore, the obtaining process is directly correlated with the quality of the EOs.

Tansy (*Tanacetum vulgare*) is an aromatic plant that combines the smell of *Achillea millefolium* with *Artemisia absintum*, *Piper nigrum*, *Salvia mirzayanii*, and *Eucalyptus* sp. due to some common aromatic compounds. Aromatic plants are rich in essential oils. The term "essential oil" was used by Paracelsus von Hohenheim, who called the effective component of a medicine "Quinta essential". Conventional methods of obtaining essential oil include cold pressing, distillation, and solvent extraction. Supercritical and subcritical carbon dioxide (CO_2) extraction methods are more advanced and used industrially. The most efficient method, both financially and in terms of working time, is via water vapor distillation, which we conducted in this work.

Although *Tanacetum vulgare* is a plant that has been studied a lot recently due to its multiple therapeutic properties, including anti-inflammatory, antioxidant, and antibacterial activities, it still presents novelties due to its chemical compounds that vary according to environmental conditions (e.g., soil pH, light exposure, humidity, pollution) [23–25]. According to the World Checklist of Selected Plant Families, Anthos, Flora Iberica, and other databases, it has been attributed to numerous names correlated with its action/benefits, such as the gate of heaven, herb of the Mother of God, herb of the air, herb of worms, triac plant, medicinal of St. Anastasia, moss herb, St. Mark's weed, bitter weed, St. Teresa's pen, frankincense, and mugwort. However, it has been destroyed by herbicide or incineration in recent years, being considered an invasive plant.

In Romania, Tansy has a wide distribution, including all geographical areas. The best harvesting period is considered to range from July to August. The plant used herein was selected from an area with abundant growth in the Sohodol Valley area, Gorj County, Romania.

This study aims to highlight the potential of the EOs extracted from locally collected *T. vulgare* to be used as a source of antibacterial formulations or compounds. In this respect, EOs have been extracted via hydrodistillation, their main chemical constituents have been identified via gas chromatography-mass spectrometry (GC-MS), and their antibacterial properties have been investigated against clinically relevant Gram-positive and Gram-negative MDR bacterial strains, demonstrating promising activity. Thus, this study seeks to emphasize the importance of local plants for developing antimicrobial formulations against ESKAPE pathogens.

2. Results

The essential oil yield was 0.43% (w/w) after 6 h of distillation. The refractive index was determined using an Abbe Zeiss refractometer, being 1.4756. The density measured with an ISOLAB pycnometer was 0.95783 g·mL^{-1}.

Further, approximately 80 compounds were identified via GC-MS analysis (Figure 1) and summarized in Table 1 in the order of elution.

Figure 1. Chromatograph of EOs obtained from *T. vulgare*. The peaks indicate the concentration of the compounds.

Table 1. Chemical compounds of essential oil from *T. vulgare*, listed in order of elution, as identified via GC-MS analysis.

Nr. Peak	Compound	Retention Time (min)	Compound Class	Concentration (w/w %)
1	α-Thujone	4.24	MO	0.05 ± 0.02
2	α-Pinenene	4.42	MH	0.85 ± 0.03
3	Camphene	4.76	MH	0.53 ± 0.02
4	Dehydro sabinene ketone	4.83	MO	0.02 ± 0.01
5	Sabinene	5.22	MH	1.51 ± 0.01

Table 1. *Cont.*

Nr. Peak	Compound	Retention Time (min)	Compound Class	Concentration (*w*/*w* %)
6	β-Pinene	5.36	MH	0.42 ± 0.04
7	β-Mircene	5.54	MH	0.14 ± 0.03
8	2,3-Dehydro-1,8-cineole	5.61	MO	0.04 ± 0.01
9	α-Phellandrene	6.00	MH	0.03 ± 0.01
10	(+)-3-Carene	6.08	MH	0.16 ± 0.02
11	α-Terpinene	6.27	MH	0.29 ± 0.03
12	p-Cymene	6.46	MO	0.52 ± 0.01
13	D-Limonene	6.59	MH	0.62 ± 0.02
14	Eucalyptol	6.67	MO	2.47 ± 0.03
15	*Trans*-β-Ocimene	7.01	MH	0.07 ± 0.01
16	γ-Terpinene	7.37	MH	0.58 ± 0.01
17	*cis*-Sabinene hydrate	7.71	MO	0.02 ± 0.01
18	Terpinolene	8.16	MH	0.16 ± 0.02
19	Linalool	8.54	MO	0.03 ± 0.01
20	Filifolone	8.57	MO	0.33 ± 0.01
21	α-Thujone	8.76	MH	3.47 ± 0.03
22	β-Thujone	9.15	MO	30.26 ± 0.04
23	Chrysanthenone	9.22	MO	1.60 ± 0.01
24	*trans*-(2-Ethylcyclopentyl)methanol	9.32	O	0.09 ± 0.01
25	(+)-Isothujol	9.71	MO	0.19 ± 0.02
26	(−)-*cis*-Sabinol	9.78	MO	0.20 ± 0.03
27	L-*trans*-Pinocarveol	9.83	MO	0.19 ± 0.01
28	(+)-Camphor	10.00	MO	1.67 ± 0.03
29	Pinocarvone	10.48	MO	0.34 ± 0.01
30	(1S)-endo)-(−)-Borneol	10.79	MO	0.24 ± 0.01
31	*cis*-Pinocamphone	10.91	MO	0.03 ± 0.01
32	(−)-Terpinen-4-ol	11.06	MO	1.01 ± 0.02
34	α-Thujenol	11.12	MO	0.02 ± 0.01
35	1,5-Menthadien-7-ol	11.42	MO	0.05 ± 0.01
36	*cis*-Dihydrocarvone	11.52	MO	0.38 ± 0.03
37	*cis*-Dihydrocarvone	11.58	MO	0.12 ± 0.02
38	(−)-*trans*-Isopiperilenol	11.69	MO	0.02 ± 0.01
39	*trans*-Dihydrocarvone	11.80	MO	0.02 ± 0.01
40	*cis*-p-Menth-2-en-7-ol	11.90	MO	0.23 ± 0.01
41	*trans*-p-Menth-2-en-7-ol	11.95	MO	0.16 ± 0.02
42	*cis*-Carveol	12.28	MO	1.23 ± 0.02
43	*trans*-Chrysanthenyl acetate	12.68	MO	0.06 ± 0.01
44	Carveol	12.70	MO	0.79 ± 0.01
45	(−)-Carvone	13.05	MO	0.4 ± 0.02
46	Piperitone	13.24	MO	0.04 ± 0.01
47	*cis*-Chrysanthenyl acetate	13.48	MO	1.25 ± 0.03
48	*iso*-3-Thujyl acetate	13.61	MO	0.06 ± 0.01
49	(Z)-Linalool oxide acetat pvr	14.23	MO	0.02 ± 0.01
50	(−)-Bornyl acetate	14.36	MO	0.09 ± 0.01
51	*trans*-Sabinil acetate	14.49	MO	4.6 ± 0.03
52	*trans-2,trans*-4-Decadiene ∣ C10H18	15.03	MH	0.25 ± 0.02

Table 1. *Cont.*

Nr. Peak	Compound	Retention Time (min)	Compound Class	Concentration (*w/w* %)
53	Chrysanthenyl propionate	15.59	MO	0.02 ± 0.01
54	1,4-p-Menthadien-7-ol	15.81	MO	0.07 ± 0.01
55	*cis*-Carvyl acetate	15.90	MO	0.23 ± 0.01
56	α-Fenchene	16.02	MH	0.52 ± 0.02
57	Pseudolimonen	16.49	MH	0.13 ± 0.01
58	*trans*-Carveyl acetate	16.78	MO	34.44 ± 0.03
59	7-epi-Silphiperfol-5-ene	17.26	SH	0.02 ± 0.01
60	α-Copaene	17.31	MH	0.06 ± 0.01
61	Caryophylene	18.66	SH	0.25 ± 0.02
62	β-Copaene	18.97	MH	0.02 ± 0.01
63	Humulene	19.75	SH	0.09 ± 0.01
64	γ-Cardinene	20.35	SH	0.05 ± 0.01
65	Germacrene D	20.53	SH	3.03 ± 0.02
66	Bicyclogermacren	20.97	SH	0.53 ± 0.01
67	β-Cadinene	21.66	SH	0.23 ± 0.02
68	*cis*-Verbenyl angelate	21.95	SO	0.05 ± 0.01
69	Bornyl acetate, (E)-methyl tiglate	22.84	MO	0.09 ± 0.01
70	Spathulenol	23.34	SO	0.09 ± 0.01
71	Caryophylene oxide	23.49	SO	0.11 ± 0.01
72	Salvial-4(14)-en-1-one	23.80	SO	0.03 ± 0.01
73	Cedrol	24.25	SO	0.14 ± 0.02
74	10-epi-juneol	24.64	SO	0.03 ± 0.01
75	Cubenol	24.81	SO	0.05 ± 0.01
76	13-Tetradecanolide	25.38	O	0.3 ± 0.01
77	α-Cardanol	25.58	SO	0.13 ± 0.01
78	Neointermedeol	25.64	SO	0.31 ± 0.02
79	Intermedeol	25.81	SO	0.32 ± 0.01
	Total concentration			99.26

Abbreviations: MH = monoterpene hydrocarbons; MO = oxygenated monoterpenes; SH = sesquiterpene hydrocarbons; SO = oxygenated sesquiterpenes; O = others. Values are mean ± standard deviation of three different samples of *T. vulgare*, analyzed individually in triplicate. Retention time identification is based on comparing retention time with standard compounds; MS identification is based on comparing mass spectra. The amounts were calculated using calibrated curves with pure standard compounds.

The chemical and active properties of Tansy depend on several factors (e.g., plant distribution, geographical location, and environmental factors) [26], which influence the yield and quality of the plant. Thus, we made a comparison between the main compounds obtained by us and those obtained and published in the specialized literature from different geographical areas: Poland, Serbia, and Canada. The working methods for obtaining the essential oil and identifying the compounds were similar, but the reports were different, suggesting the Tansy species' variety. Table 2 summarizes these differences.

In the quantitative assay of the antimicrobial activity of the tansy EOs, all tested strains proved to be very susceptible to the tested EOs in the mass concentration range of 62.5–500 μg/mL (Figure 2). The results obtained showed that Tansy had a remarkable antibacterial effect. Tansy essential oil inhibited the growth of almost all tested bacteria at a concentration lower than 61.5 μg/mL. A higher mass concentration (23.25 mg/mL) was needed to inhibit the growth of *P. aeruginosa* (125 μg/mL).

Table 2. The main chemical compounds isolated and identified in *T. vulgare* essential oils compared to similar studies.

Identified Compound	%						
	1	2	3	4 (R)	4 (M)	4 (W)	4 (T)
Sabinene	1.51	2.02	0.1	2.09	3.39	2.36	0.24
Eucalyptol	2.47	n.d.	n.d.	n.d.	n.d.	n.d.	n.d.
Trans-β-Ocimene	0.07	n.d.	n.d.	n.d.	n.d.	n.d.	n.d.
Linalool	0.03	0.38	n.d.	0.33	0.33	0.28	0.17
Filifolone	0.33	0.15	tr	n.d.	n.d.	n.d.	n.d.
A-Thujone	3.47	0.08	0.9	n.d.	tr	0.14	n.d.
β-Thujone	30.26	3.66	66.6	n.d.	n.d.	n.d.	n.d.
Chrysanthenone	1.6	3.76	tr	n.d.	n.d.	n.d.	n.d.
(+)-Camphor	1.67	30.48	3.1	31.21	10.17	11.93	1.27
cis-Pinocamphone	0.03	n.d.	n.d.	n.d.	n.d.	n.d.	n.d.
(−)-Terpinen 4-ol	1.01	0.09	0.8	n.d.	n.d.	n.d.	n.d.
cis-Carveol	1.23	n.d.	n.d.	n.d.	n.d.	n.d.	n.d.
cis-Chrysanthenyl acetate	1.25	0.1	n.d.	0.07	0.13	1.91	0.11
(z)-Linalool oxide acetate (pyranoid)	0.01	n.d.	n.d.	n.d.	n.d.	n.d.	n.d.
trans-Sabinyl acetate	4.6	n.d.	0.1	n.d.	n.d.	n.d.	n.d.
α-Fenchene	0.52	n.d.	n.d.	n.d.	n.d.	n.d.	n.d.
trans-Carvyl acetate	34.44	n.d.	n.d.	n.d.	n.d.	n.d.	n.d.
β-Copaene	0.02	n.d.	tr	n.d.	n.d.	n.d.	n.d.
Germacrene D	3.03	0.09	0.7	0.46	0.42	0.7	0.38
Cedrol	0.14	n.d.	n.d.	n.d.	n.d.	n.d.	n.d.
Juneol	0.03	n.d.	n.d.	n.d.	n.d.	n.d.	n.d.

Abbreviations: tr—Trace amounts (<0.05%); n.d.—Not determined; 1—compounds identified in this study; 2—compounds identified by Coté et al. [24]; 3—compounds identified by Radulović et al. [27]; 4—compounds identified by Nurzyńska-Wierdak et al. [23] from several sites: R—reclaimed site; M—the meadow near the river; W—ruderal site; T—plants growing along the road.

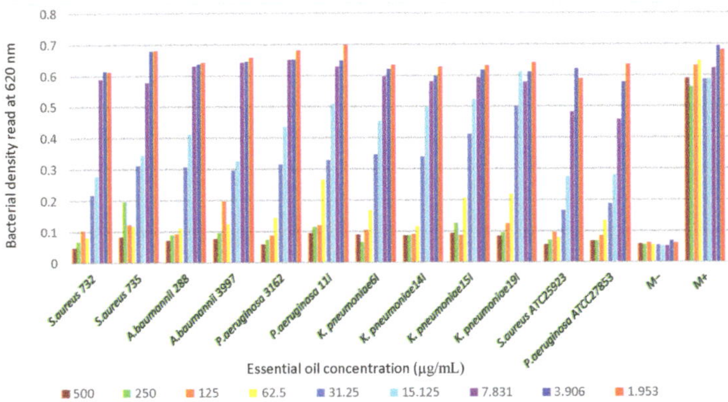

Figure 2. Graphic representation of the antibacterial activity of tansy EOs against the MDR strains. On the ordinate is written the value of the optical density of the cultures measured indirectly viaoptical density at 620 nm with a UV-vis spectrometer (Lambda25, PerkinElmer, Inc., Waltham, MA, USA), and on the abscissa is written the mass concentration of the Tansy extract (µg/mL). The best activity was recorded against the *S.aureus* strain isolated from wound secretions (31.25 µg/mL). M+ positive control (bacterial culture without extract addition) and M− (sterile culture medium). Experiments were performed in triplicate (n = 3), and results were expressed as means ± SD. Statistical analyses were performed using GraphPad Prism 7. If the probability of the difference was less than $p < 0.05$, it was deemed to be statistically significant.

The *T. vulgare* extract had a different effect on the activity of the tested antibiotics, depending on the bacterial strain and the antibiotic. Table 3 summarizes the obtained results regarding the synergism of tansy EOs with the tested antibiotics. Each experiment was repeated three times, the diameter of the inhibition zone being the arithmetic mean of these values. The tolerance was ±0.5 mm.

Table 3. Growth inhibition zone diameters obtained for beta-lactam antibiotics tested in association with Tansy EO against the Gram-negative bacterial strains.

Strain	Diameter (mm)																								
	Tv	TPZ (100 + 10 µg)	TPZ + Tv	PIP (75 µg)	PIP + Tv	SAM (10 + 10 µg	SAM + Tv	CAZ (10 µg)	CAZ + Tv	ATM (30 µg)	ATM + Tv	IPM (10 µg)	IPM + Tv	MEM (10 µg)	MEM + Tv	GM (10 µg)	GM + Tv	TOB (10 µg)	TOB + Tv	LVX (5 µg)	LVX + Tv	CIP (5 µg)	CIP + Tv
*Pa*ATC	21	20(S)	21(S)	30(S)	28(I)	20(S)	20(S)	17(S)	21(S)	16(I)	20(S)	20(S)	21(S)	24(S)	28(S)	20(S)	22(S)	18(S)	20(S)	24(S)	28(S)	20(S)	28(S)
*Pa*3162	19	6(R)	12(S)	6(R)	14(I)	8(R)	19(S)	6(R)	17(S)	6(R)	16(S)	6(R)	12(S)	10(R)	19(S)	6(R)	18(S)	6(R)	19(S)	6(R)	19(S)	6(R)	14(I)
*Pa*11I	18	6(R)	10(S)	6(R)	15(I)	10(R)	20(S)	8(R)	19(S)	6(R)	18(S)	6(R)	10(S)	8(R)	21(S)	6(R)	20(S)	6(R)	20(S)	6(R)	18(S)	6(R)	15(I)
*Ab*3997	20	6(R)	17(S)	10(R)	18(S)	6(R)	20(S)	6(R)	20(S)	6(R)	19(S)	6(R)	17(S)	6(R)	19(S)	6(R)	17(S)	6(R)	20(S)	10(R)	18(S)	10(R)	18(S)
*Ab*288	22	6(R)	20(S)	8(R)	20(S)	6(R)	22(S)	6(R)	14(S)	14(I)	20(S)	6(R)	20(S)	8(R)	24(S)	6(R)	20(S)	6(R)	22(S)	6(R)	20(S)	8(R)	20(S)
*Kp*6I	21	6(R)	19(S)	8(R)	17(S)	6(R)	19(S)	14(R)	20(S)	6(R)	21(S)	6(R)	19(S)	6(R)	19(S)	6(R)	19(S)	6(R)	19(S)	6(R)	17(S)	8(R)	17(S)
*Kp*14I	18	6(R)	17(S)	6(R)	19(S)	10(R)	18(S)	6(R)	19(S)	6(R)	19(S)	6(R)	17(S)	8(R)	18(S)	6(R)	17(S)	10(R)	18(S)	6(R)	19(S)	6(R)	19(S)
*Kp*15I	22	6(R)	18(S)	8(R)	21(S)	10(R)	20(S)	6(R)	21(S)	14(I)	20(S)	6(R)	18(S)	10(R)	20(S)	6(R)	18(S)	10(R)	20(S)	10(R)	21(S)	6(R)	21(S)
*Kp*19I	22	6(R)	20(S)	12(R)	18(S)	6(R)	18(S)	6(R)	17(S)	10(R)	20(S)	6(R)	20(S)	6(R)	18(S)	6(R)	20(S)	6(R)	18(S)	12(R)	18(S)	12(R)	18(S)

Abbreviations: *Pa* = *P. aeruginosa*, *Kp* = *K. pneumoniae*, *Ab* = *A. baumannii*, *Tv* = *T.vulgare*, TPZ = Piperacillin + Tazobactam, PIP = Piperacillin, SAM = Ampicillin + Sulbactam, CAZ = Ceftazidime, ATM = Aztreonam, IMP = Imipenem, MEM = Meropenem, GN = Gentamicin, TOB = Tobramycin, LEV = Levofloxacin, CIP = Ciprofloxacin. w/w %Tansy = 125 µg/mL; S = Susceptible; I = Intermediate; R = Resistant. Diameter of inhibition zones (mm), including disc diameter of 6 mm. Values are mean ± standard deviation of three different samples of each *T. vulgare*, analyzed individually in triplicate.

As shown in Table 4, the Tansy EOs exhibited a synergic effect on all tested antibiotics in the case of *A. baumannii* and *K. pneumoniae* strains and on at least one antibiotic from each of the tested class in the case of *P. aeruginosa* strains (Table 3).

Table 4. The number of Gram-negative strains out of the total number of strains from each species for which a synergism with *Tv* EOs was noted.

Antibiotic Class	Antibiotics	*Pseudomonas aeruginosa*	*Acinetobacter baumannii*	*Klebsiella pneumoniae*
Penicilins/+clavulanic acid or sulbactam	TPZ	2/3	2/2	4/4
	PIP	3/3	2/2	4/4
	SAM	2/3	2/2	4/4
Cephalosporins	CAZ	2/3	2/2	4/4
Monobactams	ATM	2/3	2/2	4/4
Carbapenems	IMP	1/3	2/2	4/4
	MEM	3/3	2/2	4/4
Aminoglycosides	GN	1/3	2/2	4/4
	TOB	3/3	2/2	4/4
Quinolones	LEV	3/3	2/2	4/4
	CIP	2/3	2/2	4/4

Abbreviations: TPZ = Piperacillin + Tazobactam, PIP = Piperacillin, SAM = Ampicillin + Sulbactam, CAZ = Ceftazidime, ATM = Aztreonam, IMP = Imipenem, MEM = Meropenem, GN = Gentamicin, TOB = Tobramycin, LEV = Levofloxacin, CIP = Ciprofloxacin.

Plant extracts have multiple mechanisms of action on microorganisms. To better understand their mechanisms of bactericidal or bacteriostatic action, we evaluated the influence of extracts by associating them with different classes of antibiotics: aminoglycosides, β-lactams, and quinolones. In particular, the serial microdilution method was used to quantify the synergistic effect of tansy extract with antibiotics. Antibiotics, in combination with the Tansy extract, demonstrated enhanced antibacterial activities (Table 5).

Table 5. Influence of Tansy extract on the antibiotic resistance profile of Gram-positive and Gram-negative strains.

Strain	The Influence of EO Tansy against Bacterial Growth in Combination with the Antibiotic (µg/mL)											
	CIP (5 µg)	CIP + *Tv*	FEP (30 µg)	FEP + *Tv*	AMC (30 µg)	AMC + *Tv*	GM (10 µg)	GM + *Tv*	IPM (10 µg)	IPM + *Tv*	TOB (10 µg)	TOB + *Tv*
S. aureus$_{732}$	128	16	256	32	128	32	128	16	128	16	256	16
S. aureus$_{735}$	256	32	512	16	64	16	256	32	256	32	512	16
A. baumannii$_{288}$	64	8	128	8	64	8	64	16	128	64	128	32
A. baumannii$_{3997}$	256	32	128	32	32	64	256	32	256	32	64	64
P. aeruginosa$_{3162}$	64	16	256	8	128	32	128	8	64	16	128	16
P. aeruginosa$_{111}$	128	64	64	32	256	64	128	16	128	32	256	8
K. pneumoniae$_{61}$	256	64	256	8	256	32	16	4	512	32	128	32
K. pneumoniae$_{141}$	128	32	128	32	128	8	128	8	256	16	256	64
K. pneumoniae$_{151}$	256	64	64	16	64	32	64	16	128	8	64	8
K. pneumoniae$_{191}$	128	32	64	8	64	16	256	8	128	16	128	8

Abbreviations: FEP = Cefepime; AMC = Amoxicillin + Clavulanic Acid; TOB = Tobramycin; *w*/*w* % Tansy = 125 µg/mL.

As observed in Table 5, regarding the synergism of the *T vulgare* extract with the antibiotic, the plant extract had a different effect on the activity of the associated antibiotic and also depending on the bacterial strain. The zones of inhibition had values between 14 and 30 mm. Each experiment was repeated three times, the diameter of the inhibition zone being the arithmetic mean of these values. The tolerance was ±0.5 mm.

The synergism of the plant extract with the antibiotic was evident for all classes of antibiotics inhibiting bacterial growth. The potentiation of antibacterial activity of antibiotics in combination with plant extracts can be correlated with the synergism of the specific mechanisms of action of antibiotics and extracts on multidrug-resistant bacteria. Specifically, in combination with the extract, antibiotics have regained their properties as bacterial inhibitors. Moreover, the synergistic action of Tansy extract with antibiotics on MDR strains suggests the complexity of the action of the compounds resulting from secondary metabolism.

3. Discussion

The list of plants with curative effects against a wide variety of organic and infectious diseases has expanded, especially in recent decades, as analytical methods have identified compounds with therapeutic effects, especially against bacterial infectious diseases, in the context of the expansion of the phenomenon of antibiotic resistance. In vitro tests have shown that some plant species used to treat non-infectious diseases have antibacterial activity. More than a quarter of the medicines administered in industrialized countries are obtained directly or indirectly from plants [15].

The antimicrobial action of plant extracts results from their complex chemical composition, the compounds acting synergistically and having multiple action targets. These preparations are generically referred to as "non-antibiotic antibacterial agents" [15] and were proven to be active against a large spectrum of bacterial and fungal strains [16].

In this context, the main objective of this study was to evaluate the antibacterial effect of Tansy EO as well as its potential synergy with antibiotics. In this regard, the first step assumed the identification of the bioactive compounds of *T. vulgare* extract, comparing them with those reported by other authors. The variation in the concentration of the compounds is correlated with the site from which the plant was harvested [23]. In more detail, the essential oil composition indicates plant adaptation to habitat conditions and stress conditions: drought, radiation, high temperature, heavy metal content, and predators [28]. Thus, essential oils change according to environmental conditions [29].

The biological activity of Tansy extract is related to the total terpene content of the essential oil. As depicted in Table 2, Radulović et al. [27] identified the presence of four different chemotypes of these species in Serbia (thujone, *trans*-chrysanthenyl acetate, chrysanthenyl, and camphoric chemotype) depending on the geographical areas. The chemotype of the species studied by Coté et al. [24] collected from Chicoutimi, Quebec City, QC, Canada, is camphoric (30.4%). The chemotype of the species studied by Nurzyńska-Wierdak et al. [23], from eastern Poland (Wohyń Commune, Radzyń Poviat, Lubelskie Voivodeship) is *trans*-chrysanthenyl (76.09%). The chemotype of our plant was *trans*-Carvyl acetate (34.44%).

The compounds identified in this study had approximately the same concentrations as those reported in the cited literature, with some differences that could influence the higher antibacterial activity. Thus, Eucalyptol, *trans*-β-Ocimene, *cis*-Pinocamphone, *cis*-Carveol, (z)-Linalool oxide acetate (pyranoid), α-Fenchene, *trans*-Carvyl acetate, β-Copaene, Cedrol, and Junelol were not identified in these studies [23,24,27]. Therefore, this article completes the knowledge regarding *T. vulgare* EO, identifying and quantifying a series of previously disregarded compounds.

Eucalyptol is an important monoterpene in this study, found in a proportion of 2.47%, being widely used in the pharmaceutical industry, having anti-inflammatory properties, and killing leukemic cells in vitro [30]. Antibacterial activity has been reported in several studies [31,32], the main mechanism of action being the penetration of the bacterial cell membrane and its lysis [33]. Trans-β-Ocimene is a terpene that establishes tri-trophic interactions [34], which was identified in a proportion of 0.07%. In addition to its quality as a food additive, it has several therapeutic properties, including anti-inflammatory, antifungal, and antiviral effects [35,36]. *Cis*-Pinocamphone is a monoterpenoid found especially in *Xylopia aromatica* and *Aloysia gratissima*. *Cis*-Carveol is a monoterpene that has the ability to cause the death of the bacterial cell via the disintegration mechanism of the cell membrane [37]. α-Fenchene is a monoterpene with a camphor-like odor. The presence of this compound in plants has a role in increasing antioxidant activity [38]. The greatest spread was found in Artemisia sp., hence the similarity of the smell of the two plants [39].

Trans-Carvyl acetate is a terpene ester with a mint flavor with a role in increasing antibacterial activity [40]. β–Copaene is a sesquiterpene used as a food additive and flavor due to its antioxidant properties [41]. Cedrol is a sesquiterpene found in conifers used in traditional medicine, especially due to its antimicrobial properties [42]. Juneol is a sesquiterpene identified in high concentrations in *Bursera graveolens*, a tree that belongs to the same family (Burseraceae) as frankincense and myrrh with several therapeutic properties, including antibacterial [43].

Concerning identified concentrations, the most abundant compounds were carvyl acetate (34.44%) and β-thujone (30.26%). Carvyl acetate is a flavonoid predominantly found in *Mentha spicata* L. with strong inhibitory potential against Gram-positive and Gram-negative bacteria and pathogenic fungi [44]. The quality of *Mentha longifolia* (L) EOs is proportional to the carveol content [45]. On the other hand, α-Thujone and β-thujone are the two stereoisomeric forms by which thujone is represented in the ketone group of bicyclic monoterpenes [46].

Plants that have significant thujone content, such as *Artemisia* sp., *Achillea* sp., *Thuja* sp., and *Salvia* sp., are often used to flavor foods and beverages. Absinthe, for example, is a well-known alcoholic drink called absinthe after the name of the plant used due to the flavor obtained by adding the extract of *Artemisia absinthium* L. Thujone has long been thought to cause adverse psychoactive effects. However, recent research has made convincing arguments for correctly identifying substances with possible side effects in absinthe, such as ethanol and other compounds used in the adulteration process [47]. In addition, α-Thujone is the active ingredient of wormwood oil and other drugs and has been reported to have antinociceptive, insecticidal, and anthelmintic activity [48]. The toxicity of thujone has been studied extensively, neurotoxicity being the main toxic outcome [49]. Regarding the degree of toxicity of the two forms of thujone, α-Thujone has a higher toxicity than β-thujone. As thujone is found in many medicinal plants to eliminate the supposed negative effect of this compound, HMPC (Committee on Herbal Medicinal Products) and EMA (European Medicines Agency) were able to set the maximum daily dose limit for thujone, which was set between 3.5 and 5.0 mg/person [50].

Thujone formation is not a universal phenomenon in plants. The indirect precursor of thujone, sabinene, is one of the most widespread monoterpene compounds in EOs. Various external and internal factors influence the accumulation of thujone. The isomerization of thujones can be explained by the presence of intermediates such as sabinol, sabinone, and related compounds in EOs [51]. The thujone pathway exists in many sabinene-containing species, but the expression of the corresponding genes is repressed due to different metabolic interactions, leading to the lack of thujone (for example, plants of the *Lamiaceae* family) [52].

It has been shown that α, β-Thujone (70% of α-thujone and 10% of β-thujone) also have anti-cancer effects against placental choriocarcinoma cells by inducing apoptosis via the mitochondrial-mediated intrinsic pathway [53]. A study by Pudełek et al. [54] highlighted the properties of α-Thujone as a potent attenuator on the proliferation and viability of glioblastoma multiforme cells, as this compound displayed anti-invasive and pro-apoptotic effects on glioblastoma multiforme cells.

Further, the obtained extract was tested on Gram-positive and Gram-negative bacterial strains that have been selected to exhibit multiple drug resistance to current antibiotics, i.e., beta-lactams, aminoglycosides, and quinolones. In order to evaluate the antibacterial effects and the potential synergism with antibiotics, qualitative and quantitative assays have been performed. *T. vulgare* extract was observed to work together with antibiotics, achieving more significant antimicrobial effects. The combination of conventional antibiotics, against which bacterial strains have been resistant, with plant extracts can restore the effectiveness of treatment due to the synergistic antibiotic-extract effect [55].

The microorganisms analyzed were strains with multiple antibiotic resistance and reference strains. To evaluate the effects of the association of plant extracts with antibiotics, we determined the MIC values of plant extracts as a reference point for defining the interactions with antibiotics. The association of antibiotics with volatile oil extract from *T vulgare* has been investigated for possible synergistic interactions. Using the "chessboard" method, the synergism is manifested by the increased sensitivity of the microorganism in the simultaneous presence of both antimicrobial agents, which is reflected by changes in the values of the zones of inhibition [56]. This can be explained by the ability of Tansy extract to enhance bacterial cell membrane permeability [57], thus allowing higher amounts of antibiotics to enter pathogenic cells and consequentially destroy them.

The antimicrobial action of plant extracts is the result of all chemical compounds that act synergistically, having multiple targets of action. The minimum inhibitory concentrations of oil Tansy extract for the bacterial strains tested varied in the range (62.5 ÷ 500) µg/mL. In the quantitative assay, the most susceptible to the tested EOs were the *S. aureus* strains (for which the MIC was 125 µg/mL for *S. aureus*$_{732}$ and *S. aureus*$_{735}$ and 62.5 µg/mL for *S. aureus*$_{ATC25923}$ compared to the results obtained by Coté et al. [24] for *S. aureus*$_{ATC25923}$, of 59 µg/mL). For Gram-negative bacteria, the MIC values were approximately the same. Further, for *P. aeruginosa*$_{11I}$, it was 125 µg/mL; for *P. aeruginosa*$_{3162}$, it was 250 µg/mL; and for *P.aeruginosa*$_{ATCC27853}$, it was 62.5 µg/mL like the one obtained by Chiavari-Frederico et al. [58]. For Gram-negative strains of *K. pneumoniae* isolated from urinary tract infections (UTI), the MIC concentrations were between 125 and 250 µg/mL, similar to those obtained by Gadisa and Tadesse [59].

4. Materials and Methods

4.1. Obtaining and Characterization of Tansy EOs

Tansy plants were harvested between July and August 2021 from the Sohodol Valley area, Gorj County. The plant was gathered from a soil covering, predominantly granitic, bordered to the southwest by a narrow, deep valley traversed by the Sohodol River. This entire area stands as an open clearing amidst a vast expanse of woodland, spanning approximately 10 hectares. The central reference coordinates are 45°11′13.7″ N 23°08′04.0″ E, with altitudes ranging between 550 and 700 m. This delineated area lies on the left slope of the Sohodol Valley. Only young inflorescences, unaffected by pests or mechanical factors, were used. The essential oil from the dried flowers of *T. vulgare* was obtained in a Neoclevenger distillery purchased from Pellet Lab, Houston, TX, USA. Extraction of essential oils via steam entrainment is the most widely used process. Volatile oils are very light at temperatures below the boiling point of water and are carried to the distillery's upper outlet areas by steam. Their low density and insolubility in water facilitate their separation.

The air-dried plants were introduced into the distillery boiler with a capacity of 20 L. The ratio of distilled water to dry plants was 6 L to a volume of 3 kg. The total working time was about 6 h. We obtained 20 mL of essential oil, which we stored in a dark-colored bottle at a temperature of 4 °C. The chemical compounds in the essential oil of *T. vulgare* were identified using the gas chromatography method (i.e., Shimadzu GC-2010 Plus method) coupled with a mass spectrometer (GC-MS), coupled with a quartz capillary column. Helium (1.0 mL/min) was used as carrier gas. Additionally, 1 µL of the samples were injected into the GC (detector temperature, 280 °C). Qualitative analysis used electron impact ionization (ionization energy, 70 eV). Essential oils were identified using a digital library of mass spectral data (NIST 8.0) and literature comparisons of retention indices [60]. Quantitative GC-FID analysis was performed using a SHIMADZU GC-2010 Plus instrument equipped with an MS quartz capillary column under the same conditions as GC-MS, except that N_2 was used as the carrier gas. The temperature of the FID detector was 250 °C. The relative concentration of the compounds was calculated by measuring the chromatographic peak areas without applying any correction factor. The applied software was AFT (Advanced Flow Technology), Fathom 9 version. The relative percentage values of separated compounds were calculated by recording the peaks in the FID chromatograms. Essential oils were identified by comparing their GC retention times on apolar and polar columns with those of the sample compounds and by comparing retention indices relative to commercial mass spectral libraries of the C6-C40 alkane series. Alkanes (C6-C40) were used as reference points to calculate relative retention indices [61–63].

4.2. Antibacterial Activity of T. vulgare EOs

For this study, we selected 2 *Staphylococcus aureus*, 2 *Acinetobacter baumannii*, 3 *Pseudomonas aeruginosa*, and 4 *Klebsiella pneumoniae* bacterial strains that were multidrug resistant, isolated from patients with different infections, hospitalized at the C.C. Iliescu Institute of Cardiovascular Diseases in Bucharest and previously characterized for their resistance phenotypes and genotypes. *S. aureus* ATCC 25923 and *P. aeruginosa* ATCC 27853 were used as control reference strains. The antibiotic susceptibility assay of the studied strains was performed using the standardized Kirby–Bauer method, according to CLSI, 2018 edition [64].

For the qualitative assay of the antibiotic-tansy EO synergisms, bacterial suspensions were made in sterile physiological water from 24 h of bacterial cultures at a density of 1.5×10^8 CFU/mL according to the McFarland 0.5 turbidity standard. Each bacterial inoculum was inoculated on a plate with Müller–Hinton medium, using the "cloth" seeding technique. After drying the plates, antibiotic discs alone, as well as those impregnated with a volume of 10 μL Tansy EOs, were placed at equal distances. For testing the tansy EOs, sterile paper disks impregnated with a volume of 10 μL tansy EOs were used. The plates were incubated for 18–24 h at 35 °C ± 2 °C. After incubation, the diameters of growth inhibition zones were measured and expressed in mm. Increasing the diameter of the inhibition zone of the antibiotic in the presence of tansy EOs by ≥5 mm was the indicator of the synergistic effect.

We used the serial microdilution method for the semi-quantitative quantification of the synergistic effect of Tansy extract with antibiotics. A conventional method (according to EUCAST/2010) to obtain different concentrations of antimicrobial agents for MIC determination is to obtain a stock solution of 10,240 mg/L. By adding a volume of 19 mL of liquid Muller–Hinton broth to 1 mL of the stock solution, a final concentration of 512 μg/mL is obtained. In this study, the antibacterial activity was quantitatively determined using binary serial microdilutions in a liquid culture medium (Muller–Hinton nutrient broth) in 96-well microplates according to CLSI 2006 [65] and 2008 [66]. For this purpose, 10 binary serial dilutions, from 500 μg/mL to 1.953 μg/mL, were performed in a ratio of 9:1 nutrient broth with tansy EOs + distilled water. Bacterial suspensions of 1.5×10^8 CFU/mL were prepared according to the McFarland 0.5 turbidity standard. The final volume per well was 200 μL, and the volume of bacterial suspension was 15 μL. Wells 11 and 12 corresponded to positive (bacterial culture) and negative (sterile culture medium) controls, respectively. The plates were incubated overnight at 37 °C. The minimum inhibitory concentration (MIC) was determined macroscopically by establishing the final concentration at which no increase in microbial growth and environmental turbidity was observed and via the spectrophotometric reading of the absorbance at 620 nm.

5. Conclusions

Our results have shown that the bioactive compounds from Tansy EOs are a rich source for developing new pharmaceuticals useful in the prophylaxis and treatment of bacterial infections produced by MDR Gram-negative and Gram-positive bacteria, as such or in combination with commonly used antibiotics. The antimicrobial action of Tansy Eos is justified by its complex chemical composition, the secondary metabolites potentially responsible for this activity being monoterpenes (Sabinene, Eucalyptol, *trans*-β-Ocimene, Linalool, Filifolone, Thujone, Camphor, *cis*-Carveol, Sabinol isovalerate), terpenoids (Chrysanthenone, Terpinen-4-ol), sesquiterpenes (Germacrenes D, Cedrol, Cubenol, ledol, Globulol, Artemisia ketone, Spirojatamol), and *trans*-Carvyl acetate. Moreover, Tansy essential oil showed MIC values ranging between 500 and 62.5 μg/mL against the tested strains, displaying synergistic activity with different classes of antibiotics. In conclusion, the presented results demonstrate that Tansy EOs hold promise for developing new antimicrobial formulations for treating active MDR bacterial infections, being a natural source of valuable bioactive compounds.

Author Contributions: Conceptualization, H.R., V.L. and M.M.M.; methodology, V.L. and M.M.M.; formal analysis, H.R., A.-G.N., V.L. and M.M.M.; investigation, H.R., A.-G.N., V.L. and M.M.M.; writing—original draft preparation, H.R., A.-G.N., V.L. and M.M.M.; writing—review and editing, H.R., A.-G.N., V.L. and M.M.M. All authors have read and agreed to the published version of the manuscript.

Funding: This research received no external funding.

Institutional Review Board Statement: Not applicable.

Informed Consent Statement: Not applicable.

Data Availability Statement: Data are contained within the article.

Acknowledgments: The authors are grateful to Anton Ficai for the help with the biological tests regarding the gas chromatography-flame ionization detection (GC-FID) system from the Faculty of Chemical Engineering and Biotechnologies, National University of Science and Technology Politehnica Bucharest. This study was carried out within the Biology and Systemic Ecology Research Platform of the Faculty of Biology, University of Bucharest, under the guidance of Marcela Popa. The study was supported by the Romanian Executive Agency for Higher Education, Research, Development, and Innovation, research project FDI 0690/2023, and the project C1.2. PFE- CDI.2021-587/contract number 41PFE/2021 (University of Bucharest, Romania).

Conflicts of Interest: The authors declare no conflict of interest.

References

1. WHO. WHO Publishes List of Bacteria for Which New Antibiotics Are Urgently Needed. Available online: https://www.who.int/news/item/27-02-2017-who-publishes-list-of-bacteria-for-which-new-antibiotics-are-urgently-needed (accessed on 18 September 2023).
2. Mulani, M.S.; Kamble, E.E.; Kumkar, S.N.; Tawre, M.S.; Pardesi, K.R. Emerging strategies to combat ESKAPE pathogens in the era of antimicrobial resistance: A review. *Front. Microbiol.* **2019**, *10*, 539. [CrossRef] [PubMed]
3. Chifiriuc, M.C.; Mihăescu, G.; Lazăr, V. Antimicrobial therapy. In *Microbiology and Medical Virology*; University of Bucharest: Bucharest, Romania, 2011; pp. 426–431.
4. World Health Organization. Global Shortage of Innovative Antibiotics Fuels Emergence and Spread of Drug-Resistance. Available online: https://www.who.int/news/item/15-04-2021-global-shortage-of-innovative-antibiotics-fuels-emergence-and-spread-of-drug-resistance (accessed on 28 June 2023).
5. Adeyemi, A.D.; Oluigbo, C.C.; Esan, A.O.; Bello, M.O.; Oladoye, S.O.; Emmanuel, C.P.; Effiong, E. Chemical Composition and Antimicrobial Activity of the Essential oils of 14 known *Ficus* species–A Concise. *Biointerface Res. Appl. Chem.* **2021**, *12*, 8003–8034.
6. Saber, M.; Harhar, H.; Bouyahya, A.; Ouchbani, T.; Tabyaoui, M. Chemical Composition and Antioxidant Activity of Essential Oil of Sawdust from Moroccan Thuya (*Tetraclinis articulata* (Vahl) Masters). *Biointerface Res. Appl. Chem.* **2020**, *11*, 7912–7920.
7. Balaban, Y.H.; Aka, C.; Koca-Caliskan, U. Liver immunology and herbal treatment. *World J. Hepatol.* **2017**, *9*, 757–770. [CrossRef]
8. Iriti, M.; Vitalini, S.; Fico, G.; Faoro, F. Neuroprotective herbs and foods from different traditional medicines and diets. *Molecules* **2010**, *15*, 3517–3555. [CrossRef]
9. Diao, W.-R.; Hu, Q.-P.; Zhang, H.; Xu, J.-G. Chemical composition, antibacterial activity and mechanism of action of essential oil from seeds of fennel (*Foeniculum vulgare* Mill.). *Food Control* **2014**, *35*, 109–116. [CrossRef]
10. Grigore, A.; Colceru-Mihul, S.; Bazdoaca, C.; Yuksel, R.; Ionita, C.; Glava, L. Antimicrobial Activity of an *Achillea millefolium* L. *Proceedings* **2020**, *57*, 34. [CrossRef]
11. Lu, Y.; Joerger, R.; Wu, C. Study of the chemical composition and antimicrobial activities of ethanolic extracts from roots of *Scutellaria baicalensis* Georgi. *J. Agric. Food Chem.* **2011**, *59*, 10934–10942. [CrossRef]
12. Petrovic, J.; Stanojkovic, A.; Comic, L.; Curcic, S. Antibacterial activity of *Cichorium intybus*. *Fitoterapia* **2004**, *75*, 737–739. [CrossRef]
13. Sati, S.C.; Joshi, S. Antibacterial activities of *Ginkgo biloba* L. leaf extracts. *Sci. World J.* **2011**, *11*, 2237–2242. [CrossRef]

14. Scavo, A.; Pandino, G.; Restuccia, C.; Parafati, L.; Cirvilleri, G.; Mauromicale, G. Antimicrobial activity of cultivated cardoon (*Cynara cardunculus* L. var. *altilis* DC.) leaf extracts against bacterial species of agricultural and food interest. *Ind. Crops Prod.* **2019**, *129*, 206–211. [CrossRef]
15. Al-Habib, A.; Al-Saleh, E.; Safer, A.M.; Afzal, M. Bactericidal effect of grape seed extract on methicillin-resistant *Staphylococcus aureus* (MRSA). *J. Toxicol. Sci.* **2010**, *35*, 357–364. [CrossRef] [PubMed]
16. Anesini, C.; Perez, C. Screening of plants used in Argentine folk medicine for antimicrobial activity. *J. Ethnopharmacol.* **1993**, *39*, 119–128. [CrossRef]
17. Gurib-Fakim, A. Medicinal plants: Traditions of yesterday and drugs of tomorrow. *Mol. Asp. Med.* **2006**, *27*, 1–93. [CrossRef] [PubMed]
18. Cimino, C.; Maurel, O.M.; Musumeci, T.; Bonaccorso, A.; Drago, F.; Souto, E.M.B.; Pignatello, R.; Carbone, C. Essential Oils: Pharmaceutical Applications and Encapsulation Strategies into Lipid-Based Delivery Systems. *Pharmaceutics* **2021**, *13*, 327. [CrossRef]
19. Korpinen, R.I.; Välimaa, A.L.; Liimatainen, J.; Kunnas, S. Essential Oils and Supercritical CO_2 Extracts of Arctic Angelica (*Angelica archangelica* L.), Marsh Labrador Tea (*Rhododendron tomentosum*) and Common Tansy (*Tanacetum vulgare*)-Chemical Compositions and Antimicrobial Activities. *Molecules* **2021**, *26*, 7121. [CrossRef] [PubMed]
20. Benkhaira, N.; Koraichi, S.I.; Fikri-Benbrahim, K. In vitro methods to study antioxidant and some biological activities of essential oils: A review. *Biointerface Res. Appl. Chem* **2022**, *12*, 3332.
21. Beigi, M.; Torki-Harchegani, M.; Ghasemi Pirbalouti, A. Quantity and chemical composition of essential oil of peppermint (*Mentha* × *piperita* L.) leaves under different drying methods. *Int. J. Food Prop.* **2018**, *21*, 267–276. [CrossRef]
22. Argyropoulos, D.; Müller, J. Changes of essential oil content and composition during convective drying of lemon balm (*Melissa officinalis* L.). *Ind. Crops Prod.* **2014**, *52*, 118–124. [CrossRef]
23. Nurzyńska-Wierdak, R.; Sałata, A.; Kniaziewicz, M. Tansy (*Tanacetum vulgare* L.)—A Wild-Growing Aromatic Medicinal Plant with a Variable Essential Oil Composition. *Agronomy* **2022**, *12*, 277. [CrossRef]
24. Coté, H.; Boucher, M.A.; Pichette, A.; Legault, J. Anti-Inflammatory, Antioxidant, Antibiotic, and Cytotoxic Activities of *Tanacetum vulgare* L. Essential Oil and Its Constituents. *Medicines* **2017**, *4*, 34. [CrossRef] [PubMed]
25. Stevovic, S.; Devrnja, N.; Calic-Dragosavac, D. Environmental impact quantification and correlation between site location and contents and structure of Tansy. *Afr. J. Biotechnol.* **2011**, *10*, 5075–5083.
26. Xu, W.; Cheng, Y.; Guo, Y.; Yao, W.; Qian, H. Effects of geographical location and environmental factors on metabolite content and immune activity of *Echinacea purpurea* in China based on metabolomics analysis. *Ind. Crops Prod.* **2022**, *189*, 115782. [CrossRef]
27. Radulović, N.S.; Genčić, M.S.; Stojanović, N.M.; Randjelović, P.J.; Stojanović-Radić, Z.Z.; Stojiljković, N.I. Toxic essential oils. Part V: Behaviour modulating and toxic properties of thujones and thujone-containing essential oils of *Salvia officinalis* L., *Artemisia absinthium* L., *Thuja occidentalis* L. and *Tanacetum vulgare* L. *Food Chem. Toxicol. Int. J. Publ. Br. Ind. Biol. Res. Assoc.* **2017**, *105*, 355–369. [CrossRef] [PubMed]
28. Abu-Darwish, M.S.; Abu-Dieyeh, Z.H.M. Essential oil content and heavy metals composition of *Thymus vulgaris* cultivated in various climatic regions of Jordan. *Int. J. Agric. Biol* **2009**, *11*, 59–63.
29. Stevovic, S.; Mikovilovic, V.S.; Dragosavac, D.C. Environmental adaptibility of tansy (*Tanacetum vulgare* L.). *Afr. J. Biotechnol.* **2009**, *8*, 6290–6294.
30. National Center for Biotechnology Information. PubChem Compound Database. Available online: https://pubchem.ncbi.nlm.nih.gov/compound/Eucalyptol (accessed on 20 September 2023).
31. Mączka, W.; Duda-Madej, A.; Górny, A.; Grabarczyk, M.; Wińska, K. Can eucalyptol replace antibiotics? *Molecules* **2021**, *26*, 4933. [CrossRef]
32. Cai, Z.-M.; Peng, J.-Q.; Chen, Y.; Tao, L.; Zhang, Y.-Y.; Fu, L.-Y.; Long, Q.-D.; Shen, X.-C. 1, 8-Cineole: A review of source, biological activities, and application. *J. Asian Nat. Prod. Res.* **2021**, *23*, 938–954. [CrossRef]
33. Zengin, H.; Baysal, A.H. Antibacterial and antioxidant activity of essential oil terpenes against pathogenic and spoilage-forming bacteria and cell structure-activity relationships evaluated by SEM microscopy. *Molecules* **2014**, *19*, 17773–17798. [CrossRef]
34. Farré-Armengol, G.; Filella, I.; Llusià, J.; Peñuelas, J. β-Ocimene, a Key Floral and Foliar Volatile Involved in Multiple Interactions between Plants and Other Organisms. *Molecules* **2017**, *22*, 1148. [CrossRef]
35. Loizzo, M.R.; Saab, A.M.; Tundis, R.; Statti, G.A.; Menichini, F.; Lampronti, I.; Gambari, R.; Cinatl, J.; Doerr, H.W. Phytochemical analysis and in vitro antiviral activities of the essential oils of seven Lebanon species. *Chem. Biodivers.* **2008**, *5*, 461–470. [CrossRef] [PubMed]
36. Cavaleiro, C.; Salgueiro, L.; Gonçalves, M.J.; Hrimpeng, K.; Pinto, J.; Pinto, E. Antifungal activity of the essential oil of *Angelica major* against *Candida*, *Cryptococcus*, *Aspergillus* and dermatophyte species. *J. Nat. Med.* **2015**, *69*, 241–248. [CrossRef] [PubMed]
37. Guimarães, A.C.; Meireles, L.M.; Lemos, M.F.; Guimarães, M.C.C.; Endringer, D.C.; Fronza, M.; Scherer, R. Antibacterial Activity of Terpenes and Terpenoids Present in Essential Oils. *Molecules* **2019**, *24*, 2471. [CrossRef] [PubMed]
38. Goodarzi, S.; Hadjiakhoondi, A.; Yassa, N.; Khanavi, M.; Tofighi, Z. Essential oils chemical composition, antioxidant activities and total phenols of *Astrodaucus persicus*. *Iran. J. Basic Med. Sci.* **2016**, *19*, 159–165. [PubMed]

39. Lopes-Lutz, D.; Alviano, D.S.; Alviano, C.S.; Kolodziejczyk, P.P. Screening of chemical composition, antimicrobial and antioxidant activities of Artemisia essential oils. *Phytochemistry* **2008**, *69*, 1732–1738. [CrossRef]
40. Samba, N.; Aitfella-Lahlou, R.; Nelo, M.; Silva, L.; Coca, R.; Rocha, P.; López Rodilla, J.M. Chemical Composition and Antibacterial Activity of *Lippia multiflora* Moldenke Essential Oil from Different Regions of Angola. *Molecules* **2020**, *26*, 155. [CrossRef]
41. Mischko, W.; Hirte, M.; Fuchs, M.; Mehlmer, N.; Brück, T.B. Identification of sesquiterpene synthases from the Basidiomycota *Coniophora puteana* for the efficient and highly selective β-copaene and cubebol production in *E. coli*. *Microb. Cell Fact.* **2018**, *17*, 164. [CrossRef]
42. Özek, G.; Schepetkin, I.A.; Yermagambetova, M.; Özek, T.; Kirpotina, L.N.; Almerekova, S.S.; Abugalieva, S.I.; Khlebnikov, A.I.; Quinn, M.T. Innate Immunomodulatory Activity of Cedrol, a Component of Essential Oils Isolated from Juniperus Species. *Molecules* **2021**, *26*, 7644. [CrossRef]
43. Nakanishi, T.; Inatomi, Y.; Murata, H.; Shigeta, K.; Iida, N.; Inada, A.; Murata, J.; Farrera, M.A.; Iinuma, M.; Tanaka, T.; et al. A new and known cytotoxic aryltetralin-type lignans from stems of *Bursera graveolens*. *Chem. Pharm. Bull.* **2005**, *53*, 229–231. [CrossRef]
44. Hussain, A.I.; Anwar, F.; Shahid, M.; Ashraf, M.; Przybylski, R. Chemical Composition, and Antioxidant and Antimicrobial Activities of Essential Oil of Spearmint (*Mentha spicata* L.) From Pakistan. *J. Essent. Oil Res.* **2010**, *22*, 78–84. [CrossRef]
45. Mathela, C.S.; Padalia, R.C.; Chanotiya, C.S.; Tiwari, A. Carvone rich *Mentha longifolia* (Linn.): Chemical Variation and Commercial Potential. *J. Essent. Oil Bear. Plants* **2005**, *8*, 130–133. [CrossRef]
46. Micali, G.; Lanuzza, F. HPLC determination of β- and β-thujone, potentially toxic components of natural flavourings, in alcoholic beverages. *Flavour Fragr. J.* **1995**, *10*, 329–333. [CrossRef]
47. Lachenmeier, D.W.; Emmert, J.; Kuballa, T.; Sartor, G. Thujone—Cause of absinthism? *Forensic Sci. Int.* **2006**, *158*, 1–8. [CrossRef]
48. Höld, K.M.; Sirisoma, N.S.; Ikeda, T.; Narahashi, T.; Casida, J.E. Alpha-thujone (the active component of absinthe): Gamma-aminobutyric acid type A receptor modulation and metabolic detoxification. *Proc. Natl. Acad. Sci. USA* **2000**, *97*, 3826–3831. [CrossRef] [PubMed]
49. Pelkonen, O.; Abass, K.; Wiesner, J. Thujone and thujone-containing herbal medicinal and botanical products: Toxicological assessment. *Regul. Toxicol. Pharmacol. RTP* **2013**, *65*, 100–107. [CrossRef] [PubMed]
50. European Medicines Agency. *Public Statement on the Use of Herbal Medicinal Products Containing Thujone*; European Medicines Agency: Amsterdam, The Netherlands, 2012.
51. Zámboriné Németh, É.; Thi Nguyen, H. Thujone, a widely debated volatile compound: What do we know about it? *Phytochem. Rev.* **2020**, *19*, 405–423. [CrossRef]
52. Mohammadian Yasuj, S.F.; Najafian, S.; Hosseinifarahi, M. Comparison monoterpene and sesquiterpene, herbage yield of Satureja hortensis, Thymus vulgaris, and Salvia officinalis from the Fars province of Iran. *Nat. Prod. Res.* **2022**, *37*, 3711–3715. [CrossRef]
53. Lee, J.Y.; Park, H.; Lim, W.; Song, G. α,β-Thujone suppresses human placental choriocarcinoma cells via metabolic disruption. *Reproduction* **2020**, *159*, 745–756. [CrossRef]
54. Pudełek, M.; Catapano, J.; Kochanowski, P.; Mrowiec, K.; Janik-Olchawa, N.; Czyż, J.; Ryszawy, D. Therapeutic potential of monoterpene α-thujone, the main compound of *Thuja occidentalis* L. essential oil, against malignant glioblastoma multiforme cells in vitro. *Fitoterapia* **2019**, *134*, 172–181. [CrossRef]
55. Teethaisong, Y.; Autarkool, N.; Sirichaiwetchakoon, K.; Krubphachaya, P.; Kupittayanant, S.; Eumkeb, G. Synergistic activity and mechanism of action of *Stephania suberosa* Forman extract and ampicillin combination against ampicillin-resistant *Staphylococcus aureus*. *J. Biomed. Sci.* **2014**, *21*, 90. [CrossRef]
56. Sibanda, T.; Okoh, A.I. In vitro evaluation of the interactions between acetone extracts of Garcinia kola seeds and some antibiotics. *Afr. J. Biotechnol.* **2008**, *7*, 1672–1678.
57. Devrnja, N.; Anđelković, B.; Aranđelović, S.; Radulović, S.; Soković, M.; Krstić-Milošević, D.; Ristić, M.; Ćalić, D. Comparative studies on the antimicrobial and cytotoxic activities of *Tanacetum vulgare* L. essential oil and methanol extracts. *S. Afr. J. Bot.* **2017**, *111*, 212–221. [CrossRef]
58. Chiavari-Frederico, M.O.; Barbosa, L.N.; dos Santos, I.C.; da Silva, G.R.; de Castro, A.F.; Bortolucci, W.d.C.; Barboza, L.N.; Campos, C.F.d.A.A.; Gonçalves, J.E.; Menetrier, J.V.; et al. Antimicrobial activity of Asteraceae species against bacterial pathogens isolated from postmenopausal women. *PLoS ONE* **2020**, *15*, e0227023. [CrossRef]
59. Gadisa, E.; Tadesse, E. Antimicrobial activity of medicinal plants used for urinary tract infections in pastoralist community in Ethiopia. *BMC Complement. Med. Ther.* **2021**, *21*, 74. [CrossRef]
60. Adams, R.P. *Identification of Essential Oil Components by Gas Chromatography/Mass Spectrometry*, 5th ed.; Texensis Publishing: Gruver, TX, USA, 2017.
61. Adams, R.P. *Identification of Essential Oils Components by Gas Chromatography/Mass Spectroscopy*, 4th ed.; Allured Publishing Corporation: Carol Stream, IL, USA, 2007.
62. NIST Chemistry WebBook. Available online: https://webbook.nist.gov/chemistry (accessed on 28 June 2023).
63. Sparkman, O.D. MassFinder 3. *J. Am. Soc. Mass Spectrom.* **2007**, *18*, 1137–1144. [CrossRef]
64. *M100*; Performance Standards for Antimicrobial Susceptibility Testing. Clinical and Laboratory Standards Institute: Wayne, PA, USA, 2018.

65. *M7-A7*; Methods for Dilution Antimicrobial Susceptibility Tests for Bacteria That Grow Aerobically. Clinical and Laboratory Standards Institute: Wayne, PA, USA, 2006.
66. *M27-A3*; Reference Method for Broth Dilution Antifungal Susceptibility Testing of Yeasts, 3rd ed. Clinical and Laboratory Standards Institute: Wayne, PA, USA, 2008.

antibiotics

MDPI

Article

Stachys Species: Comparative Evaluation of Phenolic Profile and Antimicrobial and Antioxidant Potential

Daniela Benedec [1,†], Ilioara Oniga [1], Daniela Hanganu [1,*], Brîndușa Tiperciuc [2], Adriana Nistor [1], Ana-Maria Vlase [3], Laurian Vlase [4], Cristina Pușcaș [5], Mihaela Duma [6], Cristian Cezar Login [7], Mihaela Niculae [8,†] and Radu Silaghi-Dumitrescu [5]

[1] Department of Pharmacognosy, "Iuliu Hațieganu" University of Medicine and Pharmacy, 12 I. Creanga Street, 400010 Cluj-Napoca, Romania; dbenedec@umfcluj.ro (D.B.); ioniga@umfcluj.ro (I.O.); adriana.nistor@elearn.umfcluj.ro (A.N.)
[2] Department of Pharmaceutical Chemistry, "Iuliu Hațieganu" University of Medicine and Pharmacy, 41 V. Babeş Street, 400012 Cluj-Napoca, Romania; btiperciuc@umfcluj.ro
[3] Department of Pharmaceutical Botany, "Iuliu Hațieganu" University of Medicine and Pharmacy, 12 I. Creanga Street, 400010 Cluj-Napoca, Romania; gheldiu.ana@umfcluj.ro
[4] Department of Pharmaceutical Technology and Biopharmacy, "Iuliu Hațieganu" University of Medicine and Pharmacy, 41 V. Babeş Street, 400012 Cluj-Napoca, Romania; laurian.vlase@umfcluj.ro
[5] Department of Chemistry and Chemical Engineering, Babes-Bolyai University, 11 A. Janos Street, 400028 Cluj-Napoca, Romania; cbischin@chem.ubbcluj.ro (C.P.); radu.silaghi@ubbcluj.ro (R.S.-D.)
[6] State Animal Health and Safety Veterinary Laboratory, 1 Piata Marasti Street, 400609 Cluj-Napoca, Romania
[7] Department of Physiology, "Iuliu Hațieganu" University of Medicine and Pharmacy, 1 Clinicilor Street, 400006 Cluj-Napoca, Romania; cezar.login@umfcluj.ro
[8] Department of Clinical Sciences, University of Agricultural Sciences and Veterinary Medicine Cluj-Napoca, 400372 Cluj-Napoca, Romania; mihaela.niculae@usamvcluj.ro
* Correspondence: dhanganu@umfcluj.ro
† These authors contributed equally to this work.

Abstract: This study aimed to investigate the polyphenolic composition and antioxidant and antimicrobial potential of six Romanian Stachys species: *S. officinalis*, *S. germanica*, *S. byzantina*, *S. sylvatica*, *S. palustris*, and *S. recta*. The LC-MS/MS method was used to analyze the polyphenolic profile, while the phenolic contents were spectrophotometrically determined. The antioxidant activity was evaluated using the following methods: DPPH, FRAP, nitrite-induced autooxidation of hemoglobin, inhibition of cytochrome *c*-catalyzed lipid peroxidation, and electron paramagnetic resonance spectroscopy. The in vitro antimicrobial properties were assessed using agar-well diffusion, broth microdilution, and antibiofilm assays. Fifteen polyphenols were identified using LC-MS and chlorogenic acid was the major component in all the samples (1131.8–6761.4 µg/g). *S. germanica*, *S. palustris*, and *S. byzantina* extracts each displayed an intense antiradical action in relation to high contents of TPC (6.40 mg GAE/mL), flavonoids (3.90 mg RE/mL), and caffeic acid derivatives (0.89 mg CAE/mL). In vitro antimicrobial and antibiofilm properties were exhibited towards *Candida albicans*, Gram-positive and Gram-negative strains, with the most intense efficacy recorded for *S. germanica* and *S. byzantina* when tested against *S. aureus*. These results highlighted Stachys extracts as rich sources of bioactive compounds with promising antioxidant and antimicrobial efficacies and important perspectives for developing phytopharmaceuticals.

Keywords: *Stachys*; polyphenols; cytochrome *c*; antimicrobial; antioxidant

1. Introduction

As a member of the Lamiaceae family, the *Stachys* L. genus (wound plants) has garnered scientific interest regarding its chemical composition and therapeutic properties. In fact, numerous species of this genus have been used empirically in different regions of the world for their medicinal and economic potential since ancient times [1,2].

A recently published paper reviewed the existing information on various traditional uses of 25 species and 6 subspecies of *Stachys* genus, conditioned mostly as herbal tea, infusion, and decoction, but also as extracts (oily and alcoholic) and edible food (tubers) [2]. This study also described the phytochemistry and pharmacological profile of distinct *Stachys* sp. originating from the Mediterranean region, Asia, America, and southern Africa.

Overall, a complex chemical composition including secondary metabolites such as flavonoids (baicalin, apigenin, isoscutellarein 7-*O*-β-D-glucopyranoside), phenolcarboxylic acids (caffeic, rosmarinic, chlorogenic acids), tannins, phenylethanoid glucosides (acteoside, martinosid), lignans, iridoids, diterpenes (kauran, clerodane), and triterpenes; essential oils characterize *Stachys* genus [1,2].

Moreover, several *Stachys* species have been studied in vitro and in vivo to scientifically justify their traditional use. The pharmacological assessment demonstrated important therapeutic properties, namely the following: antioxidant (*S. recta* subsp. *recta*, *S. palustris, S. byzantina, S. sylvatica*), anti-inflammatory (*S. recta, S. germanica, S. officinalis, S. alpina*), analgesic, anxiolytic, antidepressant, antiproliferative (*S. lavandulifolia*), antibacterial (*S. byzantina, S. officinalis, S. sylvatica*), renoprotective, and hepatoprotective (*S. pilifera*) [1,2].

Although *Stachys* sp. are spreading in the Romanian flora [3,4], only a few references are available [5–8]. In this regard, common and Latin names, botanical descriptions, and geographical distribution are presented for 14 species of *Stachys*, all perennial herbaceous plants, in the *Flora of Romania* [3,4]. Among these, *Stachys officinalis* (L.) Trevis. (sin. *Betonica officinalis* L.) is the only *Stachys* species documented by Romanian traditional medicine. Phytopreparations obtained from its leaves and aerial parts are mentioned for tonic, antipyretic, analgesic, and cicatrizing efficacy, and have been traditionally recommended for various disorders such as rhinitis, headache, hemoptysis, chest pain, wounds, and varicose ulcers [5,6]. Nowadays, most of the empirical therapeutic applications involve *S. officinalis* tea in atonic dyspepsia and liver disorders based on antispastic, astringent, carminative, cholagogue, digestive stimulant, emmenagogue, anthelmintic, and diuretic properties. The tea is also listed for anxiolytic and sedative effects, being able to reduce anxiety and irritability [6]. Regarding other *Stachys* species, *S. byzantine* is a very adaptable and decorative plant with brightly colored flowers and is commonly cultivated for ornamental purposes [3].

Previous studies on Romanian *Stachys* extracts addressed the following species: *S. officinalis* [8], *S. byzantina*, and *S. sylvatica* [7,8].

The current study objective was to evaluate the polyphenolic composition, antioxidant, and in vitro antimicrobial potential of *Stachys* species frequently found in the Romania flora: *S. officinalis, S. germanica, S. byzantina, S. sylvatica, S. palustris*, and *S. recta*. These data are required to complete these species' pharmacognostic profiles aiming to ensure a well-deserved place in phytotherapy. Thus, additional chemical and pharmacotherapeutic data are needed to reveal the most promising *Stachys* species for medicinal use.

2. Results and Discussions

2.1. Chromatographic Analysis

To characterize plant extracts rich in polyphenols, the most widely used technique for the separation and individual quantification of phenolic compounds is liquid chromatography coupled with tandem mass spectrometry (LC-MS/MS) [9,10]. The amounts of compounds detected in the six *Stachys* sp.-derived extracts were expressed in µg/g dry weight (dw) of vegetal product (Table 1).

Fifteen polyphenolic compounds, including ten phenolic acids (gallic, rosmarinic, protocatehuic, gentisic, caftaric, chlorogenic, vanillic, syringic, *p*-coumaric, ferulic acids) and five flavonoids (isoquercitrin, rutin, quercitrin, luteolin, apigenin), were detected by LC-MS in all *Stachys* extracts (Table 1).

Furthermore, all extracts presented high amounts of chlorogenic acid (1131.8–6761.4 µg/g dw). Chlorogenic acid with multiple therapeutic potentials (neuroprotective; cardio-, hepato-, gastro-, renoprotective; anticancer) is a phenolic acid widely distributed in many species of the *Stachys* genus [2,11]. The extracts richest in chlorogenic acid were from *S. germanica* (4205.2 µg/g dw), *S. sylvatica* (5552.7 µg/g dw), and *S. recta* (6761.4 µg/g dw). High concentrations of chlorogenic acid were measured in Turkish *S. germanica* [12], but this active principle was not found in *S. recta* [13]. The other two indigenous *Stachys*: *S. officinalis* (1131.8 µg/g dw) and *S. byzantina* (2012.1 µg/g dw) showed lower concentrations of chlorogenic acid compared to the other species, but higher than some published values [14]. The results obtained for the *S. officinalis* extract are similar to those previously reported by other authors [15].

Table 1. Phenolic compounds identified by LC-MS/MS in *Stachys* sp. extracts (µg/g dw).

Phenolic Compounds	*m/z* Value (Precursor)	*m/z* Value (Daughter Ions; Collision Energy)	tR ± SD (min)	*S. officinalis*	*S. germanica*	*S. byzantina*	*S. sylvatica*	*S. palustris*	*S. recta*
Gallic acid	169	169 (0.5 V)	1.50 ± 0.01	-	-	-	-	141.5 ± 8.4	-
Rosmarinic acid	359	160.7; 178.6; 196.7 (0.9 V)	2.20 ± 0.01	43.4 ± 0.5	7.8 ± 0.01	3.0 ± 0.02	1.9 ± 0.02	2.4 ± 0.01	2.6 ± 0.05
Protocatechuic acid	153	153 (0.5 V)	2.80 ± 0.01	94.6 ± 0.5	83.5 ± 0.4	28.6 ± 0.3	100.7 ± 9.2	94.2 ± 1.7	157.8 ± 2.1
Gentisic acid	153	108.7 (0.9 V)	3.52 ± 0.04	<0.2	<0.2	<0.2	<0.2	<0.2	<0.2
Caftaric acid	311	148.6; 178.6 (0.9 V)	3.54 ± 0.05	4.7 ± 0.2	-	-	-	-	-
Chlorogenic acid	353	178.7; 190.7 (0.9 V)	5.62 ± 0.05	1131.8 ± 15.8	4205.2 ± 44.7	2012.1 ± 37.8	5552.7 ± 47.2	3595.2 ± 24.7	6761.4 ± 58.5
Vanillic acid	167	167 (0.5 V)	6.70 ± 0.01	83.5 ± 0.7	21.1 ± 0.1	16.4 ± 0.3	16.6 ± 0.2	6.2 ± 0.08	20.3 ± 0.5
Syringic acid	197	197 (0.5 V)	8.40 ± 0.01	82.7 ± 0.2	-	7.0 ± 0.06	8.6 ± 0.1	4.4 ± 0.3	-
p-Coumaric acid	163	118.7 (0.9 V)	9.48 ± 0.08	27.8 ± 0.1	6.2 ± 0.08	4.4 ± 0.08	6.2 ± 0.3	14.0 ± 0.4	32.0 ± 0.9
Ferulic acid	193	133.7; 148.7; 177.6 (0.9 V)	12.80 ± 0.10	11.1 ± 0.4	5.0 ± 0.02	3.5 ± 0.04	3.0 ± 0.06	6.0 ± 0.2	<0.2
Isoquercitrin	463	254.9; 270.9; 300.7; 342.8 (1.2 V)	19.60 ± 0.1	18.9 ± 0.1	233.1 ± 6.8	-	86.2 ± 3.7	-	72.8 ± 2.1
Rutin	609	254.9; 270.9; 300.7; 342.8 (1.2 V)	20.20 ± 0.15	<0.2	-	-	-	-	-
Quercitrin	447	178.8; 300.7 (1.2 V)	23.64 ± 0.13	-	-	-	-	<0.2	-
Luteolin	285	150.6; 174.6; 198.6; 240.7 (1.5 V)	29.10 ± 0.19	15.7 ± 0.2	26.8 ± 0.1	12.2 ± 0.1	<0.2	3.9 ± 0.2	<0.2
Apigenin	269	148.6; 150.6; 224.7; 226.7 (1.5 V)	33.10 ± 0.15	84.2 ± 1.7	21.4 ± 0.2	27.3 ± 0.6	13.6 ± 0.2	<0.2	<0.2

"-" not found, below limit of detection. Values are the mean ± SD (n = 3).

S. officinalis presented higher amounts of vanilic acid (83.5 µg/g dw), syringic acid (82.7 µg/g dw), ferulic acid (11.1 µg/g dw), and apigenin (84.2 µg/g dw) than the other *Stachys* species. Bączek et al. determined ferulic acid and apigenin in Polish *S. officinalis* in higher concentrations [16] and Paun et al. have published lower values of apigenin than ours [17]. Regarding protocatechuic and *p*-coumaric acids, the *S. recta* extract was found to be the richest in these compounds, at 157.8 µg/g dw and 32.0 µg/g dw, respectively.

Caftaric acid was determined only in *S. officinalis* (4.7 µg/g dw) and gallic acid only in *S. palustris* (141.5 µg/g dw).

The *S. officinalis* extract (82.7 µg/g dw) was the richest in syringic acid, compared to the *S. sylvatica* (8.6 µg/g dw), *S. byzantina* (7.0 µg/g dw), and *S. palustris* (4.4 µg/g dw) extracts. Four species of *Stachys* (*S. officinalis*, *S. recta*, *S. sylvatica*, *S. germanica*) contained isoquercitrin; the richest species was *S. germanica* (233.1 µg/g dw). Isoquercitrin, also identified by other authors in *S. recta* [13], develops numerous chemoprotective effects in vitro and in vivo against oxidative stress, diabetes, allergies, cancer, etc. [17].

Rutin and quercitrin were found in very small quantities, below the limit of detection in the extracts of *S. officinalis* (rutin,) and *S. palustris* (quercitrin).

The characterization of polyphenolic profiles of the six *Stachys* species showed differences in the presence of key compounds, but also in what concerns the concentrations of individual phenols.

Numerous medicinal species in the Lamiaceae family contain rosmarinic acid (RA), a natural polyphenolic molecule with antioxidant, antidiabetic, antimicrobial, hepatoprotective, cardioprotective, nephroprotective, anti-aging, anti-inflammatory, antiviral, and anticancer therapeutic properties [18]. Data from the literature confirm the presence of RA in other species of *Stachys*: *S. thirkei* [19], *S. tmolea* [20], *S. cretica* [21], *S. lavandulifolia*, *S. byzantina* [22], and *S. officinalis* [15,23].

In this case, we chose to use the LC-MS/MS method, published by us, to determine the RA content of the six *Stachys* species [24].

The ESI source mass spectrometer, in the negative mode, was set to isolate and fragment the deprotonated RA molecule with $m/z = 359$. The quantification of RA was performed with a tR of 2.2 min. In the range of 40–640 ng/mL, a linear calibration curve was performed ($R^2 = 0.999$). The RA content values (µg/g dw) are presented in Table 1; this amount varied between 1.9–43.4 µg/g dw of vegetal product.

The *S. officinalis* extract showed a higher RA content (43.4 µg/g dw) compared to the other *Stachys* species extracts studied by us, but lower than the results published by other authors [15,16]. From the data in the literature accessed by us until now, we can say that RA was found for the first time in the extracts of *S. germanica* (7.8 µg/g dw), *S. recta* (2.6 µg/g dw), *S. palustris* (2.4 µg/g dw), and *S. sylvatica* (1.9 µg/g dw). Of the six spontaneous native species of *Stachys*, *S. officinalis* can be considered as an important source of rosmarinic acid.

The ethanolic extracts of *Stachys* sp. were examined to determine the polyphenolic TPC), flavonoid, and caffeic acid derivatives contents. The results obtained in this study were expressed as gallic acid (GA), rutin (R), and caffeic acid (CA) equivalents, respectively (Table 2).

Table 2. Polyphenolic contents of *Stachys* sp. extracts.

***Stachys* sp. Extracts**	**TPC (mg GAE/mL)**	**Flavonoids (mg RE/mL)**	**Caffeic Acid Derivatives (mg CAE/mL)**
S. officinalis (SO)	2.51 ± 0.09^{a}	1.18 ± 0.01^{d}	0.20 ± 0.01^{g}
S. germanica (SG)	5.98 ± 0.21^{a}	3.30 ± 0.11^{f}	0.88 ± 0.01^{i}
S. byzantina (SB)	6.40 ± 0.11	3.90 ± 0.21	0.89 ± 0.05
S. sylvatica (SS)	4.00 ± 0.13^{a}	$1.22 \pm 0.06^{d,f}$	0.20 ± 0.03^{h}
S. palustris (SP)	$5.35 \pm 0.29^{b,c}$	3.14 ± 0.17^{f}	$0.72 \pm 0.06^{g,i}$
S. recta (SR)	$3.78 \pm 0.17^{a,c}$	1.13 ± 0.09^{e}	$0.23 \pm 0.08^{h,i}$

Each value is the mean ± SD of three independent measurements; GAE, RE, CAE: gallic acid, rutin, caffeic acid equivalents. Lowercase letters in the same row indicate significant differences ($p < 0.05$). ^{a} $p < 0.001$ (SB vs. SO, SG, SS, SR); ^{b} $p < 0.05$ (SB vs. SP); ^{c} $p > 0.05$ (SG vs. SP, SS vs. SR); ^{d} $p < 0.001$ (SB vs. SO, SS); ^{e} $p < 0.05$ (SB vs. SR; SG vs. SR); ^{f} $p > 0.05$ (SO vs. SS, SO vs. SP, SB vs. SP, SG); ^{g} $p < 0.001$ (SB vs. SO, SP); ^{h} $p < 0.05$ (SG vs. SS, SR; SB vs. SS, SR; SS vs. SR); ^{i} $p > 0.05$ (SO vs. SP, SR, SB vs. SG, SP vs. SR).

Medicinal plants produce polyphenols with various chemical structures, such as flavonoids, phenolic acids, with important antioxidant, cytotoxic, anti-inflammatory, antihypertensive, and antidiabetic properties [25]. The TPC contents of these six *Stachys* sp. extracts, determined using the Folin−Ciocâlteu reagent [26], are shown in Table 2. According to this analysis, *S. byzantina* extract had the highest concentration of TPC (6.40 mg GAE/mL) and the *S. palustris* and *S. germanica* extracts had similar values (5.35 mg GAE/mL and 5.98 mg GAE/mL, respectively). The other three species showed lower values, between 2.51 mg/mL and 4.00 mg GAE/mL, the *S. officinalis* extract being the lowest in TPC (2.51 mg GAE/mL). In terms of TPC, the extract of *S. byzantina* was the richest in these active compounds. The statistical analysis of these data (Table 2) showed highly significant differences between *S. byzantina* (SB) and other *Stachys* sp.: SO, SG, SS, and SR ($p < 0.001$) and significant differences between *S. byzantina* (SB) and *S. palustris* ($p = 0.011$). Our results were similar to those published by other authors for *S. byzantina* and *S. germanica* species, [27,28] while other authors described lower values than ours for *S. officinalis* [15].

The total flavonoid contents were determined using the $AlCl_3$ method [29]. The highest content of flavonoids, with values between 3.14 and 3.90 mg RE/mL ($p > 0.05$), was found in ethanolic extracts of *S. palustris*, *S. germanica*, and *S. byzantina*. The other extracts of *S. officinalis*, *S. sylvatica*, and *S. recta* extracts had lower amounts of flavonoids, around 1 mg/mL (1.13, 1.18, and 1.22 mg RE/mL, respectively, in relation with *S. byzantina* ($0.001 < p < 0.05$). Comparing different studies from the literature, some authors have reported lower levels of flavonoids in *S. officinalis* [15], *S. germanica*, *S. sylvatica*, and *S. recta* [30]. Sytar et al. found higher concentrations of flavonoids in *S. byzantina* [14] compared to our results, and Nikolova recorded similar values for *S. officinalis* [30].

Caffeic acid derivatives, which are widespread in many plant species, have been extensively studied; this has revealed a wide range of potential therapeutic applications. Regarding the contents of caffeic acid derivatives for the *Stachys* sp. extracts, values ranged between 0.20–0.89 mg CAE/mL (Table 2). The highest values were obtained for the ethanolic extracts of *S. palustris* (0.72 mg CAE/mL), *S. germanica* (0.88 CAE mg/mL), and *S. byzantina* (0.89 CAE mg/mL), while the lowest were measured in the extracts of *S. officinalis* (0.20 mg CAE/mL), *S. sylvatica* (0.20 mg CAE/mL), and *S. recta* (0.23 mg CAE/mL), compared to *S. byzantina* ($0.001 < p < 0.05$). The literature provides data only for *S. germanica* caffeic acid derivatives' content; our results varied slightly compared to those published by Mitic et al. [28].

Qualitative and quantitative evaluation of the phenolic profile indicated S. *germanica*, *S. byzantina*, and *S. palustris* as the species with the richest content in these active compounds including flavonoids and caffeic acid derivatives.

2.2. Antioxidant Activity of *Stachys* sp. Extracts

Bioactive compounds of the polyphenol type are important natural antioxidants due to their redox characteristics, as a result of hydroxyl groups that facilitate the elimination of free radicals and thus offer many benefits to human health [25]. In this regard, extracts of *Stachys* sp. with polyphenols, have been evaluated by several antioxidant methods: the DPPH radical scavenging method, the FRAP test (the ferric-reducing ability of plasma), nitrite-induced autooxidation of hemoglobin (NHA), inhibition of cytochrome *c*-catalyzed lipid peroxidation, and EPR spectroscopy assays (Table 3).

Table 3. Antioxidant activity of *Stachys* sp. extracts.

***Stachys* sp. Extracts**	**DPPH (IC_{50} µg/mL)**	**FRAP (µM TE/mL)**	**NHA mg CATE/g**
S. officinalis	139.16 ± 3.80 [a]	280.17 ± 1.83 [b]	23.44 ± 3.24
S. germanica	54.18 ± 1.16 [a]	688.21 ± 5.91	66.59 ± 5.37
S. byzantina	53.61 ± 1.19 [a]	354.88 ± 3.11 [b]	27.06 ± 3.00
S. sylvatica	76.04 ± 0.35 [a]	218.01 ± 0.98 [b]	20.01 ± 6.78
S. palustris	54.82 ± 1.33 [a]	502.43 ± 5.56 [b]	59.38 ± 2.54
S. recta	84.94 ± 1.45 [a]	305.15 ± 2.84 [b]	37.49 ± 1.96
Trolox	11.19 ± 0.09	-	-

Each value is the mean ± SD of three independent measurements; IC_{50}: half-maximal inhibitory concentration; TE: Trolox equivalents; NHA: nitrite-induced hemoglobin autooxidation; CATE: Catechin equivalents. Lowercase letters in the same row indicate statistical differences: [a] $p < 0.001$ (Trolox vs. SO, SG, SB, SS, SP, SR); [b] $p < 0.001$ (SG vs. SO, SB, SS, SP, SR).

The results of DPPH scavenging activity revealed that five *Stachys* extracts presented high antioxidant activity: *S. byzantina* (IC_{50} = 53.61 µg/mL), *S. germanica* (IC_{50} = 54.18 µg/mL) and *S. palustris* (IC_{50} = 54.82 µg/mL) extracts, followed by extracts of *S. sylvatica* (IC_{50} = 76.04 µg/mL) and *S. recta* (IC_{50} = 84.94 µg/mL), but lower compared to Trolox ([a] $p < 0.001$). In contrast, the *S. officinalis* extract showed a higher value of IC_{50} (139.16 µg/mL), which indicates a lower activity. Other authors have obtained IC_{50} values higher than ours (*S. officinalis*, *S. germanica*, *S. sylvatica*, *S. byzantina*) [13,30]. Similar results were obtained for *S. officinalis* from Romania [15], as well as for the Bulgarian *S. recta* species [30].

The FRAP values for the investigated extracts were reported in Table 3, so that *S. germanica* and *S. palustris* extracts showed antioxidant activity (688.21 and 502.43 μM TE/mL), in relation to high polyphenol contents (5.77 and 5.56 mg GAE/mL), but also with the values obtained by the DPPH method (53.83 and 55.66 μg/mL). For the other four *Stachys* sp. extracts, lower values were obtained (between 218.17and 354.88 μM TE/mL) than *S. germanica* (^{b} $p < 0.001$). The NHA results on all *Stachys* extracts offer values in the same order and proportion as the FRAP results (e.g., highest results for *S. germanica* and lowest results— for *S. sylvatica*, by about three times). This excellent agreement between FRAP and NHA was not mirrored by the DPPH results. Thus, in the DPPH measurements *S. sylvatica* was far from being the weakest antioxidant, while *S. germanica* was narrowly exceeded as the strongest oxidant by *S. byzantina*—even though the two had widely different activities in the NHA assay. Interestingly, the NHA data does not correlate with either the total phenolic of flavonoid contents or with the content of any particular component (including the major ones—rosmarinic acid, chlorogenic acid, and caffeic derivatives). The NHA assay tests a nitrosative stress process, while FRAP was based on oxidative stress agents. The excellent agreement between NHA and FRAP, together with the fact that NHA is based on a physiological reaction employing a protein from blood, may be taken as argument that these two assays have a particularly important biomedical/physiological relevance. Regarding the FRAP values published by other authors, important results were obtained for *S. germanica subsp. heldreichii* [12]; the species *S. byzantina* and *S. sylvatica* showed a lower antioxidant activity [27,31–33].

An antioxidant assay based on the inhibition of cytochrome-catalyzed lipid autooxidation was also attempted. However, in this case the *Stachys* extracts exhibited effects that were too narrowly similar to each other—although *S. germanica* was still found at the most-active end of the range, while *S. sylvatica* was at the least-active end.

Exposure of phenolic compounds to basic pH under aerobic conditions allows for the generation of phenol-based free radicals via autooxidation processes. Such radicals can be detected by EPR spectroscopy and can be used as fingerprints for assessing the dominant components in polyphenolic-containing natural extracts. Figure 1 shows that a clear complex signal was detected for all the *Stachys* extracts, which is very similar to that of pure chlorogenic acid samples. This observation was in line with the fact chlorogenic acid was by far the most abundant polyphenolic compound in these samples, that according to the chromatographic data in Table 1; while up to a sixfold difference in chlorogenic acid concentrations is seen in Table 1, Figure 1 offers a spectra of intensities that were essentially equal among all samples. A single exception exists—namely, the *S. palustris* sample, for which the EPR spectrum was no longer identical to that of chlorogenic acid. This implies that *S. palustris* contains a unique antioxidant species, not shared with the other *Stachys* extracts. Tables 1 and 2 reveal only one such antioxidant—namely, gallic acid, which is present only in *S. palustris*. Indeed, the shape of the *S. palustris* EPR spectrum was consistent with that of a gallate radical imposed over chlorogenic acid [34].

In the present study, it was observed that the extracts of *S. germanica*, *S. palustris*, and *S. byzantina* had the highest antiradical action, in a general relation to a high content of TPC, flavonoids, and caffeic acid derivatives. The *S. recta* and *S. sylvatica* extracts with a medium content of polyphenols also presented a high antioxidant capacity. Thus, it can be concluded from the evaluation of the phenolic content and the antioxidant activity that these species of *Stachys* can be recommended as valuable natural antioxidants for various nutritional functions and to preserve health.

2.3. *Antimicrobial Activity of* Stachys *sp. Extracts*

The use of natural herbal preparations as antimicrobial agents is a therapeutic alternative, especially in the context of the increasing bacterial resistance to antibiotics. In addition, it is known from the literature that *Stachys* species have many pharmacological activities (anti-inflammatory, antianxiety, antinephritic, antioxidant, cytotoxic) [12,27,35,36] and antimicrobial properties have been demonstrated for some species, such as *S. byzantina*, *S. guyoniana*, *S. officinalis*, *S. sylvatica*, *S. cretica*, *S. scardica*, *S. recta*, and *S. germanica*. [3,23,37–41].

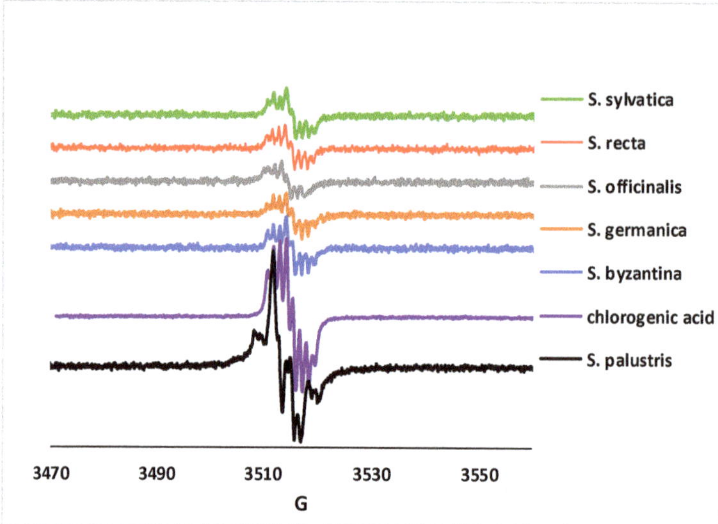

Figure 1. EPR spectra of the extracts treated with NaOH. Conditions: extracts—0.5%, NaOH—5 mM, and Et-OH—90%; G—magnetic field strength.

2.3.1. Antibacterial Activity Using the Agar-Well Diffusion Method

Using the agar-well diffusion method, we evaluated the antimicrobial susceptibility of significant bacterial isolates of the six indigenous *Stachys* species (Table 4) [42]. Our extracts showed a strong antibacterial activity, especially against *S. aureus* and *L. monocytogenes*, with areas of inhibition ranging from 14 and 20 mm, compared to gentamicin (IZD = 18 mm), used as a reference antibiotic ($0.001 < p < 0.05$). The activity on *S. aureus* was almost the same as gentamicin for *S. officinalis*, *S. sylvatica*, and *S. recta* ($p < 0.05$) and was superior for *S. germanica* and *S. byzantina* with IZD = 20 mm ($p < 0.001$). The same IZD (18 mm) was measured for the *S. palustris* extract as for the antibiotic standard ($p = 1$). All extracts showed lower activity on *L. monocytogenes* ($p < 0.001$) compared to gentamicin used as reference antibiotic.

Table 4. In vitro antibacterial activity of *Stachys* sp. ethanolic extracts by agar-well diffusion method.

	Inhibition Zone Diameter (IZD, mm)				
***Stachys* sp. Extracts**	***Staphylococcus aureus***	***Listeria monocytogenes***	***Escherichia coli***	***Salmonella enteritidis***	***Candida albicans***
S. officinalis	16 ± 0.50 [b]	14 ± 1.00 [a]	10 ± 1.00 [a]	10 ± 0.25 [a]	12 ± 0.50 [d]
S. germanica	20 ± 0.25 [a]	18 ± 0.50 [a]	8 ± 0.25 [a]	10 ± 0.50 [a]	10 ± 0.50 [d]
S. byzantina	20 ± 0.25 [a]	18 ± 0.00 [a]	8 ± 0.50 [a]	8 ± 0.50 [a]	12 ± 1.00 [d]
S. sylvatica	16 ± 0.75 [b]	16 ± 0.25 [a]	8 ± 1.00 [a]	8 ± 1.00 [a]	10 ± 0.50 [d]
S. palustris	18 ± 0.50 [c]	16 ± 1.00 [a]	8 ± 0.00 [a]	8 ± 0.25 [a]	12 ± 0.50 [d]
S. recta	16 ± 0.00 [b]	16 ± 1.00 [a]	10 ± 0.25 [a]	12 ± 0.50 [b]	12 ± 0.00 [d]
Gentamicin	18 ± 0.25	22 ± 0.50	18 ± 0.25	19 ± 1.00	-
Fluconazole	-	-	-	-	21 ± 0.00

Values are means of triplicate determination (n = 3) ± standard deviations. Lowercase letters in the same row indicate significant differences ($p < 0.05$). [a] $p < 0.001$ (extracts vs. gentamicin); [b] $p < 0.05$ (*S. sylvatica*, *S. recta* vs. gentamicin); [c] $p > 0.05$ (*S. palustris* vs. gentamicin); [d] $p < 0.001$ (extracts vs. fluconazole); gentamicin (10 μg/disk) and fluconazole (25 μg/disk) were used as positive controls.

Regarding the antibacterial activity against Gram-negative strains, *Stachys* extracts showed limited activity against *E. coli* and *S. enteritidis*, statistically lower compared to gentamicin ($p < 0.001$). These results were consistent with those published by other authors, according to which Gram-negative bacteria display less sensitivity to the effect of *Stachys* extracts compared to Gram-positive ones [3,32,38,43]. Also, similarly to previous reports, our *Stachys* extracts showed a relatively low anti-*C. albicans* activity compared to Fluconazole ($p < 0.001$), which was used as the reference antifungal [38,44].

2.3.2. Antibacterial Activity Using the Broth Microdilution Method

Moreover, the results obtained using the broth microdilution method (Table 5) showed *Stachys* extracts higher inhibitory efficacy towards Gram-positive bacteria, *S. aureus*, and *L. monocytogenes*. The lowest values of MIC were recorded for *S. germanica* and *S. byzantina*. These two extracts were found also with the lowest MBC values established against *S. aureus*, suggesting their superior bactericidal potential towards this bacterial species. All *Stachys* extracts presented in vitro inhibitory and bactericidal potential against *E. coli* and *S. enteritidis*, but only at the highest tested concentrations (Table 5). *C. albicans* growth was inhibited by all tested extracts and a two- and threefold higher fungicidal effect was noticed for MBC values than for MIC values, respectively.

Table 5. In vitro antibacterial activity of *Stachys* sp. ethanolic extracts using the broth microdilution method.

***Stachys* sp. Extracts**	***Staphylococcus aureus***		***Listeria monocytogenes***		***Escherichia coli***		***Salmonella enteriditis***		***Candida albicans***	
	MIC	**MBC**	**MIC**	**MBC**	**MIC**	**MBC**	**MIC**	**MBC**	**MIC**	**MFC**
S. officinalis	0.705	1.411	1.411	1.411	1.411	1.411	1.411	1.411	0.352	1.411
S. germanica	0.423	0.423	0.847	1.695	3.39	3.39	3.39	3.39	1.695	3.39
S. byzantina	0.468	0.468	1.875	3.75	3.75	3.75	3.75	3.75	0.937	3.75
S. sylvatica	1.20	2.40	1.20	2.40	2.40	2.40	2.40	2.40	1.20	2.40
S. palustris	0.817	1.635	1.635	3.27	3.27	3.27	3.27	3.27	0.817	3.27
S. recta	1.12	2.24	1.12	2.24	2.24	2.24	2.24	2.24	0.56	2.24
Gentamicin MIC (mg/L)	3		4		3		3		-	
Fluconazole MIC (mg/L)	-		-		-		-		8	

"-" = not active; MIC: minimum inhibitory concentration (μmol GAE/mL); MBC: minimum bactericidal concentration (μmol GAE/mL); MFC: minimum fungicidal concentration (μmol GAE/mL).

2.3.3. Antibiofilm Activity

The inhibitory activity of *Stachys* sp. extracts against biofilm formation is presented in Table 6.

Table 6. Antibiofilm activity of *Stachys* sp. ethanolic extracts.

***Stachys* sp. Extracts**	**% Inhibition**									
	Staphylococcus aureus		***Listeria monocytogenes***		***Escherichia coli***		***Salmonella enteriditis***		***Candida albicans***	
	T0	**T24**	**T0**	**T24**	**T0**	**T24**	**T0**	**T24**	**T0**	**T24**
S. officinalis	+	-	+	-	+	-	-	+	++	+
S. germanica	++	++	++	+	+	-	-	+	+	+
S. byzantina	++	++	+	+	+	-	-	++	++	+
S. sylvatica	++	+	+	+	++	+	-	-	++	-
S. palustris	++	+	++	+	+	-	-	+	++	-
S. recta	+	+	+	-	+	-	-	-	++	-
Gentamicin	+	++	+	++	-	++	-	++	-	-
Fluconazole	-	-	-	-	-	-	-	-	++	++

The extracts antibiofilm activity was described based on the inhibition (%) calculated values, as good (above 50%, ++), poor (0–50%, +), and no inhibition, or enhancement of biofilm development and growth (<0, -) [45].

Both the biofilm attachment (T0) and destruction of 24 h pre-formed biofilm (T24) were inhibited by certain extracts, the most intense effect (++) was still noticed against the planktonic cells. The highest efficacy was recorded for *S. germanica*, *S. byzantina*, *S. sylvatica*, and *S. palustris*-derived extracts.

According to the literature, *S. byzantina*, *S. officinale*, and *S. sylvatica* showed strong antibacterial activity, *S. aureus* being very susceptible to these extracts [3,32,38]. The antibacterial activity of the *Stachys* sp. extracts could be due to the presence of chlorogenic acid, which is found in large quantities in our extracts and according to studies can increase the permeability of the outer membrane and plasma and thus lead to the loss of the barrier function. It also depletes intracellular potential and releases cytoplasmic macromolecules, which can lead to bacterial cell death [46,47].

The results of this study pointed out that *Stachys* extracts were able to display an important in vitro antimicrobial potential against Gram-positive strains, with the extracts of *S. germanica*, *S. byzantina*, and *S. palustris* achieving very good antistaphylococcal activity. This aspect is relevant as *S. aureus* is regarded worldwide as one of the most important human bacteria, with both colonizing and opportunistic pathogen valences and elevated levels of multidrug resistance [48]. In this regard, the results indicated *S. germanica* and *S. byzantina* extracts for their superior antibiofilm properties against *S. aureus*.

3. Materials and Methods

3.1. Plant Material

The aerial parts from six *Stachys* species: *S. officinalis*—SO, *S. germanica*—SG, *S. byzantina*—SB, *S. sylvatica*—SS, *S. palustris*—SP, and *S. recta*—SR (Voucher numbers: 106-111) were collected from the spontaneous flora of Cluj County, Romania (Podeni village: 46°41′4″ N 23°1′45″ E), during the flowering period. The plant material was identified by Ph.D. A. Mocanu ("Iuliu Haţieganu" University of Medicine and Pharmacy Cluj-Napoca).

3.2. Chemicals

All high-quality purity chemicals (substances and reagents) used in this study were acquired from the following companies: Sigma, St. Louis, MO, USA (chlorogenic, cafeic, *p*-coumaric acids, isoquercitrin, quercitrin, hyperoside, rutin, apigenin, myricetin, quercetin, kaempferol, fisetin); Roth, Karlsruhe, Germany (sinapic, ferulic, gallic, gentisic, rosmarinic acids, patuletin, luteolin); Dalton, Toronto, ON, Canada (caftaric, cichoric acids); Alfa-Aesar, Karlsruhe, Germany (sodium hydroxide, sodium carbonate, and iron (III) chloride); Sigma-Aldrich, Steinheim, Germany (soy lecithin, bovine hemoglobin, protocatechuic, vanillic and syringic acids, (−)-epicatechin, (+)-catechin), 6-hydroxy-2,5,7,8-tetramethylchroman-2-carboxylic acid (Trolox), 2,4,6-Tris (2-pyridyl)-s-triazine (TPTZ), sodium acetate buffer solution); Merck, Darmstadt, Germany (Arnow's reagent, Folin−Ciocâlteu reagent, methanol, ethanol, aluminum chloride, sodium acetate, hydrochloric acid, 2,2-diphenyl-1-picrylhydrazyl; the methanol, acetonitrile, ammonium acetate, and acetic acid were all of the HPLC grade).

The Gram-positive bacteria: *Staphylococcus aureus* (ATCC 6538P) and *Listeria monocytogenes* (ATCC 13932); Gram-negative bacteria: *Escherichia coli* (ATCC 25922) and *Salmonella typhimurium* (ATCC14028); and one fungal strain, *Candida albicans* (ATCC 10231), were distributed by MicroBioLogics®, St. Cloud, MN, USA.

The spectrophotometric data were acquired using a Jasco V-530 UV–Vis spectrophotometer (Jasco International Co., Ltd., Tokyo, Japan).

3.3. Preparation of *Stachys* sp. Extracts

Ten grams of each powdered plant material was extracted with 100 mL of 70% ethanol using ultrasound (Polsonic Palczyski Sp. J., Sonic 3, Warsaw, Poland) at 60 °C, for 30 min. The ethanolic extracts were filtered through paper filters into 100 mL flasks and then centrifuged (at 4500 rpm, 10 min) and the supernatant solutions were collected [29,49].

3.4. LC-MS/MS Analysis of Polyphenols

The study of flavonoids, as well as of the phenolic acids present in the six extracts of *Stachys* species was performed using the LC-MS/MS analysis on an Agilent 1100 HPLC Series system (Agilent, Santa Clara, CA, USA) equipped with: degasser (G1322A), binary gradient pump (G13311A), autosampler (G1313A), column thermostat, and UV detector (G1316A) that was coupled with an Agilent Ion Trap 1100 SL mass spectrometer (LC/MSD Ion Trap VL), according to the method previously published [24,50]. The standards used were from the class of phenolic acids (caftaric, gentisic, caffeic, chlorogenic, p-coumaric, ferulic, synapic acids), but also from the class of flavonoids (rutin, hyperoside, isoquercitrin, quercitrin, quercetin, myricetol, fisetin, patuletin, luteolin, kaempferol, apigen). The following parameters were used to separate the polyphenolic principles from plant extracts: a reversed-phase HPLC columns (Zorbax Agilent, Santa Clara, CA, USA, SB-C18, 100 mm × 3.0 mm id, 3.5 µm), mobile phase with methanol: 0.1% acetic acid (*v*/*v*), and a binary solvent gradient; the detection was performed using UV and MS with an electrospray ion source in negative mode. Other HPLC parameters: flow rate = 1 mL/min, injection volume = 5 µL, and column temperature = 48 °C with combined detection: UV (330 nm, 370 nm) and MS mode. The quantitative results were processed using the Agilent ChemStation software B01.03 and DataAnalysis version 5.3.

Next, another previously described LC-MS method was used to determine 6 other polyphenols: epicatechin, catechin, syringic, gallic, protocatechuic, and vanillic acids [51]. The separation of the phenolic components was performed under the same chromatographic conditions mentioned above but with a different binary gradient, starting with 3% methanol and increasing to 8% in 3 min, 20% methanol for 8.5 min to 10 min, and finally, 3% methanol to re-equilibrate the column. An electrospray ion source operating in negative mode was used by the MS system in both analyses.

The polyphenolic substances in the *Stachys* extracts were identified by comparing their retention times and recorded electrospray mass spectra with those of the standards under the same conditions. Subsequently, the phenolic compounds were measured using their peak area and the matching standard's calibration curve. The results were calculated in µg polyphenol/g dry weight (dw) of vegetal product.

3.5. LC-MS/MS Analysis of Rosmarinis Acid

Rosmarinic acid (RA) was quantified by the LC-MS/MS method described by Prof. L. Vlase [24]. An Agilent 1100 HPLC Series system (Agilent, Santa Clara, CA, USA) equipped as in Section 3.4 was used. The mobile phase used was different and prepared with acetonitrile and ammonium acetate in water (1 mM), the gradient elution: start with 5% acetonitrile and 3.3 min 25% acetonitrile. The flow rate was 1 mL/min. The autosampler injection volume was set at 25 µL. The results obtained were expressed as µg RA/g dry weight (dw) of vegetal product.

3.6. Total Polyphenols Content

Spectrophotometry is one of the most used methods for quantifying phenolic compounds in medicinal plants. The total polyphenol (TPC) contents of the seven Stachys extracts were measured by the Folin–Ciocâlteu method, according to the European Pharmacopoeia [52]. A similar method has been described previously [53]. Brief method: the extracts were treated with the Folin–Ciocâlteu reagent, and after dilution with distilled water, with a solution of sodium carbonate (290 g/L). After 30 min, the absorbance was measured at 760 nm. After performing the gallic acid calibration curve (R^2 = 0.999), the results were calculated and expressed as mg of gallic acid equivalent (GAE)/mL plant extract [26,52]. Absorbance readings were taken in triplicates.

3.7. Flavonoid Content

The total flavonoid contents were spectrophotometrically determined, using a method previously described by us and based on the color reaction of the flavonoids with the aluminum chloride reagent (25 g/L). The absorbance of the yellow solution was measured at 430 nm [29]. Using a calibration curve (R^2 = 0.999), the results were presented as mg of rutin equivalents (RE)/mL plant extract. Absorbance readings were taken in triplicates.

3.8. Caffeic Acid Derivative Content

The quantification of caffeic acid derivatives can be evaluated by colorimetric method with Arnow's reagent (10.0 g sodium nitrite and 10.0 g sodium molybdate), according to the rules of the Romanian Pharmacopoeia X edition [31]. Absorbance was measured at 500 nm with the values of phenolic acids content of the *Stachys* extracts, expressed as caffeic acid equivalent (mg CAE/mL plant extract), using an equation derived from the calibration curve of caffeic acid (R^2 = 0.994). Absorbance readings were taken in triplicates [29,53].

3.9. Antioxidant Activity

The antioxidant activity of the six *Stachys* extracts was examined by several methods: the DPPH radical scavenging method, the FRAP test (the ferric-reducing ability of plasma), nitrite-induced autooxidation of hemoglobin (NHA), inhibition of cytochrome *c*-catalyzed lipid peroxidation, and an electron paramagnetic resonance (EPR) spectroscopy assay [9,54,55].

3.9.1. DPPH Radical Scavenging Assay

The antioxidant potentials of the *Stachys* sp. extracts were evaluated according to the DPPH method previously described by the authors [56,57]. This method measures the ability to remove stable free radicals DPPH by the natural antioxidant compounds (e.g., polyphenols) from plant extracts. A stock solution of 0.10 g/L DPPH in methanol (purple color) was prepared and 2.0 mL of this solution was added to 2.0 mL of extract solution (or standard) in methanol at different concentrations (12.50–250 µg/mL; yellow color). The absorbance of the *Stachys* extracts (As) and the control solutions (Ac = absorbance of DPPH with methanol, containing all reagents except the extracts) were spectrophotometrically measured at 517 nm, after 30 min (three replicates per treatment). Trolox was used as an antioxidant reference. The total antioxidant activity of the six extracts was expressed as IC_{50} (µg/mL): the concentration of plant material required to cause a 50% DPPH inhibition. The % of inhibition was plotted against concentration, and from the graphs, IC_{50} (R^2: 0.999, 0.997, 0.996, 0.998, 0.999, 0.997) was calculated.

3.9.2. FRAP Assay

The antioxidant capacity of the *Stachys* extracts was measured using the FRAP method [54,56,58]. After the preparation and treatment of the FRAP reagent with the samples, the absorbance of the obtained solutions was measured at 450 nm. The results were calculated in µmol Trolox Equivalent/mL *Stachys* sample.

3.9.3. Nitrite-Induced Autooxidation of Hemoglobin

Hemoglobin and nitrite's reaction was measured at 540 nm in a 50 mM pH 7 phosphate buffer. A total of 166 µM nitrite and 40 µM oxyhemoglobin were combined together with the samples. Origin 8 was utilized to calculate the inflection time (ti). The results are given in mg CAE/g (chlorogenic acid) plant for *Statcys* extracts. The linearity of the calibration curve is very good for chlorogenic acid (R^2 = 0.99) as well as for catechin (R^2 = 0.98) [59].

3.9.4. Inhibition of Lipid Peroxidation Catalyzed by Cytochrome *c*

By sonication of lecithin (5.0 mg/mL) solubilized in 10 mM phosphate and at neutral pH, liposomes were produced. They were mixed with cytochrome *c* (2.0 µM) and *Stachys* extract (8.3 µg/mL). The reaction was monitored at 235 nm [60].

3.9.5. Free Radical Generation Experiment

For the EPR experiment, the extracts were diluted at 0.05% and then mixed with 5 mM NaOH, in EtOH—90%. With a Bruker ELEXSYS E580 spectrometer (Bruker BioSpin

GmbH, Rheinstetten, Germany) operating at room temperature and recording continuous waves at the X band, the EPR spectra were obtained [60].

3.10. Determination of Antimicrobial Activity

3.10.1. Agar-Well Diffusion Method

The *Stachys* ethanolic extracts were evaluated for in vitro antibacterial and antifungal activities using the agar-well diffusion method [42]. These extracts were tested against five reference strains of microorganisms including two Gram-positive (*S. aureus, L. monocytogenes*), two Gram-negative (*S. enteritidis, E. coli*) bacteria and one yeast (*C. albicans*). Mueller–Hinton (MH) and Sabouraud dextrose (SD) broth and agar were used for bacteria and *C. albicans*, respectively. The plates containing specific agar were inoculated with a standardized inoculum prepared from pure colonies that were suspended in sterile broth to obtain a turbidity equivalent to 0.5 McFarland (1.0×10^6 CFU/mL) standard (bio-Meriuex, Marcy l'Etoile, France). Six-millimeter diameter wells were cut from the inoculated agar plates using a sterile cork borer to allow the addition of tested extracts (50 μL) (three wells for each extract). After incubation at 37 °C for 24 h for bacteria and 48 h for *C. albicans*, the growth inhibition zones diameters were measured. Tests were conducted in triplicate, and clear halos greater than 10 mm were considered positive results. Gentamicin (10 μg) and fluconazole (25 μg) commercial disks were included as positive controls (standard antibiotics and antifungals agents). The negative control was 70% methanol with a diameter = 6 mm.

3.10.2. Broth Microdilution Method

The in vitro antimicrobial efficacy was further investigated in terms of minimum inhibitory (MIC), bactericidal (MBC), and fungicidal (MFC) concentrations performing the broth microdilution method [45,58,61]. To determine these concentrations, each *Stachys* sp. extract was subjected to twofold serial dilutions using 100 μL of specific broth (MH and SD for bacteria and *C. albicans*, respectively). Each dilution was placed in two wells of sterile flat-bottomed 96-well microtiter plates (Deltalab, Barcelona, Spain) and incubated with a volume of 5.0 μL microorganism inoculum for 24 h at 37 °C. At the end of the incubation period, the wells were visually examined compared to the controls (the two types of broths used to culture bacterial and fungal species (MH and SD, respectively). No turbidity indicated an inhibitory effect, with the highest dilution associated with it determined as the MIC value. Next, a volume of 10.0 μL from each well was cultured on the corresponding agar plates. No visible growth on these plates after 24 h and 48 h for bacteria and *C. albicans*, respectively, pointed out the MBC and MFC values. This assay included controls such as gentamicin 50 mg/mL (Sigma-Aldrich, St. Louis, MO, USA), and fluconazole (10–1000 μM) (Sigma-Aldrich, St. Louis, MO, USA) and was performed in duplicates for each tested product.

3.10.3. Anti-Biofilm Assay

The inhibitory activity of *Stachys* sp. extracts against two stages of biofilm formation, biofilm attachment (T0) and destruction of 24 h pre-formed biofilm (T24), respectively, was investigated using previously reported protocols [45,61,62]. The bacterial and fungal inoculums were prepared as presented for the disk diffusion; for T0 the inoculums were placed in sterile flat-bottomed 96-well microtiter plates to be incubated with equal volumes (100 μL) of each *Stachys* extract for 24 h at 37 °C without shaking. In the case of T24, each inoculum was initially cultured for 24 h to obtain the biofilm and further treated with equal volumes of each *Stachys* extract. Controls such as organisms + specific broth, bacteria + MH broth + gentamicin, *C. albicans* + SD broth + fluconazole were included. Following 24 h incubation, the biofilm biomass was quantified using the crystal violet staining (CVS) assay. The content of each well was removed and the 96-well microtiter plates were washed three times using sterile distilled water, a step required to remove the unattached microorganism cells. The plates were dried and added with 96% methanol (150 μL) for 20 min and the fixed adhered cells were stained with 100 μL of 0.1% crystal violet solution (Sigma-Aldrich,

St. Louis, MO, USA) for 20 min at room temperature. The plates were washed five times with sterile distillated water. The crystal violet stain bound to the adherent cells of each well was re-solubilized with 150 µL of 100% ethanol. After gentle shaking, the plates' absorbance (optic density, OD) was read at 490 nm using a microplate reader Sunrise™ (Tecan, Männedorf, Switzerland). and the results were expressed as percentage inhibition using the equation below [45].

Inhibition (%) = (ODcontrol − ODExtract)/ODcontrol × 100. Based on the inhibition (%) calculated values, the tested extract activity was described as good (above 50%, ++), poor (0–50%, +), and no inhibition, or enhancement of biofilm development and growth (<0, -) [45].

3.11. Statistical Data Analysis

All experiments were performed in triplicate or more and all data were expressed as mean ± standard deviation using the Excel software package 2016. The statistical analysis of differences was performed using one-way analysis of variance (ANOVA), with $p < 0.05$ as the threshold value for statistical significance: very significant ($p < 0.001$), significant ($0.001 < p < 0.05$), and insignificant ($p > 0.05$).

4. Conclusions

This is a detailed report on the phytochemical composition and antioxidant and antimicrobial properties of extracts obtained from six medicinal species of *Stachys* from Romania: *S. officinalis*, *S. germanica*, *S. byzantina*, *S. sylvatica*, *S. palustris*, and *S. recta*. Fifteen phenolic compounds were found in the six species using LC-MS, of which seven substances were common: protocatechuic acid, rosmarinic acid, gentisic acid, vanillic acid, *p*-coumaric acid, ferulic acid, luteolin, and apigenin. Chlorogenic acid was found in large amounts; the most abundant species were *S. germanica* (4205.2 µg/g) *S. sylvatica* (5552.7 µg/g), and *S. recta* (6761.4 µg/g). Furthermore, significant antioxidant properties were demonstrated using conventional and innovative methods for *S. byzantina*, *S. germanica* and *S. palustris*-derived extracts. These extracts also displayed the most intense in vitro antimicrobial potential. These results provide a scientific foundation and open important perspectives for developing phytopharmaceuticals indicated in various pathologies that involve antioxidant and antimicrobial mechanisms.

Author Contributions: Conceptualization, D.B.; methodology, D.B., C.P., R.S.-D., L.V., A.-M.V., D.H., B.T., I.O., M.N. and M.D.; experimental work, D.B., C.P., R.S.-D., L.V., A.-M.V., D.H., B.T., A.N., M.N., I.O. and M.D.; software, D.B., C.P., R.S.-D., C.C.L. and L.V.; validation, D.B.; formal analysis, D.B., C.C.L. and B.T.; resources, D.B., R.S.-D., L.V., D.H. and M.D.; writing—original draft preparation, D.B., C.P., R.S.-D. and L.V.; writing—review and editing, D.B., C.P., R.S.-D., L.V., M.N., D.H. and I.O.; supervision D.B.; project administration, D.B., L.V., D.H., R.S.-D. and M.D.; funding acquisition, D.B. All authors have read and agreed to the published version of the manuscript.

Funding: This research received no external funding.

Institutional Review Board Statement: Not applicable.

Informed Consent Statement: Not applicable.

Data Availability Statement: Data are contained within the article.

Acknowledgments: We would like to thank Cezera Zagrean-Tuza (UBB Cluj) for the useful discussions, Andrei Mocan (UMF Cluj), as well as Larisa Silvia Ionaș.

Conflicts of Interest: The authors declare no conflict of interest. The funders had no role in the design of the study; in the collection, analyses, or interpretation of data; in the writing of the manuscript; or in the decision to publish the results.

References

1. Kanjevac, M.; Zlatić, N.; Bojović, B.; Stanković, M. Pharmaceutical and biological properties of *Stachys* species: A review. *Braz. J. Pharm. Sci.* **2022**, *58*, e20211. [CrossRef]
2. Tomou, E.M.; Barda, C.; Skaltsa, H. Genus *Stachys*: A review of traditional uses, phytochemistry and bioactivity. *Medicines* **2020**, *7*, 63. [CrossRef]
3. Sârbu, I.; Stefan, N.; Oprea, A. *Plante Vasculare din România. Determinator Ilustrat de Teren (Vascular Plants of Romania)*; Publishing House: Bucharest, Romania, 2013; pp. 656–660.
4. Gille, E.; Cretu, R.M.; Stefanache, C.P.; Gavril, G.L.; Sidoroff, M.E. *Medicinal and Aromatic Plants from the Wild Flora of Dobrogea (Romania)*; Piatra Neamt, Romania, Cuza University: Iassy, Romania, 2020.
5. Ardelean, A.; Mohan, G. *Flora Medicinala a Romaniei*; Editura ALL: Bucuresti, Romania, 2008; p. 20.
6. Dragulescu, C.; Marculescu, A. *Plantele in Medicina Populara Romaneasca*; Editura Universitatii Transilvania: Brasov, Romania, 2020; pp. 89–90.
7. Stegarus, D.I.; Lengyel, E.; Apostolescu, G.F.; Botoran, O.R.; Tanase, C. Phytochemical analysis and biological activity of three *Stachys* species (Lamiaceae) from Romania. *Plants* **2021**, *10*, 2710. [CrossRef]
8. Imbrea, I.; Butnariu, M.; Nicolin, A.; Imbrea, F.; Prodan, M. Valorising the species *Stachys officinalis* (L.) Trevis. from south-western Romania. *Res. J. Agric. Sci.* **2011**, *43*, 198.
9. López-Fernández, O.; Domínguez, R.; Pateiro, M.; Munekata, P.; Rocchetti, G.; Lorenzo, J. Determination of polyphenols using Liquid Chromatography-Tandem Mass Spectrometry Technique (LC–MS/MS): A Review. *Antioxidants* **2020**, *9*, 479. [CrossRef] [PubMed]
10. Muresan, M.; Benedec, D.; Vlase, L.; Oprean, R.; Toiu, A.; Oniga, I. Screening of polyphenolic compounds, antioxidant and antimicrobial properties of *Tanacetum vulgare* from Transylvania. *Stud. Univ. Babes-Bolyai Chem.* **2015**, *60*, 127–138.
11. Lu, H.; Tian, Z.; Cui, Y.; Liu, Z.; Ma, X. Chlorogenic acid: A comprehensive review of the dietary sources, processing effects, bioavailability, beneficial properties, mechanisms of action, and future directions. *Compr. Rev. Food Sci. Food Saf.* **2020**, *19*, 3130–3158. [CrossRef] [PubMed]
12. Sarikurkcu, C.; Ceylan, O.; Benabdallah, A.; Tepe, B. *Stachys germanica* subsp. *heldreichii (Boiss.) Hayek: Phytochemical analysis, antioxidant and enzyme inhibitory activities. S. Afr. J. Bot.* **2020**, *143*, 291–300. [CrossRef]
13. Vundac, V.B. Taxonomical and phytochemical characterisation of 10 Stachys taxa recorded in the Balkan Peninsula flora: A review. *Plants* **2019**, *8*, 32. [CrossRef]
14. Sytar, O.; Hemmerich, I.; Zivcak, M.; Rauh, C.; Brestic, M. Comparative analysis of bioactive phenolic compounds composition from 26 medicinal plants. *Saudi J. Biol. Sci.* **2018**, *25*, 631–641. [CrossRef]
15. Paun, G.; Neagu, E.; Moroeanu, V.; Ungureanu, O.; Cretu, R.; Ionescu, E.; Tebrencu, C.E.; Ionescu, R.; Stoica, I.; Radu, G.L. Phytochemical analysis and in vitro biological activity of *Betonica officinalis* and *Salvia officinalis* extracts. *Rom. Biotechnol. Lett.* **2017**, *22*, 12751–12761.
16. Bączek, K.; Kosakowska, O.; Przybył, J.L.; Węglarz, Z. Accumulation of phenolic compounds in the purple betony herb (*Stachys officinalis* L.) originated from cultivation. *Herba Pol.* **2016**, *62*, 7–16. [CrossRef]
17. Valentova, K.; Vrba, J.; Bancirova, M.; Ulrichova, J.; Kren, V. Isoquercitrin: Pharmacology, toxicology, and metabolism. *Food Chem. Toxicol.* **2014**, *68*, 267–282. [CrossRef]
18. Nadeem, M.; Imran, M.; Aslam Gondal, T.; Imran, A.; Shahbaz, M.; Muhammad Amir, R.; Wasim Sajid, M.; Batool Qaisrani, T.; Atif, M.; Hussain, G. Therapeutic potential of rosmarinic acid: A comprehensive review. *Appl. Sci.* **2019**, *9*, 3139. [CrossRef]
19. Ertas, A.; Yener, I. A comprehensive study on chemical and biological profiles of three herbal teas in Anatolia; rosmarinic and chlorogenic acids. *S. Afr. J. Bot.* **2020**, *130*, 274–281. [CrossRef]
20. Elfalleh, W.; Kirkan, B.; Sarikurkcu, C. Antioxidant potential and phenolic composition of extracts from *Stachys tmolea*: An endemic plant from Turkey. *Ind. Crops Prod.* **2019**, *127*, 212–216. [CrossRef]
21. Carev, I.; Sarikurkcu, C. LC-MS/MS profiles and in vitro biological activities of extracts of an endemic species from Turkey: *Stachys cretica* ssp. *anatolica*. *Plants* **2021**, *10*, 1054. [CrossRef]
22. Bahadori, M.B.; Zengin, G.; Dinparast, L.; Eskandani, M. The health benefits of three Hedgenettle herbal teas (*Stachys byzantina, Stachys inflata,* and *Stachys lavandulifolia*)-profiling phenolic and antioxidant activities. *Eur. J. Integr. Med.* **2020**, *36*, 101134. [CrossRef]
23. Paun, G.; Neagu, E.; Moroeanu, V.; Albu, C.; Ursu, T.M.; Zanfirescu, A.; Radu, G.L. Anti-inflammatory and antioxidant activities of the *Impatiens noli-tangere* and *Stachys officinalis* polyphenolic-rich extracts. *Rev. Bras. Farmacog.* **2018**, *28*, 57–64. [CrossRef]
24. Vlase, L.; Benedec, D.; Hanganu, D.; Damian, G.; Csillag, I.; Sevastre, B.; Mot, A.C.; Silaghi-Dumitre scu, R.; Tilea, I. Evaluation of antioxidant and antimicrobial activities and phenolic profile for *Hyssopus officinalis*, *Ocimum basilicum* and *Teucrium chamaedrys*. *Molecules* **2014**, *19*, 5490–5507. [CrossRef]
25. Rana, R.; Samtiya, M.; Dhewa, T.; Mishra, V.; Aluko, R.E. Health benefits of polyphenols: A concise review. *Food Biochem.* **2022**, *46*, e14264. [CrossRef]
26. Singleton, V.L.; Orthofer, R.; Lamuela-Raventos, R.M. Analysis of total phenols and other oxidation substrates and antioxidants by means of Folin-Ciocalteu reagent. *Methods Enzymol.* **1999**, *299*, 152–178. [CrossRef]
27. Khanavi, M.; Hajimahmoodi, M.; Cheraghi-Niroomand, M.; Kargar, Z.; Ajani, Y.; Hadjiakhoondi, A.; Oveisi, M.R. Comparison of the antioxidant activity and total phenolic contents in some *Stachys* species. *Afr. J. Biotechol.* **2009**, *8*, 1143–1147.

28. Mitic, S.S.; Stojkovic, M.B.; Pavlovic, J.L.; Mitic, M.N.; Stojanovic, B.T. Antioxidant activity, phenolic and mineral content of *Stachys germanica* L. (Lamiaceae). *Oxid. Commun.* **2012**, *35*, 1011–1020.
29. Romanian Pharmacopoeia Commission National Medicines Agency. *Romanian Pharmacopoeia*, 10th ed.; Medical Publishing House: Bucharest, Romania, 1993; p. 335.
30. Nikolova, M. Screening of radical scavenging activity and polyphenol content of Bulgarian plant species. *Pharmacogn. Res.* **2011**, *3*, 256–259. [CrossRef] [PubMed]
31. Hajimehdipoor, H.; Gohari, A.R.; Ajani, Y.; Saeidnia, S. Comparative study of the total phenol content and antioxidant activity of some medicinal herbal extracts. *Res. J. Pharmacog. (RJP)* **2014**, *1*, 21–25.
32. Toplan, G.G.; Taşkin, T.; Mataraci, K.E.; Genc, G.E. Antioxidant, and antimicrobial activities of various extracts from *Stachys cretica* subsp. *bulgarica Rech.f., Stachys byzantina K. Koch and Stachys thirkei K. Koch. Istanb. J. Pharm.* **2021**, *51*, 341–347. [CrossRef]
33. Hajdari, A.; Novak, J.; Mustafa, B.; Franz, C. Essential oil composition and antioxidant activity of *Stachys sylvatica* L. (Lamiaceae) from different wild populations in Kosovo. *Nat. Prod. Res.* **2012**, *26*, 1676–1681. [CrossRef] [PubMed]
34. Zagrean-Tuza, C.; Dorneanu, S.; Mot, A.C. The strange case of polyphenols inhibiting the Briggs-Rauscher reaction: PHmodulated reactivity of the superoxide radical. *Free Radic. Biol. Med.* **2020**, *46*, 189–197. [CrossRef] [PubMed]
35. Rabbani, M.; Sajjadi, S.E.; Zarei, H.R. Anxiolytic effects of *Stachys lavandulifolia* Vahl on the elevated plus-maze model of anxiety in mice. *J. Ethnopharmacol.* **2003**, *89*, 271–276. [CrossRef] [PubMed]
36. Hayashi, K.; Nagamatsu, T.; Ito, M.; Hattori, T.; Suzuki, Y. Acotoside, a component of *Stachys sieboldii* MIQ, may be a promising antinephritic agent. 1) Effects of acetoside on crescentic-type anti-GBM nephritis in rats. *Jpn. J. Pharmacol.* **1994**, *65*, 143–151. [CrossRef]
37. Lazarevic, J.S.; Đordevic, A.S.; Kitic, D.V.; Zlatkovic, B.K.; Stojanovic, G.S. Chemical composition and antimicrobial activity of the essential oil of *Stachys officinalis* (L.) Trevis. (Lamiaceae). *Chem. Biodivers.* **2013**, *10*, 1335–1349. [CrossRef] [PubMed]
38. Saeedi, M.; Morteza-semnani, K.; Mahdavi, M.R.; Rahimi, F. Antimicrobial studies on extracts of four species of *Stachys*. *Indian J. Pharm. Sci.* **2008**, *70*, 403–406. [CrossRef]
39. Serbetci, T.; Demirci, B.; Güzel, C.B.; Kültür, S.; Ergüven, M.; Baser, K.H. Essential oil composition, antimicrobial and cytotoxic activities of two endemic *Stachys cretica* subspecies (Lamiaceae) from Turkey. *Nat. Prod. Commun.* **2010**, *5*, 1369–1374. [CrossRef] [PubMed]
40. Skaltsa, H.D.; Demetzos, C.; Lazari, D.; Sokovic, M. Essential oil analysis and antimicrobial activity of eight *Stachys* species from Greece. *Phytochemistry* **2003**, *64*, 743–752. [CrossRef]
41. Ferhat, M.; Erol, E.; Beladjila, K.A.; Çetintaş, Y.; Duru, M.E.; Öztürk, M.; Kabouche, A.; Kabouche, Z. Antioxidant, anticholinesterase, and antibacterial activities of *Stachys guyoniana* and *Mentha aquatica*. *Pharm. Biol.* **2017**, *55*, 324–329. [CrossRef] [PubMed]
42. Reeves, D.S.; White, L.O. Principles of methods of assaying antibiotics. In *Pharmaceutical Microbiology*, 3rd ed.; Hugo, W.B., Russel, A.D., Eds.; Blackwell Scientific Publication: Oxford, UK, 1983; pp. 140–162.
43. Napolitano, A.; Di Napoli, M.; Castagliuolo, G.; Badalamenti, N.; Cicio, A.; Bruno, M.; Piacente, S.; Maresca, V.; Cianciullo, P.; Capasso, L.; et al. The chemical composition of the aerial parts of *Stachys spreitzenhoferi* (Lamiaceae) extract growing in Kythira Island (Greece) and its antioxidant, antimicrobial, anti-inflammatory and antiproliferative properties. *Phytochemistry* **2022**, *203*, 113373. [CrossRef]
44. Dulger, G.; Aki, C. Antimicrobial activity of the leaves of endemic *Stachys pseudopinardii* in Turkey. *Trop. J. Pharm. Res.* **2009**, *8*, 371–375. [CrossRef]
45. Olawuwo, O.S.; Famuyide, I.M.; McGaw, L.J. Antibacterial and antibiofilm activity of selected medicinal plant leaf extracts against pathogens implicated in poultry diseases. *Front. Vet. Sci.* **2022**, *9*, 820304. [CrossRef]
46. Lou, Z.; Wang, H.; Zhu, S.; Ma, C.; Wang, Z. Antibacterial activity and mechanism of action of chlorogenic acid. *J. Food Sci.* **2011**, *76*, 98–403. [CrossRef]
47. Kabir, F.; Katayama, S.; Tanji, N.; Nakamura, S. Antimicrobial effects of chlorogenic acid and related compounds. *J. Korean Soc. Appl. Biol. Chem.* **2014**, *57*, M359–M365. [CrossRef]
48. Cheung, G.Y.C.; Bae, J.S.; Otto, M. Pathogenicity and virulence of *Staphylococcus aureus*. *Virulence* **2021**, *12*, 547–569. [CrossRef] [PubMed]
49. Hanganu, D.; Olah, N.K.; Mocan, A.; Vlase, L.; Benedec, D.; Raita, O.; Toma, C. Comparative polyphenolic content and antioxidant activities of two Romanian *Lysimachia* species. *Rev. Chim.* **2016**, *67*, 227–231.
50. Gligor, O.; Clichici, S.; Moldovan, R.; Muntean, D.; Vlase, A.M.; Nadăș, G.C.; Matei, I.A.; Filip, G.A.; Crișan, G. The effect of extraction methods on phytochemicals and biological activities of green coffee beans extracts. *Plants* **2023**, *12*, 712. [CrossRef]
51. Rusu, M.; Gheldiu, A.-M.; Mocan, A.; Moldovan, C.; Popa, D.-S.; Tomuta, I.; Vlase, L. Process optimization for improved phenolic compounds recovery from walnut (*Juglans regia* L.) septum: Phytochemical profile and biological activities. *Molecules* **2018**, *23*, 2814. [CrossRef]
52. Council of Europe. *European Pharmacopoeia*, 5th ed.; Council of Europe: Strasbourg, France, 2005; p. 221.
53. Oniga, I.; Vlase, L.; Toiu, A.; Benedec, D.; Duda, M. Evaluation of phenolic acid derivatives and essential oil content in some *Melissa officinalis* L. varieties. *Farmacia* **2010**, *58*, 764–769.
54. Benzie, I.F.F.; Strain, J.J. The ferric reducing ability of plasma (FRAP) as a measure of "Antioxidant Power": The FRAP Assay. *Anal. Biochem.* **1996**, *239*, 70–76. [CrossRef]

55. Slinkard, K.; Singleton, V.L. Total phenol analyses: Automation and comparison with manual methods. *Am. J. Enol. Vitic.* **1977**, *28*, 49–55. [CrossRef]
56. Thaipong, K.; Boonprakob, U.; Crosby, K.; Cisneros-Zevallos, L.; Hawkins Byrne, D. Comparison of ABTS, DPPH, FRAP, and ORAC assays for estimating antioxidant activity from guava fruit extracts. *J. Food Compos. Anal.* **2006**, *19*, 669–675. [CrossRef]
57. Vundac, V.B.; Brantner, A.H.; Miško, P. Content of polyphenolic constituents and antioxidant activity of some *Stachys* taxa. *Food Chem.* **2007**, *104*, 1277–1281. [CrossRef]
58. Niculae, M.; Hanganu, D.; Oniga, I.; Benedec, D.; Ielciu, I.; Giupana, R.; Sandru, C.D.; Ciocârlan, N.; Spinu, M. phytochemical profile and antimicrobial potential of extracts obtained from *Thymus marschallianus* Willd. *Molecules* **2019**, *24*, 3101. [CrossRef] [PubMed]
59. Hathazi, D.; Scurtu, F.; Bischin, C.; Mot, A.; Attia, A.; Kongsted, J.; Silaghi-Dumitrescu, R. The Reaction of oxy hemoglobin with nitrite: Mechanism, antioxidant-modulated effect, and implications for blood substitute evaluation. *Molecules* **2018**, *23*, 350. [CrossRef]
60. Obasi, T.C.; Benedec, D.; Hanganu, D.; Gheldiu, A.M.; Vlase, L.; Oniga, I.; Pușcaș, C.; Silaghi-Dumitrescu, R.; Oprean, R. Free radical scavenging activity and total polyphenol content of *Securidaca Longipedunculata* roots and leaves extracts. *Farmacia* **2020**, *68*, 116–120. [CrossRef]
61. Soliman, S.S.M.; Semreen, M.H.; El-Keblawy, A.A.; Abdullah, A.; Uppuluri, P.; Ibrahim, A.S. Assessment of herbal drugs for promising anti-Candida activity. *BMC Complement. Altern. Med.* **2017**, *17*, 257. [CrossRef]
62. Meccatti, V.M.; Santos, L.F.; de Carvalho, L.S.; Souza, C.B.; Carvalho, C.A.T.; Marcucci, M.C.; Abu Hasna, A.; de Oliveira, L.D. Antifungal action of herbal plants' glycolic extracts against *Candida* species. *Molecules* **2023**, *28*, 2857. [CrossRef] [PubMed]

antibiotics

MDPI

Article

Applications of Romanian Propolis in Phyto-Inhibitory Activity and Antimicrobial Protection: A Comparative Study

Ramona Cristina Heghedűş-Mîndru [1], Mirel Glevitzky [2,*], Gabriel Heghedűş-Mîndru [1], Gabriela-Alina Dumitrel [3], Maria Popa [2], Doriana Maria Popa [4], Isidora Radulov [1] and Mihaela Laura Vică [5]

[1] Faculty of Food Engineering, University of Life Science "King Mihai I", 300645 Timișoara, Romania; ramonaheghedus@usab-tm.ro (R.C.H.-M.); gabrielheghedus@usab-tm.ro (G.H.-M.); isidoraradulov@yahoo.com (I.R.)

[2] Faculty of Exact Science and Engineering, "1 Decembrie 1918" University of Alba Iulia, 510009 Alba Iulia, Romania; mpopa@uab.ro

[3] Faculty of Industrial Chemistry and Environmental Engineering, Politehnica University of Timisoara, 300223 Timișoara, Romania; alina.dumitrel@upt.ro

[4] Clinical Emergency Hospital for Children Cluj Napoca, 400398 Cluj-Napoca, Romania; popa.dorianaa@yahoo.com

[5] Department of Cellular and Molecular Biology, "Iuliu Hațieganu" University of Medicine and Pharmacy, 400012 Cluj-Napoca, Romania; mvica@umfcluj.ro

* Correspondence: mirel_glevitzky@yahoo.com; Tel.: +40-740-076-768

Abstract: Propolis use in medicine, pharmaceutical, cosmetic, and food industries is well known. This study aimed to investigate propolis' phyto-inhibitory and antimicrobial potential. Nine propolis samples obtained from distinct Romanian regions and characterized in terms of physical–chemical parameters, phenols and flavonoid contents, and antioxidant properties were prepared as dry propolis and aqueous extracts. The phyto-inhibitory effect was comparatively tested on different cereals: hexaploid bread wheat (*Triticum aestivum*), maize (*Zea mays* L.), oats (*Avena sativa* L.), and barley (*Hordeum vulgare* L.), while their in vitro antimicrobial activity was evaluated against bacterial and fungal strains specific to cereals: *Bacillus subtilis*, *B. cereus*, *Proteus mirabilis*, *Fusarium oxysporum*, *Penicillium chrysogenum*, and *Aspergillus niger*. All propolis samples showed a phyto-inhibitory effect on the cereals, the most pronounced being corn and oats. Propolis powder samples displayed a lower phyto-inhibitory activity than propolis extracts. Also, all tested products showed inhibitory efficacy against both bacteria and fungi. Furthermore, principal component analysis showed differences between the samples' phyto-inhibitory and antimicrobial properties depending on the geographical origin. Positive correlations were found between the polyphenols, flavonoid content, and antioxidant activity, respectively. These data support propolis' phyto-pharmaceutical potential related to its use in plant crop management as an alternative in ecological agriculture.

Keywords: chemical analysis; phyto-inhibitory activity; antimicrobial activity; propolis; cereals

1. Introduction

Bees are important to agriculture and the environment because they contribute to plant reproduction through pollination [1]. The products obtained from bees, besides honey, are propolis, pollen, royal jelly, and beeswax [2]. Propolis is a natural aromatic, resinous substance produced by bees to cover the cracks in the inner walls of the hive and other living things that enter it [3]. It has bactericidal therapeutic properties [4], antiviral [5], antifungal [6], anti-inflammatory, anesthetic, analgesic, regenerative, and antitoxic [7], among other biological activities. Propolis also has a strong bioactive action and is a natural medicine used since ancient times. The medicinal properties were known by the Greeks and Romans, and it was used as an antiseptic and cicatrizing agent in the treatment of wounds [8]. Propolis is a resinous vegetable substance that bees create by mixing their own saliva with beeswax, to which they add components derived from plants and trees [9]. More than 500 chemical compounds have been identified in propolis to date: flavonoids, terpenoids, phenolic and fatty acids, vitamins, amino acids, sugars, proteins, and minerals [10,11].

Over time, most research has focused on potentially treating various acute and chronic diseases with propolis produced by bees as alternative complementary medicines [12]. But there are also studies that show that propolis can be used in agriculture, especially in the control of phytopathogens in crops. Moraes et al. [13] studied the use of propolis in tomato crops to control phytopathogens. With the same aim, other studies highlighted the use of propolis in the cultures of coffee [14], beans [15], cucumbers [16], and grapes [17].

Although propolis can be used as a powder in agriculture, it is often necessary for it to be in the form of a concentrated solution of propolis (aqueous, alcoholic extract–tincture). The use of propolis in agriculture is relatively recent, especially due to the promotion of organic agriculture [18]. In the scientific literature, a series of extraction methods (maceration, ultrasound, and microwave applications) in different solvents (ethanol and water) are described [19].

Propolis can protect plants as an alternative that can be applied in crop systems to avoid or reduce pesticide use that harms plants, the environment, and the population [11]. Natural production methods from organic farming encourage the use of propolis in agriculture. If it is widely incorporated in crop management, its bioactive and economic importance will increase in the future because foods produced using propolis are qualitatively different from foods produced using conventional methods. When considering natural products, certain aspects of the sustainability and quality of organic food are highlighted [20]. The bioactive compounds of propolis must be extracted from it so that the final solution can be applied to the crops. Due to the large number of chemicals, some of its compounds are soluble in water or alcohol or both solvents [21].

The multitude of bioactive components of propolis has determined its use in various fields such as medicine, pharmaceuticals, cosmetics, and food industries [22]. Although the antimicrobial effect has been intensively studied, most studies have been conducted on a limited number of strains or strains pathogenic to humans and less on microorganisms affecting plants.

The flavonoids and phenols in propolis help prevent and eliminate microbial and fungal infections that can affect grains, such as molds and pathogenic bacteria [23,24] and can increase plant resistance to abiotic stresses, such as drought, soil salinity, or extreme temperatures. These compounds can help regulate plant physiological processes to better cope with these extreme conditions [25]. So, propolis can have a good effect on grains, providing protection against pathogens, helping them cope with difficult environmental conditions, and contributing to good growth.

Additional research is required for the development of commercial products based on propolis–ethanolic and aqueous extracts at different concentrations with applicability in agriculture. The present study highlights the physico–chemical parameters of propolis collected from the regions of Romania and the effect of propolis powder or aqueous extracts on different crops. At the same time, the antimicrobial effect of propolis on some strains of microorganisms specific to cereals is presented.

2. Results and Statistical Analysis

2.1. Samples Characterization

The values of the physico–chemical parameters for the nine propolis samples collected from different regions of Romania are presented in Table 1.

The values obtained for water activity are between 0.62 and 0.78. Regarding the hygroscopicity, the value for all samples ranges between 12.6 and 14.7 g of absorbed water per 100 g of propolis. The water solubility of propolis samples is between 8.26 and 13.43%. In the case of the total phenolic content of all nine propolis samples, the values ranged from 102.7 (sample 6 from the Muntenia region) to 189.4 mg (sample 7 from the Dobruja region) of GAE/g. In contrast, the total flavonoid content was quantified between 65.30 (sample

6 from the Muntenia region) and 85.19 mg (sample 7 from the Dobruja region) of QE/g. The maximum number of phenols and flavonoid amounts was recorded in samples 1 and 7 from Alba and Constanța County, and the lowest value was in sample 6 from Dâmbovița County. The DPPH and FRAP assays estimate the antioxidant activities of propolis samples collected from all areas of Romania. Samples of propolis showed high antioxidant capacity.

Table 1. The values of the physical–chemical parameters for the analyzed propolis samples.

Sample No.	a_w	Hygroscopicity (g of Absorbed Water/ 100 g Propolis)	Water Solubility (%)	Phenols (mg GAE */g)	Flavonoids (mg QE **/g)	FRAP (mmol Fe^{2+}/g)	DPPH (mg GAE */g)
S1	0.71 ± 0.22	14.1 ± 0.9	9.12 ± 0.27	189.4 ± 5.82	84.31 ± 0.09	1.44 ± 0.31	16.44 ± 0.2
S2	0.69 ± 0.15	13.5 ± 0.8	8.98 ± 0.66	172.9 ± 3.25	78.55 ± 0.08	0.98 ± 0.02	15.08 ± 0.2
S3	0.62 ± 0.17	13.1 ± 0.6	8.74 ± 0.50	152.2 ± 6.80	70.10 ± 0.16	1.02 ± 0.06	13.50 ± 0.3
S4	0.74 ± 0.09	12.9 ± 0.9	9.52 ± 0.32	144.0 ± 2.09	81.09 ± 0.98	1.04 ± 0.06	13.92 ± 0.5
S5	0.72 ± 0.18	13.2 ± 0.5	8.26 ± 0.41	138.2 ± 3.06	77.62 ± 0.20	1.15 ± 0.15	12.30 ± 0.4
S6	0.65 ± 0.11	14.7 ± 0.7	11.31 ± 0.58	102.7 ± 2.43	65.30 ± 0.11	0.80 ± 0.09	11.70 ± 0.2
S7	0.78 ± 0.12	12.8 ± 0.6	9.07 ± 0.63	189.0 ± 4.55	85.19 ± 0.07	1.46 ± 0.11	18.30 ± 0.6
S8	0.63 ± 0.16	12.6 ± 0.5	13.43 ± 0.34	126.3 ± 3.14	82.36 ± 0.09	1.22 ± 0.09	15.06 ± 0.4
S9	0.67 ± 0.14	13.3 ± 0.8	12.66 ± 0.75	150.1 ± 4.37	79.54 ± 0.13	1.07 ± 0.07	14.32 ± 0.2

* Gallic acid equivalent. ** Quercetin equivalent.

2.2. *Phyto-Inhibitory Activity of Propolis Samples*

In Supplementary Tables S1–S8, the plume lengths for 13 days (growth rate) are presented comparatively for wheat, corn, barley, and oat samples, over which different quantities of powdered propolis were applied (1, 5, and 10 g), and aqueous extracts of propolis at different concentrations (1%, 5%, and 10%). The samples were collected from the nine regions of Romania. The control sample (M) is the one for which propolis was not applied.

In the case of the average plumule growth lengths for the wheat samples (Supplementary Table S1), it is found that the slowing down of plant growth is directly proportional to the amount of propolis applied over time. After 13 days, for the doses of 1 g and 10 g, samples S4 from Timiș County and S9 from Suceava had the lowest growth. Also, when 5 g of propolis is applied, sample S4 records the lowest plume growth at the end of the monitoring period. In the wheat samples, the radicle and the plumule are visible even from the first days, except for the samples in which 10 g of propolis was applied. The control sample, without propolis inhibitor, has the fastest growth.

The wheat samples treated with different concentrations of aqueous propolis extracts (Supplementary Table S2) have a similar tendency to inhibit grain growth as those treated with propolis powder. In the case of wheat samples, the plume growth speeds are relatively close for all nine propolis samples. Samples S4 and S9 show the most pronounced inhibitory effect. Plumule growth lengths are comparatively smaller when using concentrations of aqueous propolis extracts of 1%, compared to the 10% solution.

From the results obtained, it can be seen that the phyto-inhibitory activity is higher when propolis powder is applied than when aqueous solutions are used.

As with wheat, the plume growth trend is similar in the case of corn samples treated with propolis powder (Supplementary Table S3). However, the smallest increases in the plume are recorded in the case of samples S7 (Constanța County) and S9 (Suceava County) for the samples to which 1 g of propolis was applied, respectively, S8 (Vaslui County) and S9 (Suceava County) to which was applied a 10 g propolis powder. In the case of corn samples, the plume growth values are similar in the case of dosing 1 g and 5 g of propolis powder as an inhibitor, the difference compared to the control sample being insignificant for all nine propolis samples. The plume growth rate is significantly reduced when 10 g of propolis powder is dosed into corn samples. There is a similarity between the samples to which powder propolis was applied and the case of using aqueous solutions (Supplementary

Table S4) of the same inhibitor. However, it is obvious that the propolis solution applied to corn samples has a much stronger inhibitory effect than the powder one.

Among the propolis samples collected from different regions of Romania, there were no large variations in the growth speed of the barley seed plume for doses of 1 g and 5 g. These are more obvious when applying the dose of 10 g, where the maximum difference is 11 mm between sample S4 (Timiș County) with the lowest growth and sample S2 (Bihor County) with the highest growth (Supplementary Table S5). In the case of barley samples, plumule growth lengths are not significantly reduced when treated with inhibitor solutions of different concentrations: 1%, 5%, and 10% (Supplementary Table S6). Overall, plume growth rates are slightly below the control sample (M).

In the case of oat samples (Supplementary Tables S7 and S8), when applying 10 g inhibitory propolis, after 13 days, samples S3 (Maramureș County) and S4 (Timiș County) have the lowest average increase in plumule lengths. In the case of oats, a similar evolution of the plume lengths is constant as in the case of the other cereals but with growth values similar to those of the corn samples. In general, all propolis samples studied inhibited germination significantly compared to the control sample.

2.3. Antimicrobial Activity of Propolis Samples

The antimicrobial effect of the nine aqueous extracts of propolis collected from all regions of Romania against six microbial (bacterial and fungal) strains specific to cereals are presented in Table 2.

Table 2. The diameters of the inhibition zones (mm) for the nine propolis samples collected from regions of Romania.

Strain	Sample									Ciprofloxacin, 5 µg	Voriconazole, 1 µg
	S1	S2	S3	S4	S5	S6	S7	S8	S9		
B. subtilis	28 * ± 1.71	25 * ± 0.00	26 ± 0.57	26 ± 0.57	27 ± 1.14	25 * ± 0.00	26 ± 0.57	26 ± 0.57	25 ± 0.57	30 ± 0.00	-
B. cereus	25 ± 1.14	26 ± 1.14	27 ± 1.14	26 ± 0.57	27 ± 0.57	28 * ± 1.71	25 * ± 0.00	26 * ± 0.00	27 * ± 1.71	29 ± 0.00	-
P. mirabilis	29 * ± 1.71	24 * ± 0.00	25 * ± 0.00	27 * ± 1.14	28 * ± 1.71	25 * ± 0.00	27 * ± 1.14	25 ± 0.57	24 * ± 0.00	28 ± 0.00	-
F. oxysporum	28 * ± 1.14	24 ± 0.57	27 ± 0.57	22 * ± 0.00	26 ± 0.57	23 ± 0.57	25 * ± 0.00	24 * ± 0.00	22 ± 0.57	-	29 ± 0.00
P. chrysogenum	22 ± 0.57	17 * ± 0.00	19 * ± 0.57	17 * ± 0.00	18 * ± 0.00	16 * ± 0.00	19 * ± 0.57	17 * ± 0.00	18 * ± 0.57	-	18 ± 0.00
A. niger	24 ± 0.57	19 ± 0.57	16 * ± 0.00	16 * ± 0.00	17 ± 0.57	18 * ± 0.00	17 * ± 0.00	18 * ± 0.00	16 * ± 0.00	-	45 ± 0.00

Note: Values are means ± SD of three independent experiments. * The *p*-values of one-way ANOVA indicate no significant differences ($p > 0.05$) among groups.

As shown in Table 2, all propolis extracts showed antibacterial activity against all strains tested, with the diameters of the inhibition zones varying between 16 and 29 mm. Sample S1 (from Transylvania) had the strongest inhibitory effect, and the most sensitive strain was that of *B. cereus*.

The extracts obtained from sample S1 displayed an intense antimicrobial efficacy, with the values of the inhibition zone diameter comparable to those recorded for the positive control ($p > 0.05$).

In the case of bacteria, it can be observed that for *B. subtilis* and *B. cereus*, the diameters of the inhibition zones produced by propolis were smaller than in the case of the antibiotic, but in the case of *P. aeruginosa* sample S1 showed a larger diameter of inhibition than that produced by ciprofloxacin.

All propolis extracts are presented in vitro antifungal activity against *F. oxysporum*, *P. chrysogenum*, and *A. niger*. The diameters of the inhibition zones are smaller than in the case of the antifungal, except for *P. chrysogenum*, where samples S1, S3, and S7 showed larger inhibition zones.

The comparative effect of Romanian propolis and its aqueous extracts on cereals and the species selected in the research has not been extensively studied.

2.4. Analysis of statistical data

2.4.1. Principal Component Analysis

Principal component analysis (PCA) was performed in two steps. In the first stage, the amounts of propolis powder C(1 g), C(5 g), C(10 g), and the control were used as input data (variables). The analysis (PCA) aimed to evaluate the phyto-inhibitory effect of propolis powder, in different amounts, on the four cereal samples, wheat, corn, barley, and oat, after 3, 5, 7, 9, 11, and 13 days.

Principal components were obtained based on the values of the correlation matrix. The eigenvalues were 3.64, 0.28, 0.057, and 0.013 for PC1–PC4. Figure 1 shows that the first two PCs explain 98.23% of the total data variance, PC1—91.20% and PC2—7.02%. In the second step, concentrations of propolis extracts, C(1%), C(5%), C(10%), and control were used as input data (variables). The purpose of the analysis (PCA) of this paper was to evaluate the phyto-inhibitory effect of propolis extracts of different concentrations on the four samples of cereals, wheat, corn, barley, and oats after 3, 5, 7, 9, 11, and 13 days. The eigenvalues were 3.81, 0.14, 0.035, and 0.0077 for PC1–PC4. In Figure 2, it can be seen that the first two PCs explain 98.91% of the total data variance. PC1—95.32 and PC2—3.59%.

Figure 1 shows observations and PCs obtained from the analyzed data. The first step is the use of propolis powder in the treatment of cereal samples. The scores graph of PC1 versus PC2 shows the formation of two groups of cereal samples. The first group, marked with a blue color and located at the top right, is composed of oat and barley samples after 9, 11, and 13 days of treatment with propolis powder. The second group, marked with a green color and located at the bottom right, is composed of corn and wheat samples after 9, 11, and 13 days of treatment with propolis powder. In the left center of the score graph, marked with a red color, cereal samples that showed a lower response in the first 3 to 7 days to treatment with propolis powder appear.

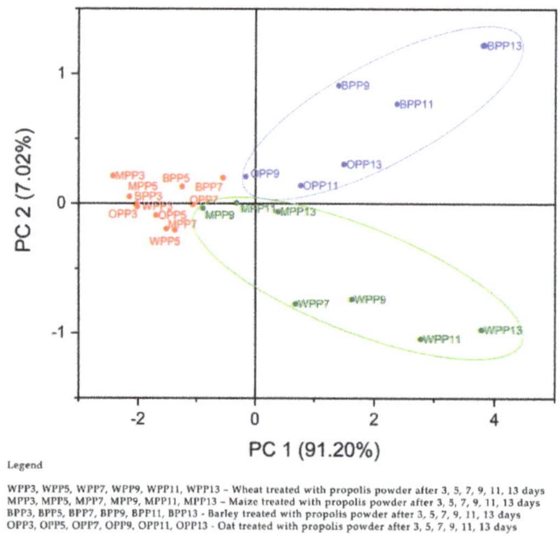

Figure 1. Scores plot of PCA scores of the four cereal samples according to their responses to propolis powder C(1 g), C(5 g), C(10 g), and the control sample.

Figure 2 shows observations and PCs obtained from the analyzed data. Step two shows the use of propolis extract in the treatment of cereal samples. Score plot PC1 versus PC2 shows the formation of the same cereal groups. The first group, marked with a blue color and located at the top right, is composed of oat and barley samples after 9, 11, and 13 days of treatment with propolis extract. The second group, marked with a green color located at the bottom right, is composed of corn samples after 9, 11, and 13 days and wheat after 7, 9, 11, and 13 days of treatment with propolis extract. At this stage, cereal samples, marked with a red color, located in the left central part, treated for 3–7 days with propolis extract did not show a favorable response to the phyto-inhibitory effect, except for the WPE7 sample.

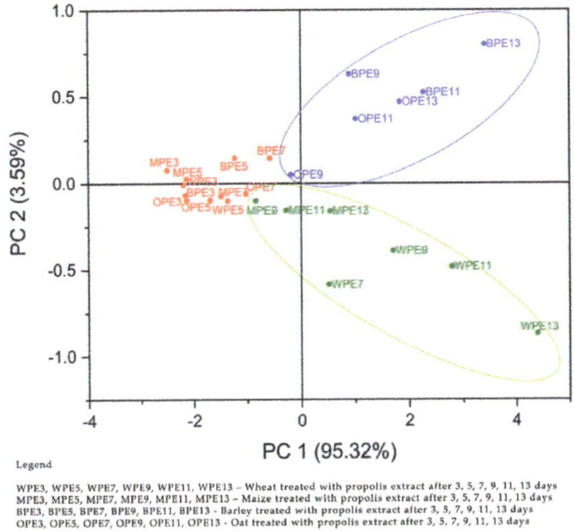

Figure 2. Scores plot for PCA analysis of the four cereal samples according to their responses to propolis extract C(1%), C(5%), C(10%), and the control sample.

It can be concluded that the values of the variables represented by the amount of propolis powder C 1 g, C 5 g, and C10 g, in the first stage and the concentrations of propolis extracts C1%, C5%, and C10% in the second stage (Figures S1 and S2), are useful in separating grain groups. For the cereal group consisting of oat and barley samples after 9, 11, and 13 days, the variables responsible for the classification were the amount of propolis powder of 10 g and the concentration of 10% propolis extract. For the cereal group consisting of corn and wheat samples after 7, 9, 11, and 13 days, responsible for the classification were the variables represented by the amount of propolis powder of 1 g and 5 g and the concentrations of 1% and 5% propolis solution. Regarding the treatment of cereal samples with propolis extract, it can be stated that it had a greater influence on the inhibition, the WPE7 sample being located in the lower right group of the score graph.

2.4.2. Analysis of Variance (ANOVA)

A two-way ANOVA is used to estimate if the geographical origin of Romanian propolis (nine samples) and the type of strain used (six strains) affect the diameter of the inhibition zone.

Table 3 shows the values obtained related to the dispersion analysis with two inputs for the two-way ANOVA.

Table 3. Bifactorial variance analysis for propolis samples and different microbial strains.

Dispersion Sums of the Diameters of Inhibition Zones	Quadratic Sum	Degrees of Freedom ν	Variance	$F_{computed}$	$F_{0.05}$
Between the propolis samples	70.15	5	14.03	6.69	2.45
Between strains	732.81	8	91.60	43.70	2.18
Residual, S_r	83.85	40	2.10	-	-

Because both in the case of propolis samples and the types of strains $F_{computed} > F_{0.05}$, we will reject the null hypothesis and conclude that the geographical origin of Romanian propolis and the type of strain used have a significant influence on the diameter of the zone of inhibition at a significance level $\alpha = 0.05$.

2.4.3. Pearson Correlation

A Pearson's correlation attempts to assess the relationship between the flavonoid and phenol content of propolis samples and the microbial strains used. The Pearson correlation coefficients are presented in Table 4.

Table 4. Pearson correlation coefficients and the interpretation of correlation for the relation of flavonoid and phenol content of propolis samples with microbial strain type.

Microbial Strains	Flavonoids		Phenols	
	Pearson	**Strength and Direction**	**Pearson**	**Strength and Direction**
B. subtilis	0.43	low positive	0.40	low positive
B. cereus	−0.88	high negative	−0.82	high negative
P. mirabilis	0.43	low positive	0.36	low positive
F. oxysporum	0.09	negligible	0.47	low positive
P. chrysogenum	0.45	low positive	0.74	high positive
A. niger	0.29	negligible	0.42	low positive

There was a statistically significant correlation between the flavonoid content and the diameter of the inhibition zone for the following strains: *B. subtilis* and *P. mirabilis*. A strong correlation is noticed between the phenols content and the diameter of the inhibition zone for the *P. chrysogenum* strain. The correlations between the diameter of the inhibition zone of the strains used and the content of phenols are stronger than in the case of flavonoids.

3. Discussion

The results of the physico–chemical properties of propolis from different regions of Romania showed differences between the samples, depending on the geographical origin with its specific flora. The water activity of sample S3 (from the Maramureș region) was 0.62 and 0.78 for S7 (Dobrogea region, Constanța County). According to Sunil et al. [26], samples with high humidity (water content) also show a higher water activity. The Indian crude propolis samples have an a_w between 0.68 and 0.73. Brazilian propolis a_w was 0.76 for red, 0.8 for green, and 0.87 for brown [27]. Hygroscopicity was relatively low, between 12.6 in S8 from Vaslui County (Moldavia region) and 14.7 g absorbed water/100 g sample in S6 from Dâmbovița County (Muntenia region), and coincides with the research of da Silva et al. [28] where the value is 13.1 g of adsorbed moisture per 100 g of dry solids.

Aqueous extracts of propolis usually contain up to 10 times lower amounts of active ingredients than alcoholic extracts due to the poor solubility of propolis and its bioactive compounds [29]. The water solubility of propolis samples from the regions of Romania varies between 8.26 and 13.43%, having values close to those obtained for Indian propolis, which varies from 8.71 to 19.28% [30].

Propolis has more than 300 natural chemical compounds [31]. Mainly, propolis contains flavonoids, phenolic acids, and their esters. For example, the total phenolic content of Polish propolis ranged from 150.05 to 197.14 mg/g GAE, while the total flavonoid content was 35.64–62.04 mg/g QE [32]. The phenolic content of propolis from Türkiye is 16.73 to 125.83 mg GAE/g sample, while the number of total flavonoids varied from 57.98 to 327.38 mg QE/g sample [33], depending on different geographical origins. The samples taken from all the regions of Romania accumulate large amounts of phenolic compounds

(189.4 mg of GAE/g in sample 7 from the Dobruja region), while the highest total flavonoid content was determined for the same sample and is 85.19 mg QE/g.

The antioxidant activity of the propolis was determined using the method with diphenylpicrylhydrazyl (DPPH) and ferric-reducing antioxidant power (FRAP). The results of the two methods used seem to be well correlated [34]. Other research [35,36] indicates that FRAP and DPPH values for propolis analyzed from other countries are compatible with our findings.

The phyto-inhibitory effect of propolis refers to its ability to inhibit seed germination and plant root growth. This effect is due to its high content of bioactive compounds, such as flavonoids and phenolic acids [37], which can interfere with the physiological processes of plants. Although propolis can be used as a natural treatment for weed control in agricultural practice, it must be considered that its use can negatively affect crop plants, depending on the dosage and the application method. For example, doses that are too high may result in plant death, while doses that are too low may have an insignificant effect. The antigerminative activity of propolis has been mentioned in the past [38–40], being considered a property attributed to the presence of an antibiotic factor in the composition. Studies targeting the germination percentage and cell division of wheat roots treated with propolis ethanolic extracts significantly inhibited the germination percentage compared to distilled water and control samples [41].

Regarding the effects of propolis on human health, its antioxidant, antimicrobial, anti-inflammatory, and anti-carcinogenic properties have been extensively studied. Studies have shown that flavonoids and other compounds in propolis can help reduce inflammation and protect against cell damage caused by free radicals [42]. Further investigations are needed to understand the exact health effects of propolis and the optimal doses for its use. When using products with propolis for therapeutic purposes, interactions with other drugs or food supplements may occur.

Compared to non-propolis-treated maize grains, the larger grain borer LGB population was lower in propolis-treated grains at all concentrations examined. Propolis's greatest benefits were observed at a 20% concentration [43].

A positive correlation was found between the amount of total polyphenols and flavonoid content and the DPPH radical scavenging activity and FRAP values of propolis samples. The relationship between the total phenol and flavonoid content and the antioxidant potential of propolis samples assessed using DPPH and FRAP is shown in Figures 3–6.

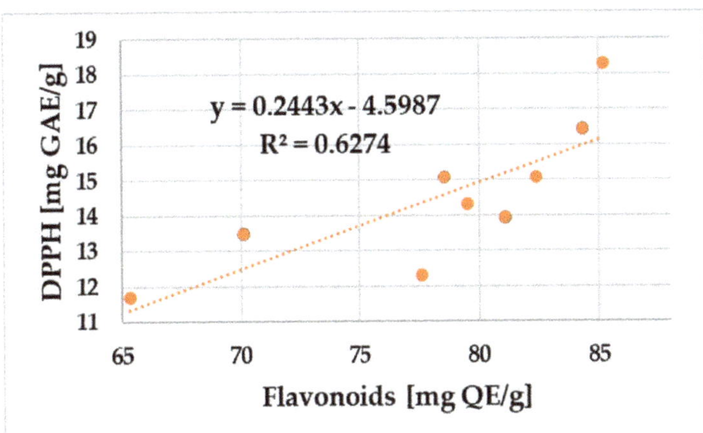

Figure 3. Correlation of total flavonoid content and DPPH free radical scavenging activity of the propolis samples.

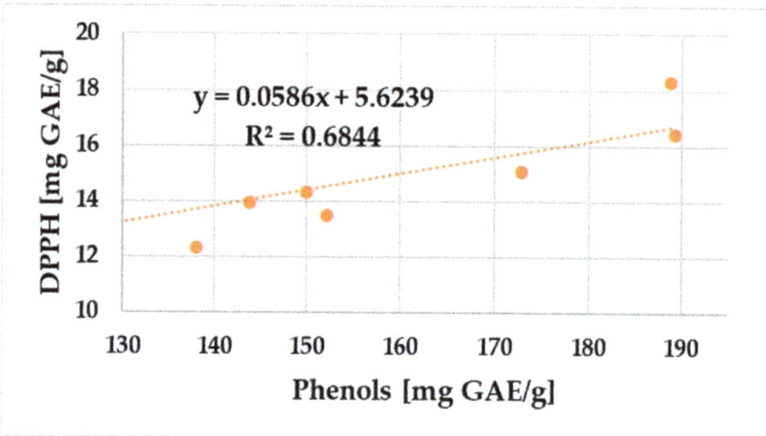

Figure 4. Correlation of total phenolic content and DPPH free radical scavenging activity of the propolis samples.

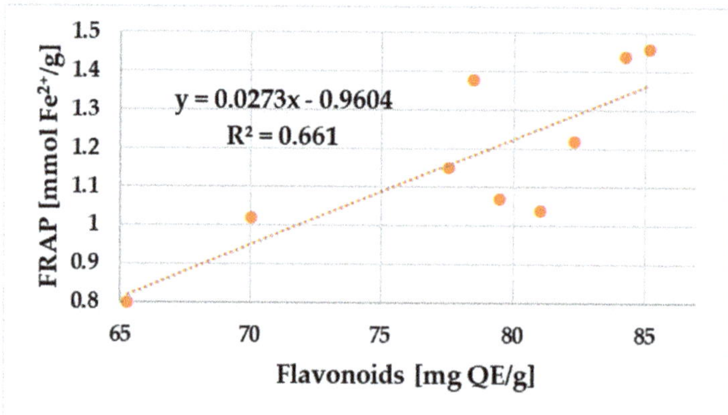

Figure 5. Correlation between total flavonoid content and FRAP in the propolis samples.

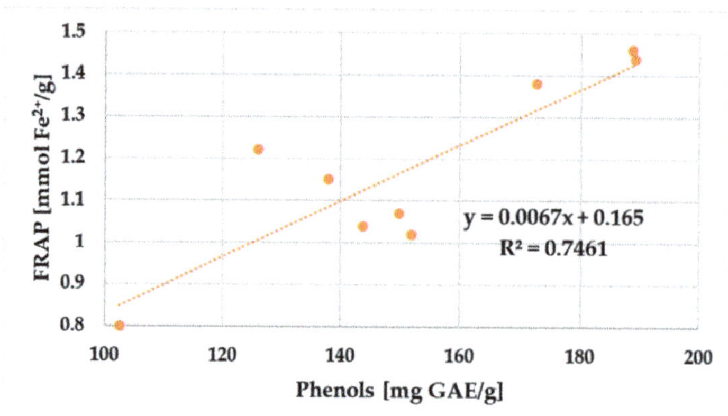

Figure 6. Correlation between total phenolic contents and FRAP in the propolis samples.

Figures 5 and 6 show that both total flavonoids (R^2 = 0.66) and phenolics (R^2 = 0.75) were moderate and very strongly correlated with FRAP antioxidant activity.

There is not enough scientific evidence to prove that propolis can be used as a natural treatment to combat weeds in agricultural practice. Most of the studies on the properties and benefits of propolis focus on its use in the food, pharmaceutical, or cosmetic industries. However, some research has shown that propolis can inhibit the growth of some species of bacteria and fungi that can affect plants. A study shows that propolis can have an antifungal effect against a fungus that affects potato crops [44,45].

In the case of the nine samples, a significant correlation (R^2 = 0.63) between the flavonoid content and the free radical scavenging assays was obtained. The total phenolics were also essentially correlated with DPPH antioxidant activity in Figure 4 (R^2 = 0.68).

In his research, Gonnet [46] demonstrated the phytotoxic and photo-inhibitory properties of propolis applied by bees on potatoes, which exhibited permanent inhibition. In addition, some studies have shown that propolis can have antimicrobial and antifungal properties, making it useful in controlling certain diseases and plant infections. However, these studies were conducted in the laboratory, and more research is needed to evaluate the effectiveness of propolis in agricultural practice.

In general, most of the research on the antimicrobial properties of propolis has been performed in vitro on microorganisms that affect human health, and few studies have focused on the antibacterial or antifungal effect of propolis against species that affect plants used as a food source. For example, a study that tested the antifungal effect of different concentrations of propolis extracts on some species that can affect plants showed that the most affected microorganisms at all propolis concentrations among the tested fungi were *Alternaria alternata* and *Penicillium digitatum* [47]. The results of another study showed that Colombian propolis extracts could act as antifungal agents against *Colletotrichum gloeosporioides* and *Botryodiplodia theobromae*, species that affect food products of vegetable origin [48].

Regarding Romanian propolis, some studies have tried to investigate its antimicrobial activity, confirming its antibacterial effect. Thus, a study on ethanolic extracts of propolis from Transylvania found a better sensitivity of the Gram-positive bacteria (*Staphylococcus aureus*, *Bacillus cereus*, and *Listeria monocytogenes*). At the same time, for *P. aeruginosa*, a total resistance was noticed, and inhibition zone diameters for *Candida albicans* showed a large variation [49]. Another study that investigated the antifungal activity of propolis fractions and ethanolic extracts of propolis from different regions of Romania showed that they exhibited antifungal and antibiofilm activity against all tested *Candida albicans* strains [50]. It was also observed that Romanian propolis ethanolic extracts showed strong antimicrobial efficacy against *E. coli* strains, positively correlated with chemical composition, along with an interesting synergistic interaction with antibiotics [51]. In contrast to these studies that investigated alcoholic propolis extracts, our study used aqueous extracts and demonstrated the antimicrobial activity of propolis.

Socio-economic development in recent years has influenced food contamination with fungi, thus creating the need for new antifungal agents to provide safer food. Our study showed that propolis is one of the promising natural antifungal agents and phyto-inhibitors.

4. Materials and Methods

4.1. Propolis Samples

Raw brown propolis samples were obtained directly from beekeepers. These were taken from wooden beehives. Sampling was performed by scraping the lid and entering the hives with a stainless steel spatula. The samples were taken during the same period of the year, between June and July 2021, from nine regions of Romania (Transylvania, Banat, Crișana, Maramureș, Oltenia, Muntenia, Dobruja, Moldavia, and Bukovina). The samples were kept at −18 °C in the dark until analysis.

Table 5 shows the number of samples, the region, the county, and the relief form related to where the sample was taken.

Table 5. The area, origin, and the landform form where the propolis samples were collected.

Sample	Region	County of Origin	Landforms
S1	Transilvania (Transylvania)	Alba	Mountainous
S2	Crișana	Bihor	Hilly
S3	Maramureș	Maramureș	Mountainous
S4	Banat	Timiș	Plain
S5	Oltenia (Lesser Wallachia)	Golj	Sub-mountainous
S6	Muntenia (Greater Wallachia)	Dâmbovița	Hilly
S7	Dobrogea (Dobruja)	Constanța	Plain
S8	Moldova (Moldavia)	Vaslui	Hilly
S9	Bucovina (Bukovina)	Suceava	Mountainous

Figure 7 shows the map and the regions of Romania, highlighting the counties where the samples were taken.

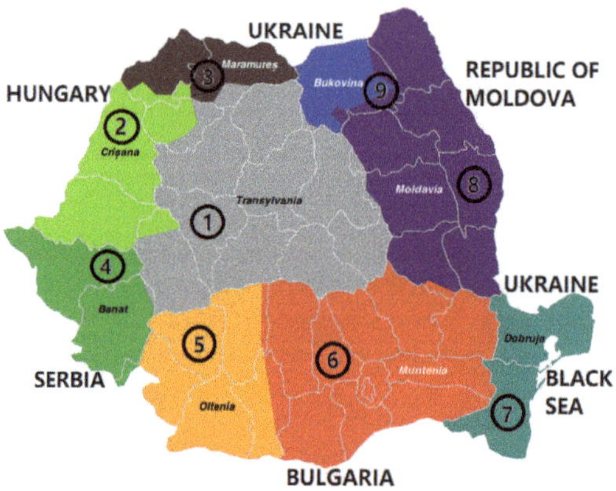

Figure 7. Map of the regions of Romania with propolis sampling points.

The numbers from 1 to 9 in Figure 7 represent the areas where the samples from S1 to S9 were taken (Table 5).

4.2. Cereal Samples

Table 6 shows the cereals used to determine the phyto-inhibitory activity of propolis and their characteristics. The temperature of the grains used was 26.5 °C.

Table 6. Cereals used and their characteristics.

Cereal Type	Scientific Name	Moisture (%)	Standard Mass Per Storage Volume (kg/hL)
Hexaploid bread wheat	*Triticum aestivum*	13.8	77.1
Maize	*Zea mays* L.	14.4	73.8
Oats	*Avena sativa* L.	12.9	41.1
Barley	*Hordeum vulgare* L.	14.2	63.7

4.3. Physico–Chemical Analysis

The water activity (a_w) of propolis was measured at 25 °C using the Aquaspector apparatus AQS-2-TC (Nagy Messsysteme GmbH, Gäufelden, Germany) [52].

Hygroscopicity. The method for determining hygroscopicity proposed by Cai and Corke [53] was used. A total of 10 g of propolis in 100 mL ultra-pure water was centrifuged

(70 rpm) in a centrifuge Centra CL2 (Thermo Fisher Scientific Inc., Waltham, MA, USA). The solutions were filtered using Whatman Filter Paper Grade No. 1 (Whatman International Ltd., Maidstone, UK), and the purified propolis extract was frozen at −50° C. The drying of the frozen propolis was performed in a condenser-type freeze dryer (TOPT-12A vacuum freeze dryer, Xi'an, China). A total of 2 g of propolis powder was kept at 25° C in a container with a saturated Na_2SO_4 solution (81% RH) for 7 days and then weighed. The hygroscopicity was expressed as g of absorbed water/100 g of propolis.

Water solubility. The Cano-Chauca et al. standard procedure [54] was applied. A total of 2 g of a propolis sample was spun (at 5000 rpm) for 5 min in a Centra CL2 centrifuge (Thermo Fisher Scientific Inc., Waltham, MA, USA) with twenty milliliters of distilled water. A total of 5 mL of the aliquot was dried at 105 °C in an oven. Solubility was measured using the sample's mass both before and after drying.

Determination of Total Phenolic Content (TPC). The Folin–Ciocalteu reagent technique [55,56] was applied. The TPC was calculated at 760 nm by interpolating propolis absorbance using a calibration curve made with standard gallic acid, 98%. The propolis samples' total phenolic content was expressed as the gallic acid equivalent (GAE) in one gram of raw propolis.

Determination of Total Flavonoid Content (TFC). A total of 2.5 mL of 96% ethanol and 1 g of finely ground propolis were centrifuged for 24 h at 200 rpm in a Centra CL2 centrifuge (Thermo Fisher Scientific Inc., Waltham, MA, USA). A 25 mL ethanol 80% adjustment was made to the mixture. A total of 0.1 mL of 10% $AlCl_3$, 1.5 mL of 95% ethanol, 0.1 mL of CH_3COO-K 1M, and 2.8 mL of distilled water were added separately. The mixture was kept in the dark for thirty minutes. The absorbance was measured at 425 nm using the Lambda 20—Perkin Elmer UV/VIS Spectrophotometer (Waltham, MA, USA). The TFC was calculated using a standard quercetin solution and a calibration curve. The TFC was expressed in mg of quercetin equivalents (QE)/100 g of propolis [57].

Ferric Reducing Antioxidant Power (FRAP). The 2,4,6-tripyridyl-S-triazine solution 10 mM (2.5 mL), $FeCl_3 \cdot 6H_2O$ solution 20 mM (2.5 mL), and 25 mL of 300 mM acetate buffer (pH 3.6) were used to prepare the FRAP reagent. In addition, 200 μL of propolis methanolic extracts (1 g in 7 mL methanol) was added along with 1.5 mL of a freshly made FRAP reagent, and the mixture was then maintained at 37 °C for four minutes. After the spectrophotometer calibration with 200 μL of distilled water, the absorbance was measured at 593 nm using the Lambda 20—Perkin Elmer UV/VIS (Waltham, MA, USA). The $FeSO_4$ (151.5–9.5 mg/mL) and the FRAP reagent were reacted to create the standard curve. [58,59].

The Antioxidant Activity of Propolis (RSA). In order to prepare the maceration, raw propolis was extracted using a 70% ethanol solution (1:100 *w*/*v*), homogenized continuously for 24 h, and then evaporated until it was completely dry. A mixture of 2,2-diphenyl-1-picrylhydrazyl (DPPH) 0.1 mM ethanoic solution and 0.6 mg/mL propolis solution was produced. The absorbance was measured at 515 nm using the Lambda 20—Perkin Elmer UV/VIS Spectrophotometer (Waltham, MA, USA). At the start of the reaction, as well as after 10 and 20 min, the absorbance (A) was measured. Using DPPH, one can calculate antioxidant activity as follows: % of antioxidant activity (RSA) = $(A_{DPPH} - A_{sample})/A_{DPPH} \times 100$ [60,61].

4.4. The Phyto-Inhibitory Activity of Propolis

The phyto-inhibitory effect was determined by assessing the germination duration (inhibiting growth) of specific cereal samples with physico–chemical attributes in standard systems, both with and without the controlled inclusion of propolis [62,63]. In Petri dishes (20 cm^2) containing a layer of hydrophilic wool, varying amounts of propolis (powder) or aqueous solutions at concentrations of 1%, 5%, and 10% were introduced—this process involved monitoring the selected cereals in the established environment every two days over a 13-day period, with statistical evaluations (averages) conducted on 10 germinated plants.

To produce the aqueous propolis extract, 50 g of propolis was finely chopped and ground into particles, after which 250 mL of distilled water was added, and the mixture was refluxed for 1 h in a round-bottomed flask equipped with a condenser. The resulting heterogeneous mixture underwent centrifugation (~4500× *g*) using a Centra CL2 centrifuge (Thermo Fisher Scientific Inc., Waltham, MA, USA), followed by coarse filtration through a vacuum-connected filter (Merck KgaA, Darmstadt, Germany). Subsequently, another centrifugation at ~4000× *g* took place, and the solution was further filtered (under vacuum) through a low-porosity surface. The final step involved heating at 100 °C until only 20% of the initial quantity remained [64].

4.5. Antimicrobial Activity of Propolis

The antibacterial efficacy of aqueous propolis extracts was assessed using three bacterial strains commonly found as contaminants in cereals: *Bacillus subtilis* (ATCC 6633), *Bacillus cereus* (ATCC 11788), and *Proteus mirabilis* (ATCC 7002). Additionally, the antifungal activity was determined against three fungal strains known to contaminate the cereals investigated in our study: *Fusarium oxysporum* (ATCC 48112), *Penicillium chrysogenum* (ATCC 10106), and *Aspergillus niger* (derived from ATCC 16888). All bacterial and fungal strains were procured from MicroBioLogics Inc. (St. Cloud, MN, USA) and Thermo Fisher Scientific Inc. (Waltham, MA, USA). The bacterial and fungal cultures were prepared by diluting overnight cultures in sterile normal saline, and the turbidity of cell suspensions was adjusted to 0.5 McFarland using a McFarland densitometer (Mettler Toledo, Columbus, OH, USA).

The antimicrobial attributes of propolis extracts were examined using the disk diffusion method in accordance with the procedures recommended by CLSI [65]. The diameters of the inhibition zones generated by microorganisms were regarded as a semi-quantitative indicator of the antimicrobial activity. A Mueller–Hinton agar (Merck KgaA, Darmstadt, Germany) was used as the culture medium for bacterial strains, while a Sabouraud 4% dextrose agar (Merck KgaA) was employed for fungal strains. Petri dishes containing culture media were inoculated by flooding with 1 mL of each culture, evenly spreading it across the entire surface.

For the test, 6 mm filter paper discs with 50 µL of each propolis aqueous extract (0.1 g/mL), obtained as described earlier, were utilized. The discs were aseptically positioned on the culture medium surface at approximately equal distances. Discs containing 5 µg ciprofloxacin (Bio-Rad, Marnes-la-Coquette, France) served as a positive control for bacterial growth, while discs with 1 µg voriconazole (Bio-Rad, France) acted as a positive control for fungal growth. Following a 2 h storage at 5 °C, the Petri dishes underwent incubation for 24 h at 37 °C for bacterial growth and 5 days at 25 °C for fungal growth. The measurement of inhibition zone diameters (in mm) was conducted using a DIN 862 ABS digital caliper (Fuzhou Conic Industrial Co., Ltd., Fuzhou, China). All experiments were conducted in triplicate, by the same operator, and under identical laboratory conditions, with the results expressed as the average of the three tests.

4.6. Statistical Analysis

Using a two-way analysis of variance (ANOVA), the significance of the variation in inhibition zone diameters was assessed based on the strain type tested and the propolis's geographic point of origin. In order to examine the relationship between the diameter of the inhibition zone and the flavonoid and phenol content of propolis samples, as well as the germination periods of cereal samples treated with propolis, this study used principal component analysis (PCR) and the Pearson correlation coefficient.

5. Conclusions

The bioactive properties of propolis result from the collective action of its various constituents, including flavonoids and phenolic compounds, found in appreciable quantities in propolis from all the regions of Romania. The highest content of phenols and flavonoids was found in propolis samples from Alba and Constanța Counties.

The propolis samples had a phyto-inhibitory effect on the germination of cereal seeds depending on the way they were used (powder or aqueous extract), the concentration used, and the geographical area where they were taken. The propolis samples present antimicrobial activity against all studied bacterial and fungal strains, making them useful in controlling certain plant diseases and infections.

Due to its properties, Romanian propolis can be integrated with other ecological control methods to manage the infestation of cereal crops. Propolis can be used to manage plant crops in the fight against some microorganisms as an alternative to the intensive, conventional practice in ecological agriculture.

Supplementary Materials: The following supporting information can be downloaded at https://www.mdpi.com/article/10.3390/antibiotics12121682/s1, Figure S1: Explanation of the total variance of the PCs, respectively the eigenvariance for each of the PCs in the case of the first stage PCA analysis; Figure S2. Explanation of the total variance of the PCs, respectively the eigenvariance for each of the PCs in the case of the second stage PCA analysis; Table S1: Plumule growth lengths (mm) for wheat samples treated with different amounts of propolis powder in time; Table S2: Plumule growth lengths (mm) for wheat samples treated with different concentrations of propolis extract in time; Table S3: Plumule growth lengths (mm) for corn samples treated with different amounts of propolis powder in time; Table S4: Plumule growth lengths (mm) for corn samples treated with different concentrations of propolis extract in time; Table S5: Plumule growth lengths (mm) for barley samples treated with different amounts of propolis powder in time; Table S6: Plumule growth lengths (mm) for barley samples treated with different concentrations of propolis extract in time; Table S7: Plumule growth lengths (mm) for oat samples treated with different amounts of propolis powder in time; Table S8: Plumule growth lengths (mm) for oat samples treated with different concentrations of propolis extract in time.

Author Contributions: Conceptualization, M.G. and M.L.V.; methodology, R.C.H.-M.; software, G.H.-M.; validation, G.-A.D., I.R. and M.P.; formal analysis, D.M.P.; investigation, R.C.H.-M., M.G. and M.L.V.; resources, M.G.; data curation, G.H.-M.; writing—original draft preparation, M.G.; writing—review and editing, M.L.V.; visualization, I.R.; supervision, M.P.; project administration, D.M.P.; funding acquisition, G.-A.D., M.L.V. and I.R. All authors have read and agreed to the published version of the manuscript.

Funding: This research paper is supported by the project "Increasing the impact of excellence in research on the capacity for innovation and technology transfer within USAMVB Timisoara", project code 6PFE, submitted in the competition Program 1—Development of the national system of research-development, Subprogram 1.2—Institutional performance, Institutional development projects—Development projects of excellence in R.D.I.

Institutional Review Board Statement: Not applicable.

Informed Consent Statement: Not applicable.

Data Availability Statement: Data are contained within the article and supplementary materials.

Acknowledgments: We thank the research team from all involved universities for their good collaboration and valuable contributions during the critical stages of the experiments and analyses. Gratitude to the Romanian beekeepers who made the propolis available to us and the constant and essential work of colleagues in the laboratory, which involved a large number of determinations.

Conflicts of Interest: The authors declare no conflict of interest.

References

1. Khalifa, S.A.M.; Elshafiey, E.H.; Shetaia, A.A.; El-Wahed, A.A.A.; Algethami, A.F.; Musharraf, S.G.; AlAjmi, M.F.; Zhao, C.; Masry, S.H.D.; Abdel-Daim, M.M.; et al. Overview of Bee Pollination and Its Economic Value for Crop Production. *Insects* **2021**, *12*, 688. [CrossRef] [PubMed]
2. Pasupuleti, V.R.; Sammugam, L.; Ramesh, N.; Gan, S.H. Honey, Propolis, and Royal Jelly: A Comprehensive Review of Their Biological Actions and Health Benefits. *Oxid. Med. Cell. Longev.* **2017**, *2017*, 1259510. [CrossRef] [PubMed]
3. Saccardi, L.; Brümmer, F.; Schiebl, J.; Schwarz, O.; Kovalev, A.; Gorb, S. Interaction between honeybee mandibles and propolis. *Beilstein J. Nanotechnol.* **2022**, *13*, 958–974. [CrossRef] [PubMed]
4. Przybyłek, I.; Karpiński, T.M. Antibacterial Properties of Propolis. *Molecules* **2019**, *24*, 2047. [CrossRef] [PubMed]

5. Schnitzler, P.; Neuner, A.; Nolkemper, S.; Zundel, C.; Nowack, H.; Sensch, K.H.; Reichling, J. Antiviral activity and mode of action of propolis extracts and selected compounds. *Phytother. Res.* **2010**, *24*, 632. [CrossRef]
6. Ahlam, A.G.; Youssf, A.E.; Omnia, A.E.; Taha, M. Antimicrobial Activity of Propolis Against Some Bacteria and Fungi. *Zag. Vet. J.* **2013**, *41*, 81–97.
7. Castaldo, S.; Capasso, F. Propolis, an old remedy used in modern medicine. *Fitoterapia* **2002**, *73*, S1–S6. [CrossRef]
8. Golder, W. Proopolis—Das Kittharz der Bienen im Schrifttum der Antike [Propolis. The bee glue as presented by the Graeco-Roman literature]. *Wurzbg. Medizinhist. Mitt.* **2004**, *23*, 133–145.
9. Gniewosz, M.; Pobiega, K.; Olbryś, N.; Kraśniewska, K.; Synowiec, A. The Effect of Ethanol Propolis Extracts on Inhibition of Growth of Fusarium solani on Hen Eggs. *Appl. Sci.* **2023**, *13*, 315. [CrossRef]
10. Hossain, R.; Quispe, C.; Khan, R.A.; Saikat, A.S.M.; Ray, P.; Ongalbek, D.; Yeskaliyeva, B.; Jain, D.; Smeriglio, A.; Trombetta, D.; et al. Propolis: An update on its chemistry and pharmacological applications. *Chin. Med.* **2022**, *17*, 100. [CrossRef]
11. De Carvalho, G.J.L.; Sodré, G.S. Application of propolis in agriculture. *Arq. Inst. Biol.* **2021**, *88*, e0632019. [CrossRef]
12. Braakhuis, A. Evidence on the Health Benefits of Supplemental Propolis. *Nutrients* **2019**, *11*, 2705. [CrossRef] [PubMed]
13. Moraes, W.B.; Jesus Jr, W.C.; Belan, L.L.; Peixoto, L.A.; Pereira, A.J. Aplicação foliar de fungicidas e produtos alternativos reduz a severidade do oídio do tomateiro. *Nucleus* **2011**, *8*, 57–68. [CrossRef]
14. dos Santos Pereira, A.; Seixas, F.R.M.S.; de Aquino Neto, F.R. Própolis: 100 anos de pesquisa e suas perspectivas futuras. *Quím. Nova* **2002**, *25*, 321–326. [CrossRef]
15. Pereira, C.S.; Maia, L.F.P.; de Paula, F.S. Aplicação de extrato etanólico de própolis no crescimento e produtividade do feijoeiro comum. *Rev. Ceres* **2014**, *61*, 98–104. [CrossRef]
16. Pereira, C.S.; Matte, W.D.; Venâncio, P.H.B. Aplicação de extrato de própolis na agricultura. *Rev. Ciênc. Agro-Ambient.* **2016**, *14*, 143–156.
17. Marini, D.; Mensch, R.; Freiberger, M.B.; Dartora, J.; Franzener, G.; Garcia, R.C.; Stangarlin, J.R. Efeito antifúngico de extratos alcoólicos de própolis sobre patógenos da videira. *Arq. Inst. Biol.* **2012**, *79*, 305–308. [CrossRef]
18. Atikovic, A.; Salkic, B.; Imsirovic, E. Impact of propolis on the occurrence and development of phytopathogenic fungi. *Int. J. Adv. Res.* **2020**, *8*, 982–990. [CrossRef]
19. Yıldırım, H.K. Assessment of Propolis Treated by Different Extraction Methods. *Braz. Arch. Biol. Technol.* **2022**, *65*, e22210251. [CrossRef]
20. Pereira, C.S.; Guimarães, R.J.; Pozza, E.A.; Silva, A.A. Controle da cercosporiose e da ferrugem do cafeeiro com extrato etanólico de própolis. *Rev. Ceres Viçosa* **2008**, *55*, 369–376.
21. Mello, B.C.B.S.; Petrus, J.C.C.; Hubinger, M.D. Desempenho do processo de concentração de extratos de própolis por nanofiltração. *Food Sci. Technol.* **2010**, *30*, 166–172. [CrossRef]
22. Pobiega, K.; Kraśniewska, K.; Gniewosz, M. Application of propolis in antimicrobial and antioxidative protection of food quality—A review. *Trends Food Sci. Technol.* **2019**, *83*, 53–62. [CrossRef]
23. Curifuta, M.; Vidal, J.; Sánchez-Venegas, J.; Contreras, A.; Salazar, L.A.; Alvear, M. The in vitro antifungal evaluation of a commercial extract of Chilean propolis against six fungi of agricultural importance. *Agric. Nat. Resour.* **2012**, *39*, 347–359. [CrossRef]
24. Vica, M.L.; Glevitzky, M.; Dumitrel, G.A.; Bostan, R.; Matei, H.V.; Kartalska, Y.; Popa, M. Qualitative characterization and antifungal activity of Romanian honey and propolis. *Antibiotics* **2022**, *11*, 1552. [CrossRef]
25. Desoky, E.S.M.; Elrys, A.S.; Mansour, E.; Eid, R.S.M.; Selem, E.; Rady, M.M.; Ali, E.F.; Mersal, G.A.M.; Semida, W.M. Application of biostimulants promotes growth and productivity by fortifying the antioxidant machinery and suppressing oxidative stress in faba bean under various abiotic stresses. *Sci. Hortic.* **2021**, *288*, 110340. [CrossRef]
26. Sunil, L.S.; Vignesh, S.; Meenatchi, R. Physicochemical properties and antimicrobial activity of Indian propolis. *J. Pharm. Innov.* **2021**, *10*, 1660–1664.
27. Devequi-Nunes, D.; Machado, B.A.S.; Barreto, G.A.; Rebouças Silva, J.; da Silva, D.F.; da Rocha, J.L.C.; Brandão, H.N.; Borges, V.; Umsza Guez, M.A.A. Chemical characterization and biological activity of six different extracts of propolis through conventional methods and supercritical extraction. *PLoS ONE* **2018**, *13*, e0207676. [CrossRef]
28. da Silva, F.C.; Favaro-Trindade, C.S.; de Alencar, S.M.; Thomazini, M.; Balieiro, J.C.C. Physicochemical properties, antioxidant activity and stability of spray-dried propolis. *J. ApiProd. ApiMed. Sci.* **2011**, *3*, 94–100. [CrossRef]
29. Juodeikaitė, D.; Žilius, M.; Briedis, V. Preparation of Aqueous Propolis Extracts Applying Microwave-Assisted Extraction. *Processes* **2022**, *10*, 1330. [CrossRef]
30. Pant, K.; Thakur, M.; Chopra, H.K.; Nanda, V.; Ansari, M.J.; Pietramellara, G.; Pathan, S.I.; Alharbi, S.A.; Almoallim, H.S.; Datta, R. Characterization and discrimination of Indian propolis based on physico-chemical, techno-functional, thermal and textural properties: A multivariate approach. *J. King Saud Univ. Sci.* **2021**, *33*, 101405. [CrossRef]
31. Anjum, S.I.; Ullah, A.; Khan, K.A.; Attaullah, M.; Khan, H.; Ali, H.; Bashir, M.A.; Tahir, M.; Ansari, M.J.; Ghramh, H.A.; et al. Composition and functional properties of propolis (bee glue): A review. *Saudi J. Biol. Sci.* **2019**, *26*, 1695–1703. [CrossRef]
32. Socha, R.; Gałkowska, D.; Bugaj, M.; Juszczak, L. Phenolic composition and antioxidant activity of propolis from various regions of Poland. *Nat. Prod. Res.* **2015**, *29*, 416–422. [CrossRef]
33. Altuntaş, Ü.; Güzel, İ.; Özçelik, B. Phenolic Constituents, Antioxidant and Antimicrobial Activity and Clustering Analysis of Propolis Samples Based on PCA from Different Regions of Anatolia. *Molecules* **2023**, *28*, 1121. [CrossRef]

34. Okuyan, S.; Mehmetoglu, S.; Çakici, N. Antioxidant Variability of Propolis Collected from Different Zones in Hives. *Bee Stud.* **2020**, *12*, 1–4. [CrossRef]
35. Hernández Zarate, M.S.; Abraham Juárez, M. del R.; Cerón García, A.; Ozuna López, C.; Gutiérrez Chávez, A.J.; Segoviano Garfias, J.deJ.N.; Avila Ramos, F. Flavonoids, phenolic content, and antioxidant activity of propolis from various areas of Guanajuato, Mexico. *Food Sci. Technol.* **2018**, *38*, 210–215. [CrossRef]
36. Mihai, C.M.; Mărghitaş, L.A.; Dezmirean, D.S.; Bărnuţiu, L. Correlation between Polyphenolic Profile and Antioxidant Activity of Propolis from Transylvania. *J. Anim. Sci. Biotechnol.* **2011**, *44*, 100–103.
37. Marghitas, L.A. *Albinele și Produsele lor*, 2nd ed.; Ceres Press: Bucuresti, Romania, 2008; pp. 168–175. (In Romanian)
38. Lavie, P. Les substances antibactériennes dans la colonie d'abeilles (*Apis mellifica* L.). *Les Annales de l'Abeille* **1960**, *3*, 103–183.
39. Marchenko, A.I. L'usage de la Propolis en Stomatology. Ph.D. Thesis, Leningrad State University, Leningrad, Russia, 1960; pp. 57–58. (In Russian).
40. Derevici, A.; Popesco, A.; Popesco, N. Recherches sur certaines propriétés biologiques de la propolis. *Ann. Abeille* **1964**, *7*, 191–200. [CrossRef]
41. Sorkun, K.; Bozcuk, S.; Gomurgen, A.N.; Tekin, F. An Inhibitory Effect of Propolis on Germination and Cell Division in the Root Tips of Wheat Seedlings. In *International Conference on Bee Products: Properties, Applications, and Apitherapy*; Springer: Boston, MA, USA, 1996.
42. Gulcin, I.; Bursal, E.; Sehitoglu, M.H.; Bilsel, M.; Goren, A.C. Polyphenol contents and antioxidant activity of lyophilized aqueous extract of propolis from Erzurum, Turkey. *Food Chem. Toxicol.* **2010**, *48*, 2227–2238. [CrossRef]
43. Osipitan Adebola, A.; Ogunbanwo Ibikunle, A.; Adeleye Issa, G.; Adekanmbi Dende, I. Propolis production by honey bee *Apis mellifera* (*Hymenoptera: Apidae*) and its potential for the management of the larger grain borer *Prostephanus truncates* (*Horn*) (*Coleoptera: Bostrichidae*) on maize grains. *J. Plant Prot. Res.* **2010**, *50*, 61–66.
44. Mercan, N.; Guvensen, A.; Çelik, A.; Katırcıoğlu, H.T. Antimicrobial activity and pollen composition of honey samples collected from different provinces in Turkey. *Nat. Prod. Res.* **2007**, *21*, 187–195. [CrossRef]
45. Sallemi, S.; Lekired, A.; Korbi, N.; Saadouli, I.; Cherif, A.; Zidi, I.; Klibi, N.; Ouzari, H.I.; Mosbah, A. Fungal Community Investigation from Propolis Natural Products: Diversity and Antibacterial Activities Evaluation. *Evid.-Based Complement. Altern. Med.* **2022**, *2022*, 7151655. [CrossRef]
46. Gonnet, M. Propriétés phytoinhibitrices de la colonie d'abeilles (*Apis mellifica* L.). Il-action de la propolis et de quelques autres produits de la ruche sur la croissance chez "*Solanum tuberosum*". *Les Annales de l'Abeille* **1968**, *11*, 105–116.
47. Özcan, M. Antifungal Properties of Propolis. *Grasas y Aceites* **1999**, *50*, 395–398. [CrossRef]
48. Meneses, E.A.; Durango, D.L.; García, C.M. Antifungal activity against postharvest fungi by extracts from Colombian propolis. *Quím. Nova* **2009**, *32*, 2011–2017. [CrossRef]
49. Marghitas, L.A.; Mihai, C.M.; Chirila, F.; Dezmirean, D.S.; Fit, N.I. The Study of the Antimicrobial Activity of Transylvanian (Romanian) Propolis. *Not. Bot. Horti Agrobot. Cluj-Napoca* **2010**, *38*, 40–44.
50. Stan, T.; Teodor, E.D.; Gatea, F.; Chifiriuc, C.M.; Lazăr, V. Antioxidant and antifungal activity of Romanian propolis. *Rom. Biotechnol. Lett.* **2017**, *22*, 13116–13124.
51. Niculae, M.; Stan, L.; Pall, E.; Paștiu, A.I.; Balaci, I.M.; Muste, S.; Spînu, M. In vitro Synergistic Antimicrobial Activity of Romanian Propolis and Antibiotics against *Escherichia coli* Isolated from Bovine Mastitis. *Not. Bot. Horti Agrobot. Cluj-Napoca* **2015**, *43*, 327–334. [CrossRef]
52. AOAC. *978.18 Water Activity. Official Methods of Analysis of the Association of Official Analytical Chemist*, 16th ed.; Association of Official Analytical Chemists: Washington, DC, USA, 1995.
53. Cai, Y.Z.; Corke, H. Production and properties of spray-dried Amaranthus betacyanin pigments. *J. Food Sci.* **2000**, *65*, 1248–1252. [CrossRef]
54. Cano-Chauca, M.; Stringheta, P.C.; Ramos, A.M.; Cal-Vidal, J. Effect of the carriers on the microstructure of mango powder obtained by spray drying and its functional characterization. *Innov. Food Sci. Emerg. Technol.* **2005**, *6*, 420–428. [CrossRef]
55. Bogdanov, S. *Harmonised Methods of the International Honey Commission*; Swiss Bee Research Centre, FAM: Liebefeld, Switzerland, 2009; p. 63.
56. Singleton, V.L.; Orthofer, R.; Lamuela-Raventós, R.M. Analysis of total phenols and other oxidation substrates and antioxidants by means of Folin-Ciocalteu reagent. *Methods Enzymol.* **1999**, *29*, 10–18.
57. Chang, C.C.; Yang, M.H.; Wen, H.M.; Chern, J.K. Estimation of Total Flavonoid Content in Propolis by Two Complementary Colorimetric Methods. *J. Food Drug Anal.* **2002**, *10*, 178–182.
58. Ahmed, M.; Imtiaz Shafiq, M.; Khaleeq, A.; Huma, R.; Abdul Qadir, M.; Khalid, A.; Ali, A.; Samad, A. Physiochemical, biochemical, minerals content analysis, and antioxidant potential of national and international honeys in Pakistan. *J. Chem.* **2016**, *2016*, 8072305. [CrossRef]
59. ALaerjani, W.M.A.; Khan, K.A.; Al-Shehri, B.M.; Ghramh, H.A.; Hussain, A.; Mohammed, M.E.A.; Imran, M.; Ahmad, I.; Ahmad, S.; Al-Awadi, A.S. Chemical Profiling, Antioxidant, and Antimicrobial Activity of Saudi Propolis Collected by Arabian Honey Bee (*Apis mellifera jemenitica*) Colonies. *Antioxidants* **2022**, *11*, 1413. [CrossRef] [PubMed]
60. Mărghitas, L.A.; Dezmirean, D.; Moise, A.; Mihai, C.; Laslo, L. DPPH method for evaluation of propolis antioxidant activity. *Bull. Univ. Agric. Sci.* **2009**, *66*, 253–258.

61. Popova, M.; Bankova, V.; Butovska, D.; Petkov, V.; Nikolova-Damyanova, B.; Sabatini, A.G.; Marcazzan, G.L.; Bogdanov, S. Validated methods for the quantification of biologically active constituents of poplar type propolis. *Phytochem. Anal.* **2004**, *15*, 235–240. [CrossRef]
62. Biron, R.C.; Hegheduş-Mîndru, G.; Hădărugă, N.G.; Jianu, C.; Ştef, D.; Jianu, I. Activitatea Fitoinhibitorie a Propolisului Recoltat din Zona de Vest a României—Partea I—Vol. 50, Seria Agronomie, Supplement. Lucrări Ştiinţifice, Universitatea de Ştiinţe Agricole şi Medicină Veterinară Iaşi. 2007, pp. 462–467. Available online: https://www.uaiasi.ro/revagrois/PDF/2007s_462.pdf (accessed on 14 March 2023). (In Romanian).
63. Kirby, L.T.; Styles, E.D. Flavonoids associated with specific gene action in maize and the role of light in substituting for the action of a gene. *Can. J. Genet. Cytol.* **1970**, *12*, 934–940. [CrossRef]
64. Vică, M.L.; Glevitzky, M.; Tit, D.M.; Behl, T.; Heghedus-Mîndru, R.C.; Zaha, D.C.; Ursu, F.; Popa, M.; Glevitzky, I.; Bungau, S. The antimicrobial activity of honey and propolis extracts from the central region of Romania. *Food Biosci.* **2021**, *41*, 101014. [CrossRef]
65. Clinical and Laboratory Standard Institute. Performance Standards for Antimicrobial Susceptibility Testing. 2020. Available online: https://clsi.org/media/3481/m100ed30_sample.pdf (accessed on 2 November 2023).

antibiotics

MDPI

Article

Specific Antimicrobial Activities Revealed by Comparative Evaluation of Selected Gemmotherapy Extracts

Melinda Héjja [1,2], Emőke Mihok [2,3], Amina Alaya [2,3], Maria Jolji [1,2], Éva György [4], Noemi Meszaros [5], Violeta Turcus [5,6], Neli Kinga Oláh [7,8] and Endre Máthé [2,5,*]

1 Doctoral School of Nutrition and Food Science, Faculty of Agricultural and Food Sciences and Environmental Management, University of Debrecen, Böszörményi Str. 128, 4032 Debrecen, Hungary; hejja.melinda@agr.unideb.hu (M.H.); maria.jolji@agr.unideb.hu (M.J.)

2 Institute of Nutrition Science, Faculty of Agricultural and Food Sciences and Environmental Management, University of Debrecen, Böszörményi Str. 128, 4032 Debrecen, Hungary; mihokemoke@uni.sapientia.ro (E.M.); aleya.amina@agr.unideb.hu (A.A.)

3 Doctoral School of Animal Science, Faculty of Agricultural and Food Sciences and Environmental Management, University of Debrecen, Böszörményi Str. 128, 4032 Debrecen, Hungary

4 Department of Food Science, Faculty of Economics, Socio-Human Sciences and Engineering, Sapientia Hungarian University of Transylvania, Libertății sq. 1., 530104 Miercurea Ciuc, Romania; gyorgyeva@uni.sapientia.ro

5 Department of life Sciences, Faculty of Medicine, Vasile Goldis Western University of Arad, L. Rebreanu Str. 86, 310414 Arad, Romania; noe.meszaros@gmail.com (N.M.); violeta_buruiana@yahoo.com (V.T.)

6 CE-MONT Mountain Economy Center, Costin C. Kirițescu National Institute of Economic Research, Romanian Academy, Petreni Str. 49, 725700 Suceava, Romania

7 Department of Pharmaceutical Chemistry, Faculty of Pharmacy, Vasile Goldis, Western University of Arad, L. Rebreanu Str. 86, 310414 Arad, Romania; neli.olah@plantextrakt.ro

8 PlantExtrakt Ltd., No. 46, 407059 Cluj, Romania

* Correspondence: endre.mathe@agr.unideb.hu; Tel.: +36-305396075

Abstract: Nowadays, unprecedented health challenges are urging novel solutions to address antimicrobial resistance as multidrug-resistant strains of bacteria, yeasts and moulds are emerging. Such microorganisms can cause food and feed spoilage, food poisoning and even more severe diseases, resulting in human death. In order to overcome this phenomenon, it is essential to identify novel antimicrobials that are naturally occurring, biologically effective and increasingly safe for human use. The development of gemmotherapy extracts (GTEs) using plant parts such as buds and young shoots has emerged as a novel approach to treat/prevent human conditions due to their associated antidiabetic, anti-inflammatory and/or antimicrobial properties that all require careful evaluations. Seven GTEs obtained from plant species like the olive (*Olea europaea* L.), almond (*Prunus amygdalus* L.), black mulberry (*Morus nigra* L.), walnut (*Juglans regia* L.), blackberry (*Rubus fruticosus* L.), blackcurrant (*Ribes nigrum* L.) and bilberry (*Vaccinium myrtillus* L.) were tested for their antimicrobial efficiency via agar diffusion and microbroth dilution methods. The antimicrobial activity was assessed for eight bacterial (*Bacillus cereus*, *Staphylococcus aureus*, *Salmonella enterica* subsp. *enterica*, *Proteus vulgaris*, *Enterococcus faecalis*, *Escherichia coli*, *Pseudomonas aeruginosa* and *Listeria monocytogenes*), five moulds (*Aspergillus flavus*, *Aspergillus niger*, *Aspergillus ochraceus*, *Penicillium citrinum*, *Penicillium expansum*) and one yeast strain (*Saccharomyces cerevisiae*). The agar diffusion method revealed the blackberry GTE as the most effective since it inhibited the growth of three bacterial, four moulds and one yeast species, having considered the total number of affected microorganism species. Next to the blackberry, the olive GTE appeared to be the second most efficient, suppressing five bacterial strains but no moulds or yeasts. The minimum inhibitory concentration (MIC) and minimum bactericidal concentration (MBC) were then determined for each GTE and the microorganisms tested. Noticeably, the olive GTE appeared to feature the strongest bacteriostatic and bactericidal outcome, displaying specificity for *S. aureus*, *E. faecalis* and *L. monocytogenes*. The other GTEs, such as blueberry, walnut, black mulberry and almond (the list indicates relative strength), were more effective at suppressing microbial growth than inducing microbial death. However, some species specificities were also evident, while the blackcurrant GTE had no significant antimicrobial activity. Having seen the antimicrobial properties of the analysed GTEs, especially the olive and black mulberry GTEs, these could be envisioned as potential antimicrobials that might enhance antibiotic therapies efficiency, while the blackberry GTE would act as an antifungal agent. Some of the GTE mixtures analysed have shown interesting antimicrobial synergies, and all the antimicrobial effects observed argue for extending these studies to include pathological microorganisms.

Keywords: gemmotherapy extracts; antimicrobial activity; antifungal activity; *Morus nigra; Juglans regia; Prunus amygdalus; Olea europaea; Ribes nigrum; Rubus fruticosus; Vaccinium myrtillus*

1. Introduction

Many studies claim that antimicrobial resistance (AMR) is one of the major public health problems and that, if nothing is done, AMR could be one of the leading causes of mortality by 2050 [1]. To this day, an estimated 700,000 people die yearly from AMR-related diseases, and without an effective plan, an estimated 10 million people could die from the same causes by the year 2050. This is not only a scientifically challenging task but also bears an enormous economic cost, by some estimates at around USD 100 trillion of worth [2]. One of the main reasons for this happening is the liberal use of antibiotics, as well as the relatively limited number of available types of antibiotics, leading to an ever-increasing number of drug-resistant processes in bacteria [3]. It is a relatively well-known fact that pathogenic bacteria adapt to different antibacterial agents, and these can be divided into four major categories: drug uptake limitation, drug target modification, drug inactivation and active drug efflux. Drug resistance processes can also vary based on the type of bacteria (Gram-negative or Gram-positive), changing their structures. Out of the thirty-two types of antibacterial agents in development in 2019, only six were considered novel by the WHO, and, as such, the development of a very good quality antimicrobial drug remains a major problem. Recently, there has been an increasing interest in natural substance-based antibiotics. While the existing types of antimicrobial agents remain in use, albeit with reduced effectiveness, and there are some new types of synthetically manufactured drugs, one can argue that natural substances show great promise in this regard [2].

These natural substances also showed potential in preventing diseases caused by drug-tolerant and resistant strains of microorganisms. There are several studies that prove that plant extracts have antimicrobial effects against multidrug-resistant bacteria. For example, Mascarello et al. (2018) reported that eight compounds isolated from mulberry root barks were capable of *M. tuberculosis* protein tyrosine phosphatase inhibition, a bacterium that increased the number of cases in multidrug-resistant tuberculosis [4]. Walnut bark and leaf extracts were effective against methicillin-resistant *Staphylococcus aureus* [5,6], *Salmonella enterica* serovar Typhi, *Enterobacter cloacae* [5] and *Pseudomonas aeruginosa* [5,7]. Ildiz et al. (2021) reported that bilberry fruit extracts have antimicrobial effects against multidrug-resistant *Escherichia coli* and *Pseudomonas aeruginosa* [8]. There are approximately 374,000 plant species in the world [9] that produce many phytochemicals as secondary metabolites to protect themselves against biotic and abiotic stresses [10]. It has been suggested that the most important categories of chemical compounds found in plants with proven antimicrobial activity are terpenoids, alkaloids, sulphur-containing compounds and polyphenols. Not only do they provide defence against various microorganisms, but also show anti-fungal, anticancer and antioxidant properties as well [11]. It is assumed that the structural arrangement of the different compounds found in these plants influences the effectiveness of the antimicrobial property; one such structure is the hydroxyl (-OH) group of a phenol compound. It is a known fact that this group can directly disrupt a microbial membrane structure and cause leakages [12]. A number of documented chemical compounds, such as flavonoids, quinones, tannins, lignans and other polyphenols, are also effective as antifungal agents [13]. These compounds are also potentially effective in food preservation, as they are not only considered nutritionally safe and easily digestible but also have proven health benefits [14,15].

Most of the research focuses on the extracts made from differentiated tissues, but in recent years, there have been more and more studies based on meristematic tissues. This type of tissue contains many phytonutrients, and they are used for the preparation of so-called gemmotherapy extracts (GTEs) that are more complex and potentially more effective than adult plant parts [16]. Besides the secondary metabolites, these GTEs usually contain proteins, amino acids, hormones, vitamins, growth factors and cytokines [17]. The best time to harvest the buds is late winter or early spring, as this is when the maximum concentration of active ingredients is present [18]. In reviewing the studies that have been carried out in this area, we conclude that there is only a small amount of research that focuses on the efficacy of the antimicrobial properties of such GTEs, so this area is largely unexplored. The application of GTEs in phytotherapy has been proposed by Pol Henry [19], and such extracts are hydroglycerine alcoholic solutions of macerated fresh buds, stems, roots, or other meristematic plant tissues, and are easy to prepare and administer, usually by dilution in water [20,21]. In the following, some of the recent results are presented concerning the studied GTEs associated antimicrobial properties.

1.1. Olive Tree (*Olea europaea* L.)

The olive (*Olea europaea* L.) belongs to the *Oleaceae* family, and it is a largely studied Mediterranean crop because of its health benefits, such as its antioxidant, antimicrobial, anticancer, antiviral and gastroprotective effects [22]. Young olive shoot extracts' antimicrobial effects were first examined in 2023 by Popović et al. [16], and according to them these extracts have inhibitory and bactericidal effects against several Gram-positive (*Staphylococcus aureus* ATCC 25923, *Bacillus cereus* ATCC 14579, *Listeria monocytogenes* ATCC 14579, *Enterococcus faecalis* ATCC 29212) and Gram-negative (*Escherichia coli* ATCC 25922, *Salmonella enteritidis* ATCC 13076) bacteria. Recent research proved that olive leaf extract might have a protective effect against the negative impacts of exposure to noise and toluene on the heart tissue, so it could be a safe and natural therapeutic option to counteract the adverse impact of environmental toxicants on cardiovascular health [23]. Another work of research claimed that olive leaf extract has wound-healing effects and can increase hair growth by detoxifying the hair follicles and promoting blood circulation in the scalp [24].

1.2. Almond (*Prunus amygdalus* L.)

The almond (*Prunus amygdalus* L.) belongs to the *Rosaceae* family, and it is cultivated in east Mediterranean countries, Australia and Africa [25]. The skin of the nut has anti-inflammatory and antioxidant activities due to the presence of nutrients, such as lipids, fatty acids, proteins, amino acids, vitamins, carbohydrates and minerals [26]. The sphingolipids isolated from nuts are capable of inhibiting the development of colon cancer and also decreasing the proportion of adenocarcinomas in mice [25]. There are no studies based on the antimicrobial effects of buds, but Ibibia (2013) [25] reported that almond leaf extracts were effective against *E. coli*, *S. aureus*, *B. subtilis*, *B. cereus* and *P. aeruginosa*. Ramachandran et al. (2020) [27] reported that almonds could be a promising agent for the treatment of polycystic ovary syndrome, as it was able to restore hormone levels in experimental animals.

1.3. Black Mulberry (*Morus nigra* L.)

The black mulberry (*Morus nigra* L.) belongs to the *Moraceae* family, and there are 24 species of *Morus* and one subspecies. The black mulberry originates from Iran, and it is one of the most important species grown in Mediterranean countries. The fruit is known not only for its nutritional qualities but also for its use in traditional medicine, as it contains a high number of bioactive compounds. The fruit is reported to have several biological activities, such as antioxidant, antidiabetic, anti-hyperlipidaemic and anti-inflammatory properties [28]. The leaves can be used for the prevention of throat infections, inflammations and irritations, and it is an anti-hyperglycemic nutraceutical food for diabetic people. The root barks have cathartic and anti-helmentic effects, while the stem barks are considered to be purgative and antidiabetic [29].

1.4. Walnut (*Juglans regia* L.)

The walnut (*Juglans regia* L.) belongs to the *Juglandaceae* family, and it originates from Central Asia, the western Himalayan chain, reaching Europe before the Roman times [30]. The walnut is rich in fats and contains valuable polyunsaturated fatty acids, proteins and minerals. Walnut-derived polyphenolic compounds have been attributed to health benefits like the ability to reduce oxidative stress and inhibit macromolecular oxidation. Regular walnut consumption reduces the risk of heart disease [31]. Oliveira et al. (2008) [32] examined the walnut's green husk antimicrobial properties, observing the growth inhibition of *B. cereus*, *B. subtilis*, *S. aureus* and *P. aeruginosa*, while walnut fruits were less effective, as reported by Pereira et al. (2008), [33]. Another study on walnut kernel extracts reported increased brain dopamine levels in rats, which were inversely correlated with oxidative stress, suggesting that such an extract could have neuroprotective effects [34].

1.5. Bilberry (*Vaccinium myrtillus* L.)

The bilberry (*Vaccinium myrtillus* L.) belongs to the *Ericaceae* family and is a wild-growing species with its most important distribution area in Northern and Eastern Europe and North Africa. These berries have been used in traditional medicine since ancient times as they have antioxidant, cardioprotective, antimicrobial, anti-inflammatory, anti-obesity and other beneficial health properties [35]. There are many studies that examine these berries and other parts of the plant for associated antimicrobial properties [36–39], but no such study was conducted for the bilberry GTE. However, some bilberry fruit extracts' specific phytonutrient profiles were determined and the antidiabetic effect was revealed through nutrigenetic studies (Neamțu et al., 2020) [40]. Habanova et al. (2016) [41] reported that even a short period of regular consumption of whole wild bilberries is associated with an improvement in the lipid profile in humans and can contribute to beneficial effects on CVD risk reduction, such as decreasing LDL-C and TG and increasing HDL-C.

1.6. Blackberry (*Rubus fruticosus* L.)

The blackberry (*Rubus fruticosus* L.) belongs to the *Rosaceae* family, and it has been collected for about two thousand years from the wild, though currently, many cultivated varieties are also available. Nowadays, the main regions for blackberry production are North America, Europe, Asia, South America, Central America and Africa [42]. The berries were used for medicinal purposes, and the plants were domesticated in the 17th century [43]. Due to their phenolic compounds, these berries have been attributed to many potential health benefits, such as the prevention of chronic and inflammatory diseases and some types of cancer, and could also reduce the changes associated with age-related neurodegenerative diseases [42].

1.7. Blackcurrant (*Ribes nigrum* L.)

The blackcurrant (*Ribes nigrum* L.) belongs to the *Glossulariaceae* family, and it is native to central Europe and northern Asia. It is also a well-studied plant; its berries have many positive effects on health, like blood glucose regulation, as well as anti-inflammatory, antioxidant, antimicrobial and anticancer properties [44]. Raiciu et al. (2010) [18] investigated the antimicrobial effects of blackcurrant bud extracts and found that they inhibited the growth of *Staphylococcus aureus* ATCC6538, *Pseudomonas aeruginosa* ATCC 9027, *Escherichia coli* ATCC 35218, *Aspergillus niger* ATCC 16,404 and *Candida albicans* ATCC 10231. Tabart et al. (2006; 2011) [45,46] compared the antioxidant capacities and profiles of different plant parts (buds, leaves and berries) from different blackcurrant cultivars, and the berries exhibited a significantly diminished phenol content compared to the buds and leaves. Kendir et al. (2019) [47] reported that blackcurrant leaf extracts had wound-healing effects, the activity of which could be attributed to phenolic compounds, especially chlorogenic acid and rutin. Another work of research showed that blackcurrant GTEs prevented neuroinflammation in rats that underwent lipopolysaccharide treatment [48].

1.8. Aim of the Research

Seven GTEs made of plant species like *Olea europaea* (OGTE), *Prunus amygdalus* (AGTE), *Morus nigra* (BMGTE), *Juglans regia* (WGTE), *Rubus fruticosus* (BkBGTE), *Ribes nigrum* (BCGTE) and *Vaccinium myrtillus* (BBGTE) were comparatively assessed for their antimicrobial properties by monitoring the growth and function of food-derived pathogens (*Escherichia coli, Pseudomonas aeruginosa, Salmonella enterica* subsp. *enterica, Proteus vulgaris, Bacillus cereus, Staphylococcus aureus, Enterococcus faecalis, Aspergillus flavus, A. niger, A. ochraceus, Penicillium citrinum, P. expansum*) and *Saccharomyces cerevisiae*. The ultimate goal was to determine which of the tested GTEs could feature antimicrobial properties and if such properties could further be influenced by combining GTEs through their synergistic, additive and/or antagonistic interactions. Therefore, if an antimicrobial interaction is detected between some GTEs, then their possible combination for other putative beneficial physiological effects should be further investigated.

2. Results

In order to gain information about the antimicrobial activity of the selected GTE Gram-positive and negative bacterial species, together with yeast and mould fungi species, were included in this study (see Section 4).

All studied GTEs were evaluated for their polyphenol contents in order to have a better characterisation of them previous to the study. The identified and quantified bioactive compounds from the studied GTEs are presented in Table 1.

Table 1. The phytochemical composition of GTEs.

Studied Components	OGTE	AGTE	BMGTE	WGTE	BBGTE	BkBGTE	BCGTE
Phenolic acids							
Caffeic acid	-	0.825 ± 0.0094	-	-	1.693 ± 0.0188	-	1.693 ± 0.0101
Chlorogenic acid	0.265 ± 0.0042	1.390 ± 0.0095	3.539 ± 0.0251	0.244 ± 0.0038	7.552 ± 0.0217	0.157 ± 0.0057	0.227 ± 0.0057
Ferulic acid	-	-	-	-	-	-	0.109 ± 0.0086
Gallic acid	-	-	-	-	-	0.049 ± 0.0010	0.049 ± 0.0008
Salicylic acid	0.053 ± 0.0012	-	-	-	0.066 ± 0.0009	0.895 ± 0.0202	0.071 ± 0.0017
Flavonoids							
Apigenin	0.055 ± 0.0021	0.017 ± 0.0009	0.103 ± 0.0025	0.002 ± 0.0001	-	0.330 ± 0.0108	0.043 ± 0.0011
Catechin	-	-	-	0.008 ± 0.0001	0.044 ± 0.0018	-	0.028 ± 0.0009
Chrysine	0.109 ± 0.0051	0.103 ± 0.0049	0.093 ± 0.0009	-	0.117 ± 0.0085	0.101 ± 0.0022	0.114 ± 0.0027
Hyperoside	0.202 ± 0.0074	1.967 ± 0.0157	0.162 ± 0.0052	1.301 ± 0.0094	0.392 ± 0.0102	0.172 ± 0.0089	0.547 ± 0.0187
Kaempferol	-	0.032 ± 0.0010	-	-	0.033 ± 0.0009	-	-
Luteolin	0.049 ± 0.0009	-	0.017 ± 0.0014	-	-	0.013 ± 0.0008	-
Luteolin-7-O-glucoside	1.777 ± 0.0257	-	0.072 ± 0.0023	0.072 ± 0.0023	-	0.078 ± 0.0012	0.074 ± 0.0021
Naringenin	0.032 ± 0.0011	0.110 ± 0.0067	0.046 ± 0.0014	0.064 ± 0.0011	0.036 ± 0.0005	0.043 ± 0.0009	-
Quercetin	0.052 ± 0.0015	0.201 ± 0.0076	-	0.313 ± 0.0092	0.989 ± 0.0118	-	0.210 ± 0.0100
Rutoside	0.416 ± 0.0201	5.506 ± 0.0051	1.367 ± 0.0204	0.103 ± 0.0024	0.105 ± 0.0028	0.278 ± 0.0047	1.662 ± 0.0198

The concentrations are expressed in mg/mL, mean ± RSD.

The presence of many polyphenols can be observed both from the phenolic acid class and flavonoids. Generally, the main compounds identified are caffeic and chlorogenic acids, respectively, and quercetin and its derivatives hyperoside and rutoside. Certainly, each GTE has its own specificity. The OGTE contains a high amount of luteolin-7-*O*-glucoside; in the meantime, the WGTE has more flavonoids and fewer phenolic acids. In the BkBGTE, we found a higher amount of salicylic acid and apigenin.

We used two types of experimental setups to assess the putative antimicrobial activity of the selected GTEs. The agar diffusion method was applied to test the extent of the selected GTE-specific antimicrobial effect. This was based on the ability of the tested GTE to diffuse in the agar medium, forming a circular zone where its concentration decreased from the centre to the periphery. The resulting concentration gradient of the putative antimicrobial GTE provides an indication of the sensitivity of a given microorganism as a function of complete or partial inhibition.

In addition to the agar diffusion method, we also analysed the antimicrobial activity in broth by means of dilutions (microbroth dilution assay). Broths containing the tested GTEs at various concentrations were inoculated with a defined amount of microbial suspension, and after incubation, the dilutions that inhibited the microorganism being tested were determined. As the microbial cells in this liquid culture media came into direct contact with the nutrient broth containing a given concentration of the antimicrobial GTE, an accurate result was obtained regarding the change in cell number (decrease, complete inhibition–destruction). Therefore, based on the broth culture, we determined the minimum inhibitory concentration (MIC) as the lowest concentration of a given GTE with antimicrobial properties that still cause a decrease in the cell number of the tested microbe. We also evaluated the minimum bactericidal concentration (MBC), which is the lowest concentration of an antimicrobial GTE that destroys 99.9–100% of the original cell's suspension. The MIC test indicates the lowest level of antimicrobial agent that strongly inhibits growth, while the MBC test indicates the lowest level of antimicrobial agent that results in microbial death.

2.1. GTEs' Antimicrobial Activity in the Context of Inhibition Zones

The antibacterial testing of selected GTEs using the agar diffusion method was continued whenever possible by evaluating the diameter of the inhibition zones. The larger the diameter of the inhibition zone, the more sensitive the microorganism tested and the lower the amount required to inhibit the microorganism (see Figure 1).

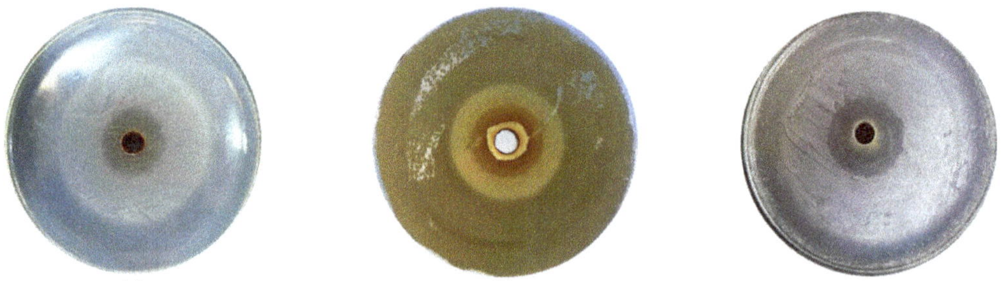

(a) (b) (c)

Figure 1. The different sizes of the inhibition zones induced by the GTEs on some microorganisms: (**a**) *L. monocytogenes—Juglans regia* 100% GTE; (**b**) *P. vulgaris—Vaccinium myrtillus* 100% GTE; and (**c**) *L. monocytogenes—Rubus fruticosus* 100% GTE.

Figure 1 The inhibition zones generated through the agar diffusion method for some of the tested microorganisms and GTEs.

Data on the inhibition zone diameters produced by the GTEs evaluated are presented in Table 2. Among the Gram-positive bacteria, *B. cereus* was the most sensitive, with the exception of blackberry and blackcurrant GTEs that showed no inhibitory effects.

The walnut GTE excelled particularly, inhibiting the growth of some microbes, even at a concentration of 20%, as the most effective against *B. cereus*, *L. monocytogenes*, and *E. faecalis*. For *S. aureus*, only the blackberry and olive GTEs produced zones of inhibition. Remarkably, for *E. faecalis*, the almond GTE looked like the most effective, followed by the blueberry and walnut GTEs.

In the case of *L. monocytogenes*, the walnut and blackberry GTEs were the most relevant, showing inhibitory effects at a wide range of 100–20% of the GTE's concentration. Interestingly, *P. vulgaris* was the only Gram-negative bacteria on which most GTEs had some effect, being mostly sensitive to the bilberry GTE, inhibiting growth even at a 30% concentration, and behaving completely resistant to blackcurrant GTE, where even the fully concentrated extract failed to inhibit growth.

Table 2. The antimicrobial effects of GTEs, concentrations and inhibition zones ($n = 3$).

Studied Microorganisms	Conc. (%)	OGTE	AGTE	BMGTE	WGTE	BkBGTE	BBGTE	BCGTE
Gram-positive bacteria								
B. cereus	100	12.34 ± 0.46 [d,e]	10.17 ± 0.92 [a,b,c,d]	9.96 ± 0.55 [a]	13.19 ± 1.17 [d,e]	nd	10.45 ± 0.55 [c,d]	nd
	90	11.59 ± 0.34 [c,d,e]	9.71 ± 0.30 [a,b]	9.67 ± 0.69 [a]	11.79 ± 0.83 [b,c,d]	nd	10.70 ± 0.85 [c,d,e,f]	nd
	80	12.54 ± 1.65 [e]	9.40 ± 0.28 [a]	10.18 ± 0.73 [a]	11.74 ± 0.59 [b,c,d]	nd	10.56 ± 0.65 [c,d,e]	nd
	70	10.59 ± 0.46 [b,c]	9.53 ± 0.27 [a,b]	9.70 ± 0.54 [a]	10.95 ± 0.82 [a,b]	nd	9.91 ± 0.57 [a,b,c]	nd
	60	10.73 ± 0.30 [b,c]	nd	nd	11.29 ± 0.49 [a,b,c]	nd	nd	nd
	50	9.68 ± 0.60 [a,b]	nd	nd	10.22 ± 0.52 [a,b]	nd	nd	nd
	40	nd	nd	nd	10.18 ± 0.33 [a]	nd	nd	nd
	30	nd	nd	nd	nd	nd	nd	nd
S. aureus	100	10.52 ± 0.18 [b,c]	nd	nd	nd	12.2 ± 0.51 [c,d]	nd	nd
	90	11.32 ± 0.31 [c,d]	nd	nd	nd	10.47 ± 0.40 [a]	nd	nd
	80	10.96 ± 0.43 [c]	nd	nd	nd	10.79 ± 1.06 [a,b,c]	nd	nd
	70	10.54 ± 0.55 [b,c]	nd	nd	nd	13.95 ± 0.63 [e,f]	nd	nd
	60	10.55 ± 0.27 [b,c]	nd	nd	nd	13.29 ± 0.65 [d,e]	nd	nd
	50	9.24 ± 0.15 [a]	nd	nd	nd	13.22 ± 0.58 [d,e]	nd	nd
	40	nd	nd	nd	nd	9.81 ± 0.56 [a]	nd	nd
	30	nd	nd	nd	nd	nd	nd	nd
E. faecalis	100	10.95 ± 0.60 [c]	13.86 ± 0.46 [m,n]	nd	10.99 ± 0.91 [a,b,c]	nd	10.91 ± 0.46 [d,e,f]	nd
	90	nd	14.17 ± 0.55 [n]	nd	10.53 ± 0.97 [a,b]	nd	10.49 ± 0.63 [c,d]	nd
	80	nd	13.30 ± 0.29 [m,n]	nd	10.09 ± 0.59 [a]	nd	9.97 ± 0.18 [a,b,c,d]	nd
	70	nd	13.03 ± 0.42 [k,l,m]	nd	nd	nd	10.00 ± 0.20 [a,b,c,d]	nd
	60	nd	12.88 ± 0.28 [k,l]	nd	nd	nd	9.84 ± 0.26 [a,b,c]	nd
	50	nd	12.75 ± 0.55 [j,k,l]	nd	nd	nd	10.14 ± 0.42 [b,c,d]	nd
	40	nd	11.88 ± 0.56 [h,i,j]	nd	nd	nd	nd	nd
	30	nd	10.11 ± 0.51 [a,b,c,d]	nd	nd	nd	nd	nd
	20	nd	nd	nd	nd	nd	nd	nd
L. monocytogenes	100	9.71 ± 0.62 [a,b]	nd	nd	21.98 ± 1.13 [i]	19.20 ± 0.87 [i]	nd	10.81 ± 0.74 [b]
	90	nd	nd	nd	17.16 ± 0.90 [g,h]	18.71 ± 0.60 [h,i]	nd	10.77 ± 0.41 [b]
	80	nd	nd	nd	18.08 ± 0.41 [h]	18.59 ± 0.41 [h,i]	nd	nd
	70	nd	nd	nd	15.53 ± 0.83 [f,g]	17.84 ± 0.71 [g,h,i]	nd	nd
	60	nd	nd	nd	16.73 ± 0.69 [g,h]	17.37 ± 2.31 [g,h]	nd	nd
	50	nd	nd	nd	14.13 ± 0.47 [e,f]	17.33 ± 0.46 [g,h]	nd	nd
	40	nd	nd	nd	15.07 ± 1.46 [f]	16.93 ± 0.68 [g]	nd	nd
	30	nd	nd	nd	13.33 ± 0.49 [d,e]	15.4 ± 0.73 [f]	nd	nd

Table 2. *Cont.*

Studied Microorganisms	Conc. (%)	OGTE	AGTE	BMGTE	WGTE	BkBGTE	BBGTE	BCGTE
L. monocytogenes	20	nd	nd	nd	12.61 ± 0.96 c,d,e	13.4 ± 0.53 d,e	nd	nd
	10	nd	nd	nd	nd	nd	nd	nd
Gram-negative bacteria								
P. vulgaris	100	11.09 ± 0.33 c	11.14 ± 0.99 e,f,g,h	10.40 ± 0.37 a,b	10.33 ± 0.34 a,b	12.77 ± 0.64 d,e	12.76 ± 0.80 h,i	nd
	90	11.05 ± 0.44 c	12.12 ± 0.84 i,j,k	10.53 ± 0.58 a,b	nd	11.18 ± 0.45 a,b,c	13.55 ± 0.75 i,j	nd
	80	10.94 ± 0.52 c	11.57 ± 0.73 f,g,h,i	11.52 ± 1.31 b	nd	10.99 ± 0.30 a,b,c	15.04 ± 1.03 k	nd
	70	11.40 ± 0.42 c,d	10.69 ± 0.64 c,d,e,f	nd	nd	nd	14.24 ± 0.86 j,k	nd
	60	9.02 ± 0.37 a	10.00 ± 0.71 a,b,c,d	nd	nd	nd	11.91 ± 0.48 g,h	nd
	50	8.78 ± 0.22 a	10.44 ± 0.33 b,c,d,e	nd	nd	nd	10.59 ± 0.38 c,d,e	nd
	40	nd	10.91 ± 0.76 d,e,f,g	nd	nd	nd	11.64 ± 0.57 f,g	nd
	30	nd	nd	nd	nd	nd	10.15 ± 0.45 b,c,d	nd
	20	nd	nd	nd	nd	nd	nd	nd
P. aeruginosa	100	nd	nd	nd	nd	nd	nd	nd
E. coli	100	nd	nd	nd	nd	nd	nd	nd
S. enterica	100	nd	nd	nd	nd	nd	nd	nd
Yeast								
S. cerevisiae	100	nd	11.76 ± 0.66 g,h,i	nd	nd	10.39 ± 0.43 a	10.84 ± 0.37 c,d,e,f	9.63 ± 0.35 a
	90	nd	11.84 ± 0.14 g,h,i,j	nd	nd	11.97 ± 0.64 b,c,d	11.68 ± 0.9 f,g	10.61 ± 0.96 a,b
	80	nd	10.20 ± 0.16 a,b,c,d,e	nd	nd	10.43 ± 0.42 a	11.52 ± 0.56 e,f,g	10.90 ± 0.20 b
	70	nd	9.95 ± 0.28 a,b,c	nd	nd	10.56 ± 0.55 a,b	9.90 ± 0.48 a,b,c	9.78 ± 0.38 a
	60	nd	9.43 ± 0.13 a	nd	nd	nd	nd	nd
	50	nd	nd	nd	nd	nd	nd	nd
Moulds								
A. niger	100	nd	nd	nd	nd	nd	nd	nd
A. flavus	100	nd	nd	nd	nd	10.4 ± 0.27	nd	nd
	90	nd	nd	nd	nd	10.13 ± 0.25	nd	nd
	80	nd	nd	nd	nd	9.76 ± 0.54	nd	nd
	70	nd	nd	nd	nd	9.42 ± 0.25	nd	nd
	60	nd	nd	nd	nd	nd	nd	nd
A. ochraceus	100	nd	nd	nd	nd	10.47 ± 0.7	nd	nd
	90	nd	nd	nd	nd	10.07 ± 0.26	nd	nd
	80	nd	nd	nd	nd	9.96 ± 0.22	nd	nd
	70	nd	nd	nd	nd	9.56 ± 0.19	nd	nd
	60	nd	nd	nd	nd	nd	nd	nd
P. citrinum	100	nd	nd	nd	nd	14.02 ± 0.64	9.34 ± 0.25	nd
	90	nd	nd	nd	nd	13.22 ± 0.32	9.09 ± 0.31	nd
	80	nd	nd	nd	nd	12.81 ± 0.36	8.83 ± 0.35	nd
	70	nd	nd	nd	nd	11.91 ± 0.24	9.00 ± 0.18	nd
	60	nd	nd	nd	nd	nd	nd	nd
P. expansum	100	nd	nd	nd	nd	9.09 ± 0.07	nd	nd
	90	nd	nd	nd	nd	8.87 ± 0.19	nd	nd
	80	nd	nd	nd	nd	8.90 ± 0.22	nd	nd
	70	nd	nd	nd	nd	8.83 ± 0.14	nd	nd
	60	nd	nd	nd	nd	nd	nd	nd

nd—not detectable. Results are expressed as the mean in mm ± SD. Inhibition zones, including the diameter of the hole (8 mm). Values with different letters ($^{a–n}$) within a column are statistically different at $p < 0.05$, according to Tukey's test.

In the case of the budding yeast, the almond GTE produced significant zones of inhibition, followed by the blackberry, blueberry and blackcurrant GTEs. Despite the fact that for moulds, no significant zones of inhibition were observed, and even colonies were found within the inhibition ring, the blackberry GTEs seemed to be an exception as they showed some inhibitory effect.

2.2. GTEs' Antimicrobial Activity as Revealed by the Agar Diffusion Method

The application of this method in the case of the GTEs under investigation showed variable antimicrobial activity. The blackberry (*Rubus fruticosus*) GTE has been shown to be effective for eight strains, the olive (*Olea europaea*) GTE and blueberry (*Vaccinium myrtillus* L.) GTE for five strains, the almond (*Prunus amygdalus* L.) GTE and walnut (*Juglans regia* L.) GTE for four, and the black mulberry (*Morus nigra* L.) GTE and blackcurrant (*Ribes nigrum* L.) GTE for only two microbial species each (see Table 3). Notably, the olive GTE was effective at inhibiting Gram-negative bacteria, albeit to a variable extent (50–100% concentration), and the blackberry GTE showed inhibitory effects against mould species such as *Aspergillus flavus* (*A. flavus*), *Aspergillus ochraceus* (*A. ochraceus*), *Penicillium citrinum* (*P. citrinum*) and *Penicillium expansum* (*P. expansum*), although at a high 70% concentration.

Table 3. The GTEs specific minimal antimicrobial concentration (%) revealed by the agar diffusion method.

Studied Microorganisms	OGTE	AGTE	BMGTE	WGTE	BBGTE	BkBGTE	BCGTE
Gram-positive bacteria							
B. cereus	50	70	70	40	70	nd	nd
S. aureus	50	nd	nd	nd	nd	40	nd
E. faecalis	100	30	nd	80	50	nd	nd
L. monocytogenes	100	nd	nd	20	nd	20	90
Gram-negative bacteria							
P. vulgaris	50	40	80	100	30	80	nd
P. aeruginosa	nd	nd	nd	nd	nd	nd	nd
E. coli	nd	nd	nd	nd	nd	nd	nd
S. enterica	nd	nd	nd	nd	nd	nd	nd
Yeast							
S. cerevisiae	nd	60	nd	nd	70	70	70
Moulds							
A. niger	nd	nd	nd	nd	nd	nd	nd
A. flavus	nd	nd	nd	nd	70	70	nd
A. ochraceus	nd	nd	nd	nd	nd	70	nd
P. citrinum	nd	nd	nd	nd	nd	70	nd
P. expansum	nd	nd	nd	nd	nd	70	nd

nd—non-detectable.

Remarkably, the most effective GTE based on the number of inhibited growths proved to be the blackberry (*Rubus fruticosus*), showing bacterial and fungal growth inhibition for eight out of the fourteen examined strains. One of the most sensitive microorganisms to the blackberry GTE proved to be the *Listeria monocytogenes* (*L. monocytogenes*), where even a 20% (v/v) extract concentration exhibited growth inhibition. In the case of *Staphylococcus aureus* (*S. aureus*), a concentration of 40% showed growth inhibition, while in the case of *Proteus vulgaris* (*P. vulgaris*), only a concentration of 80% proved effective. *Bacillus cereus* (*B. cereus*), *Pseudomonas aeruginosa* (*P. aeruginosa*), *Escherichia coli* (*E. coli*) and *Salmonella enterica* (*S. enterica*) proved to be totally resistant to the blackberry GTE. Based on the results for the microscopic fungi, all except the *Aspergillus niger* (*A. niger*) strain were sensitive to the blackberry GTE.

The second most potent antimicrobial effect was found for the GTEs of olive (*Olea europaea* L.) and bilberry (*Vaccinium myrtillus* L.). The olive GTE inhibited the growth of 5 strains out of the examined 14. It can be noted that a concentration of 50% olive

GTE was effective against *B. cereus*, *S. aureus* and *P. vulgaris*, while the concentrated GTE (100%) showed inhibition against *Enterococcus faecalis* (*E. faecalis*) and *Listeria monocytogenes* (*L. monocytogenes*). Unfortunately, it did not show any effectiveness for the rest of the Gram-negative strains, where not even the concentrated solutions showed any growth inhibition. Moreover, the olive GTE did not affect the growth of budding yeast. The bilberry (*Vaccinium myrtillus* L.) GTE inhibited the growth of five strains of microorganisms, such as *B. cereus*, *E. faecalis* and *P. vulgaris*, and was also effective against *Saccharomyces cerevisiae* (*S. cerevisiae*) and *Aspergillus flavus* (*A. flavus*). In the case of the bilberry GTE, for the tested bacteria, the effective minimum concentration varied between 30 and 70%, while for the moulds and yeast, it was 70%.

Next in line are the almond (*Prunus amygdalus* L.) and walnut (*Juglans regia* L.) GTEs, which proved effective against four tested microorganism species. The almond extract showed inhibition for *B. cereus*, *E. faecalis* and *P. vulgaris*, but also for *S. cerevisiae*. The almond GTE was effective against *E. faecalis* even at a 30% dilution, against *P. vulgaris* at 40% and against *B. cereus* at 70%. The minimum effective concentration in the case of *S. cerevisiae* was 60%. The walnut GTE was efficient against *B. cereus*, *E. faecalis*, *L. monocytogenes* and *P. vulgaris*, starting from a concentration of 20% all the way up to 100%. The walnut GTE did not show effectiveness for any of the tested fungi.

The least effective GTEs were the black mulberry (*Morus nigra* L.) and blackcurrant (*Ribes nigrum* L.), which showed efficacy against only two types of microorganisms currently assessed. The black mulberry GTE inhibited the growth of *B. cereus* at a 70% concentration and *P. vulgaris* at 80%. In the case of the blackcurrant GTE, the lowest concentration was 70% for the *S. cerevisiae*, and it showed effectiveness at a 90% concentration for *L. monocytogenes*.

Finally, it is important to mention that in our research, using the agar diffusion method, none of the studied GTEs were found to inhibit the growth of *Escherichia coli* (*E. coli*), *Salmonella enterica* subsp. *enterica* (*S. enterica* subsp. *enterica*), *Pseudomonas aeruginosa* (*P. aeruginosa*) and *Aspergillus niger* (*A. niger*). Taking together the olive, almond, black mulberry, walnut and blackcurrant GTEs, they did not feature any antimicrobial effects on the tested mould species, as revealed using the agar diffusion assay.

2.3. Revealing the Antimicrobial Efficacy of Different GTE Mixtures

As described in the Materials and Methods section, different mixtures of GTEs were prepared, and their antimicrobial activity was tested using the agar diffusion method, and the diameter of the inhibition zones was quantified. The results of these tests are presented in Table 4.

The results exhibited three types of outcomes for the mixed GTEs and their antimicrobial effectiveness based on the presence and/or the diameter of the inhibition zone generated by the tested bacterial strains. It can be reported that most of the mixed GTEs performed worse than their single-use variants, resulting in smaller inhibition zone diameters.

For *B. cereus* with a 1:1 mixture of olive and walnut GTEs, the inhibition diameter was 10.07 $\pm$ 0.61 mm, which is almost identical with 9.68 $\pm$ 0.6 mm of 50% olive GTE and 10.22 $\pm$ 0.52 mm, corresponding to the 50% walnut GTE, respectively. The olive and almond GTE mixture had an inhibition zone of 11.13 $\pm$ 0.36 mm, which is similar to the 9.68 $\pm$ 0.6 mm of the 50% olive GTE but significantly increased compared to the non-existent antimicrobial effect of the 50% almond GTE, suggesting that the almond GTE did not have any inhibitory effect on the olive GTE. Similarly, the walnut and bilberry GTE mixture induced an inhibition zone of 12.1 $\pm$ 0.66 mm that resembled 10.22 $\pm$ 0.52 mm corresponding to the 50% walnut GTE, while the 50% bilberry GTE had no detectable antimicrobial effect. The latest situation is that the blueberry GTE was not able to inhibit the antimicrobial property of the olive GTE. Furthermore, the mixture of blackcurrant and almond GTEs produced an inhibition zone of 9.16 $\pm$ 0.22 mm compared to the ineffective antimicrobial activity of the individual 50% blackcurrant and 50% almond GTEs, which is an example of a synergistic type of interaction between the above-mentioned GTEs. A similar situation was observed in the case of the mixture of blueberry and almond

GTEs, where an inhibitory zone of 9.48 ± 0.29 mm was observed, despite the fact that the individual 50% GTEs did not produce any antimicrobial effect, which, again, suggests a synergistic interaction between the blueberry and almond GTEs. Another such synergistic interaction was found for the GTE combination of the bilberry and black mulberry and the GTE mixture of the black mulberry combined with almond.

Table 4. Mixed GTEs tested antimicrobial effects on selected bacteria.

Extract Mixture	*B. cereus*	*S. aureus*	*E. faecalis*	*L. monocytogenes*	*P. vulgaris*	*P. aeruginosa*	*E. coli*	*S. enterica*
OGTE + WGTE	10.07 ± 0.61 +	nt	nt	nt	nt	nt	nt	nt
BCGTE + AGTE	9.16 ± 0.22 ++	nt	nt	nt	nt	nt	nt	-
BBGTE + WGTE	12.1 ± 0.66 +	nt	nt	nt	11.99 ± 0.3 +	-	-	nt
BBGTE + AGTE	9.48 ± 0.29 ++	16.57 ± 0.27++	-	nt	12.54 ± 0.28 +	nt	nt	nt
BBGTE + BMGTE	10.66 ± 0.33 ++	nt	nt	nt	nt	nt	nt	nt
OGTE + AGTE	11.13 ± 0.36 +	16.91 ± 1.02 ++	nt	nt	nt	-	-	-
BMGTE + AGTE	8.67 ± 0.1 ++	nt	nt	-	nt	-	-	nt
OGTE + BCGTE	-	nt	-	-	nt	nt	-	-
WGTE + BMGTE	-	13.17 ± 0.8 ++	nt	15.2 ± 0.28 +	nt	-	-	-
OGTE + BMGTE	-	nt	nt	nt	nt	nt	nt	nt
BCGTE + BkBGTE	-	nt	nt	nt	nt	-	-	-
OGTE + BkBGTE	-	12.78 ± 0.26 +	nt	nt	nt	-	-	-
WGTE + AGTE	-	nt	-	nt	nt	nt	nt	nt
WGTE + BCGTE	-	10.87 ± 0.58 ++	-	nt	-	nt	nt	nt
BBGTE + OGTE	nt	12.17 ± 0.43 +		-	nt	-	nt	nt
BkBGTE + BMGTE	nt	12.74 ± 0.96 +	-	14.86 ± 0.4 +	nt	-	nt	nt
WGTE + BkBGTE	nt	14.45 ± 0.35 +		16.2 ± 0.36 +	nt	nt	-	-
BBGTE + BCGTE	nt	-		-	11.52 ± 0.45 +	nt	nt	nt
BCGTE + BMGTE	nt	nt	-	nt	nt	-	-	-
WGTE + OGTE	nt	nt	-	10.7 ± 0.14 +	nt	nt	nt	nt
BkBGTE + AGTE	nt	nt	nt	14.53 ± 0.29 +	nt	nt	nt	nt
BBGTE + BkBGTE	nt	nt	nt	nt	nt	nt	-	-

Note: (nt)—not tested; (-) no inhibition zone; (++) synergistic antimicrobial effect; (+) basic antimicrobial effect.

Further to the *B. cereus* and in the case of *S. aureus*, synergistic interactions were found for GTE mixtures like the bilberry–almond and walnut–black mulberry combinations. The olive–almond GTE mixture induced a 16.91 ± 1.02 mm diameter that exceeded significantly the 50% olive GTE, which generated a 9.24 ± 0.15 mm diameter, while the 50% almond GTE had no inhibition zone. Seeing the extent of the olive–almond GTE mixture-associated effect, another synergistic interaction could be envisioned between the olive and almond GTEs. Again, the walnut and blackcurrant GTE mixtures could be envisioned as synergies. The olive–blackberry GTE mixture showed neither synergy nor additive effects but a basic antimicrobial effect, while the size of the inhibition zone was near that of the olive GTE. The bilberry–olive, blackberry–black mulberry and walnut–blackberry GTE mixtures showed the basic type of antimicrobial effects that were close to one of the GTE components.

One of the most interesting GTE mixtures proved to be the walnut and blackcurrant combination for *S. aureus* bacteria. Neither of these extracts showed efficacy alone, but when mixed together, their synergy resulted in an inhibition zone of 10.87 ± 0.58 mm. The same synergy could also be envisioned for the GTE mix of almond and bilberry, both of which have no effect on *S. aureus* on their own, but when mixed together, they form a zone of inhibition of 16.57 ± 0.27 mm.

2.4. Assessing GTE-Associated Minimal Inhibitory Concentrations—MIC Test

In order to further characterise the antimicrobial potential of the GTEs, we analysed the minimum inhibitory concentration (MIC), which represents the lowest concentration of a given GTE that still causes a decrease in the cell number of the tested microbe by inhibiting bacterial growth. The results of the MIC assay are presented in Table 5, where the seven evaluated GTEs and their associated MIC values are shown in concordance with the microorganisms tested.

Table 5. The GTE % corresponding to the minimum inhibitory concentration.

Studied Microorganisms	OGTE	AGTE	BMGTE	WGTE	BBGTE	BkBGTE	BCGTE
Gram-positive bacteria							
B. cereus	10	10	10	20	20	20	40
S. aureus	20	40	20	30	30	60	70
E. faecalis	20	40	50	40	30	60	-
L. monocytogenes	20	40	30	30	30	60	70
Gram-negative bacteria							
P. vulgaris	30	10	20	30	20	10	20
P. aeruginosa	40	60	40	40	50	40	50
E. coli	50	70	50	60	50	50	70
S. enterica	30	60	50	50	40	60	100
Yeast							
S. cerevisiae	50	90	40	70	60	60	80

The MIC assay is based on the colour change in the compound resazurin to resorufin [49] due to the metabolic activities of the bacterium and is a valuable non-invasive method for measuring cell numbers, as seen in Figure 2.

In the case of the MIC assay, each GTE displayed an inhibitory effect for all the tested microorganisms at different concentrations.

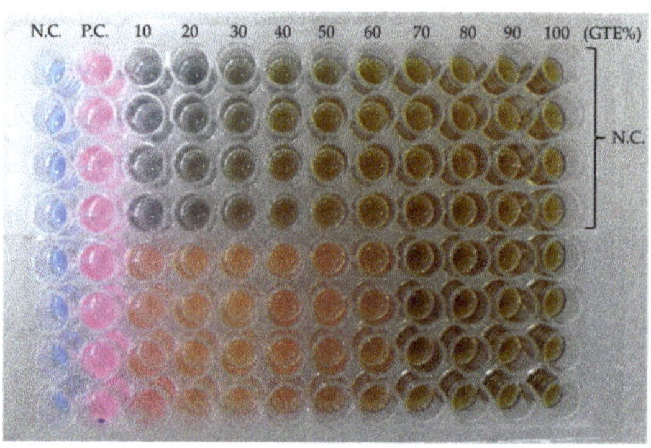

Figure 2. Picture of a microtiter plate with the various concentrations of GTEs and the microorganism in broth culture. Pink to red colour indicates bacterial growth. (N.C.—negative control, P.C.—positive control).

In the case of the olive GTE, even a 10% extract concentration showed an inhibitory effect on the *B. cereus* microbe, while for *S. aureus* and *E. faecalis*, the MIC value reached 20%. The most resistant were *E. coli* and *S. cerevisiae*; in their cases, only olive GTE concentrations above 50% inhibited reproduction.

For the almond, two bacteria, *B. cereus* and *P. vulgaris*, proved to be significantly sensitive to the 10% GTE, while *S. cerevisiae* (90%) proved to be the most resistant in this test.

It can be seen that all other Gram-positive bacteria were inhibited at medium concentrations, such as 40%, while Gram-negative bacteria showed a wider range of growth inhibition based on concentrations between 10% and 70%.

The 10% GTE concentration of the black mulberry already inhibited the *B. cereus*, while the 20% concentration was effective in the case of *S. aureus* and *P. vulgaris* bacteria. The highest concentration needed for Gram-positive bacteria was measured at 50% for *E. faecalis*, while in the case of Gram-negatives, the highest value was also 50% for *E. coli* and *S. enterica*. *S. cerevisiae* yeast proved to be more sensitive as a 40% concentration was sufficient to inhibit growth.

The walnut GTE also inhibited the microbe *B. cereus* the most at a low concentration of 20%, but *S. aureus*, *L. monocytogenes* and *P. vulgaris* also proved to be sensitive, and in their case, the inhibitions started from the 30% extract. The most resistant were *E. coli* and *S. enterica*, at 50 and 60%, while yeast also proved resistant at 70%.

In the case of bilberry GTE, *B. cereus* and *P. vulgaris* were the most sensitive since inhibition was observed at a 20% concentration. All Gram-positive bacteria were easily inhibited at a lower concentration of 30%. The Gram-negative bacteria showed higher resistance to this extract, requiring 40–50% concentrations for inhibition. *S. cerevisiae* proved to be the most resistant to this extract, requiring a 60% concentration for growth inhibition.

The blackberry GTE showed significant growth inhibition in the case of *P. vulgaris* (Gram-negative bacteria) and *B. cereus* (Gram-positive bacteria), requiring as low as a 10% and 20% GTE concentration for growth inhibition, respectively. The Gram-positive bacteria proved significantly more resistant to this extract, requiring 60% concentration for supressing growth. The remaining Gram-negative bacteria showed varied results, but still required higher concentrations, between 40 and 60%, to inhibit growth. The most resistant microbes were *S. aureus*, *L. monocytogenes* and *S. cerevisiae*.

The blackcurrant GTE showed mixed results in the MIC test, with the highest inhibition of *P. vulgaris* at 20% but no effect on *E. faecalis*. All the Gram-positive bacteria showed a high level of resistance to the extract at 70%. Gram-negative bacteria were inhibited, but also at higher concentrations, with *S. enterica* requiring a 100% concentrated GTE for inhibition. As usual, the yeast required higher concentrations for inhibition, which, in this case, was 80% GTE.

In summary, the GTEs showed bacteriostatic activity against several types of microorganisms capable of causing major human infections, including *S. aureus*, *L. monocytogenes*, *E. coli* and *S. enterica*, as inferred from the observed MIC values.

2.5. Analysis of GTE-Associated Minimal Bactericidal Concentrations—MBC Assay

The MBC test indicates the lowest level of an antimicrobial agent, which, in our case, is the GTE concentration that results in microbial death. The results of the MBC test are presented in Table 6. The analysed GTEs showed a different MBC based on their concentrations and the microorganism species assessed.

The olive (*Olea europaea*) and bilberry (*Vaccinium myrtillus* L.) GTEs showed an increased efficacy against almost identical six strains of both bacteria and yeast. Both types of GTE showed bactericidal activity against the same Gram-positive bacteria, with the exception of *Bacillus cereus*. In the case of olive GTE, the MBC with the lowest concentration was around 50% for *E. faecalis*, followed by 60% of *S. aureus* and 70% for *L. monocytogenes*. The bilberry GTE with the lowest MBC was 30% for *E. faecalis*, followed by 60% of *L. monocytogenes* and 80% for *S. aureus*. Furthermore, when the Gram-negative bacteria were analysed, both GTEs showed some effectiveness, but at much higher concentrations (70–80%). The current study revealed both *E. coli* and *S. enterica* presented an MBC value of 70% olive GTE, while the bilberry GTE had no bactericidal effect on *E. coli*. In addition, the bilberry GTE demonstrated an MBC of 70% for *P. aeruginosa* and an 80% GTE for *S. enterica*. It should be noticed that both olive and bilberry GTEs proved effective against *S. cerevisiae* but at very high concentrations of 90–100%.

Table 6. The GTE % corresponding to the minimum bactericidal concentration.

Studied Microorganisms	OGTE	AGTE	BMGTE	WGTE	BBGTE	BkBGTE	BCGTE
Gram-positive bacteria							
B. cereus	-	-	-	-	-	-	-
S. aureus	60	-	80	-	80	60	-
E. faecalis	50	70	70	90	30	70	-
L. monocytogenes	70	60	50	80	60	40	-
Gram-negative bacteria							
P. vulgaris	-	-	-	-	-	-	-
P. aeruginosa	-	100	-	-	70	-	-
E. coli	70	-	-	-	-	-	-
S. enterica	70	-	100	100	80	-	-
Yeast							
S. cerevisiae	90	-	100	-	100	100	-

In the Materials and Methods chapter, we proposed a test for verifying the authenticity of the MBC colour-changing method, and Figure 3 presents the obtained results for such a test. This figure also shows the concentration (%) used for the GTE and the initial and final number of colony-forming units.

In the case of the olive GTE, the inhibitory effects on *S. enterica* species were observed at the 30% GTE concentration, where bacteria were still able to survive, while at higher concentrations in the 60–70% range, bacterial growth inhibition was more pronounced. At even higher concentrations, like 80–100%, the olive GTE was completely bactericidal. Overall, this experiment clearly demonstrated the validity of olive GTE-specific MBC data.

The second most effective GTE was the black mulberry (*Morus nigra* L.), killing five types of microorganisms at various concentrations, starting from concentrations of 50% to 100%. The black mulberry GTE showed bactericidal effects for most of the Gram-positive bacteria, except for *B. cereus*. Among the Gram-negative bacteria, only *S. enterica* subsp. *enterica* exhibited a 100% MBC, while the yeast *S. cerevisiae* again displayed a 100% concentration-specific MBC.

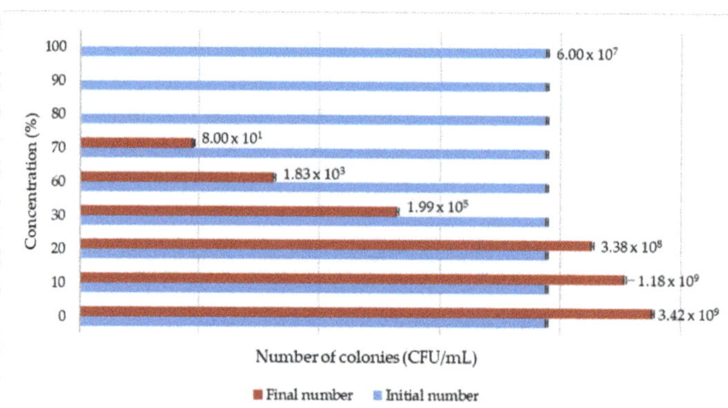

Figure 3. Olive GTE concentration with specific *Salmonella enterica* colony numbers.

The third most effective GTE for the MBC test was the blackberry (*Rubus fruticosus* L.), which demonstrated effective bactericidal power against four types of microorganisms. The blackberry GTE proved not to be effective against *B. cereus* but was efficacious against the remainder of Gram-positive bacteria, even at a concentration as low as 40% (*L. monocytogenes*). It also proved effective against the yeast *S. cerevisiae*, but only at a concentration of 100%.

The fourth most effective GTEs are almond (*Prunus amygdalus* L.) and walnut (*Ju-glans regia* L.) extracts, which showed bactericidal activity against only three types of bacterial microorganisms. The almond extract completely stopped the growth of two Gram-positive bacteria, *E. faecalis* and *L. monocytogenes*, but proved ineffective against *B. cereus* and *S. aureus*. In the case of almond GTE and Gram-negative bacteria, it was only efficacious against *P. aeruginosa* and only at a 100% concentration. The walnut GTE also proved effective against two Gram-positive bacteria, *E. faecalis* and *L. monocytogenes*, at concentrations of 90% and 80%, but showed ineffective against *B. cereus* and *S. aureus*. Among the Gram-negative strains, the walnut GTE presented an MBC only against *S. enterica* and at a 100% concentration. However, neither the almond nor the walnut GTEs featured any effectiveness for the yeast *S. cerevisiae*.

In terms of the MBC, the least effective GTE was blackcurrant (*Ribes nigrum* L.), as it had no bactericidal effect for any of the concentrations tested.

3. Discussion

In recent years, interest in natural antimicrobials has increased, and more studies are being carried out with a focus on plant extracts [50]. However, there is a paucity of data in the literature on the antimicrobial activity of plant parts, such as buds and young shoots, despite the fact that they contain many bioactive compounds and could have potent antimicrobial properties. In addition, recent studies have described the phytonutrient profile of some GTEs while also revealing their nutritional, antidiabetic and anti-inflammatory effects [40,48,51]. The phytonutrient composition of these GTEs also suggests that they may have antimicrobial properties, and this article presents relevant research data.

The phytochemical characterisation of GTEs showed that they are rich in polyphenols. Polyphenols are well known for their antioxidant activity, but they also have several other biological effects, including antimicrobial activity. Studies have shown that quercetin destroys the cell wall of bacteria, alters cell permeability, modifies protein synthesis and expression, reduces the activity of bacterial enzymes and inhibits nucleic acid synthesis, appearing effective against *Pseudomonas aeruginosa, Salmonella enteritidis, Staphylococcus aureus, Escherichia coli, Proteus* and *Aspergillus flavus* [52]. Their derivatives release quercetin in the body, which has the same effect on bacteria. Our study and the results presented in Table 1 show that hyperoside and rutoside, two of the best-known derivatives of quercetin, are the most represented flavonoids in all the GTEs studied.

Other studies have demonstrated that caffeic acid and its derivatives, alongside chlorogenic acid, could potentiate the effect of antibiotics and, in this way, be more effective in the fight against some types of resistant pathogenic bacteria like *Staphylococcus aureus* [53]. Our results show that the GTEs studied are rich in chlorogenic acid (see Table 1). However, besides the assessed polyphenols, there could be other bioactive constituents responsible for the detected antimicrobial activity.

3.1. Olive GTE Emerges as a Potent Antimicrobial against B. cereus, S. aureus and E. faecalis

As shown by the agar diffusion method, our data indicate that olive GTE inhibited the growth of *B. cereus*, *S. aureus*, *E. faecalis*, *L. monocytogenes* and *P. vulgaris* (see Table 2). The 100% concentrated olive GTE induced for *B. cereus* an inhibition zone of 12.34 ±0.46 mm, in the case of *S. aureus*, a zone of 10.52 ± 0.18 mm, for *E. faecalis*, 10.95 ± 0.5 mm, for *L. monocytogenes*, 9.71 ± 0.62 mm and for *P. vulgaris*, 11.09 ± 0.33 mm. These data suggest a certain concentration dependency that does not feature regular proportionality (see Table 2 and Figure 4). Furthermore, similar inhibition zone sizes were measured for the 50% olive GTE concentration in the case of *B. cereus*, *S. aureus* and *P. vulgaris*, for the 60% concentration in the case of *P. vulgaris* and for the 100% concentration in the case of *L. monocytogenes*. These data suggest that different olive GTE concentrations have similar inhibitory effects on different microbes. The extent of the inhibitory effect may depend on the synergetic interaction of certain olive GTE-specific phytonutrients, and the nature of this interaction is not necessarily concentration-dependent.

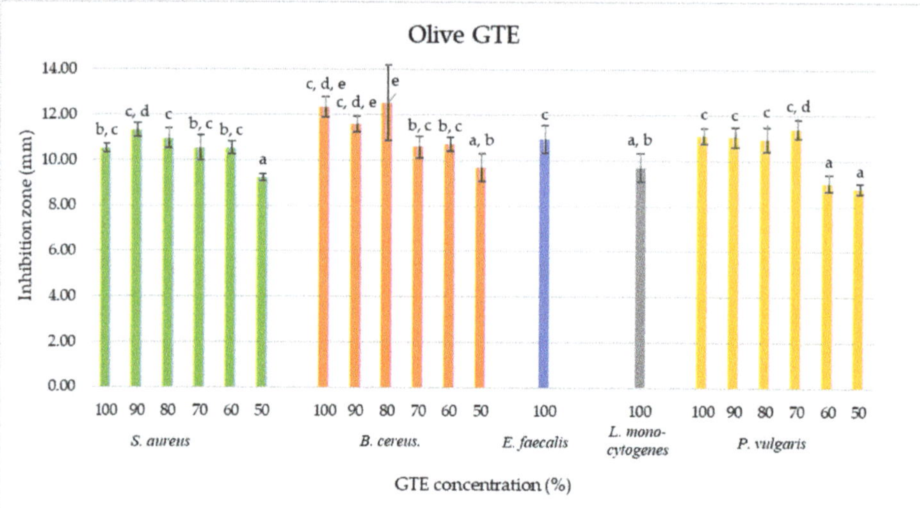

Figure 4. Inhibition zone size comparison for *Olea europaea*. Values with different letters ([a–e]) are statistically different at $p < 0.05$, according to Tukey's test.

Indeed, Aleya and colab. (2023) reported that olive GTE contains flavonoids, iridoids and polyphenols, which might confer some antimicrobial effects [51]. Aliabadi and colab. (2012) investigated the antimicrobial effect of Iranian olive leaf extracts and found that different concentrations of the extract have an inhibitory effect on *B. cereus*, *E. coli*, *Klebsiella pneumonia*, *Salmonella typhimurium* and *S. aureus* bacteria [54]. It is remarkable that the above-mentioned observations for the olive leaf extracts are in agreement with our findings for the olive GTE. Himour and colab. (2017) examined Algerian olive leaves and, in their case, the extract inhibited the bacteria *S. aureus*, *E. coli*, *Klebsiella pneumonia* and *P. aeruginosa* [55]. Nora and colab. (2012) tested the aqueous Algerian olive leaf extracts, and their effectiveness was proven against microbes like *E. coli* ATCC25922, *P. aeruginosa* ATCC10145, *Klebsiella pneumoniae*, *Enterobacter cloacae* ATCC13047, *S. aureus* ATCC6538 and ATCC25923 and *Bacillus stearothermophilus* ATCC11778 [56]. Moreover, Borges and colab. (2020) investigated the antimicrobial effect of Portuguese olive leaf extracts obtained through different methods, and in their case, the ultrasound-assisted ethanolic extract best inhibited the growth of *S. aureus* and *E. coli* microbes [57]. Furthermore, Gökmen and colab. (2014) investigated the effect of a Turkish olive leaf extract, and in their case the extract was effective against *B. cereus* (12.34 ± 0.46), *S. aureus* (18.67 ± 1.53), *Enterococcus faecalis* (19 ± 1.73), *Listeria monocytogenes* (19.33 ± 0.58), *Proteus vulgaris* (17.33 ± 1.53), *E. coli* (18 ± 1), *E. coli* O157 (17.67 ± 0.58), *Salmonella typhimurium* (13.33 ± 2.08), *Enterobacter sakazakii* (18.33 ± 1.15) and *P. aeruginosa* (18 ± 1.73), [58]. Taken together, these studies based on olive leaves indicate that the corresponding extracts contain oleuropein, hydroxytyrosol, chlorogenic acid, caffeic acid, verbascoside and rutin polyphenols [59], all of which could contribute to antimicrobial efficacy [60,61]. It is also interesting that caffeic acid was not identified in the olive GTE [51]. It is, therefore, logical that, based on the specificity of the phytonutrient profiles of the olive leaves extract and GTE, some differences are foreseen with regard to their antimicrobial activities.

In order to gain more information on the bacteriostatic and bactericidal activity of the analysed GTEs, we determined the associated MIC and MBC values (see Section 4). The MIC shows the lowest level of antimicrobial substance that strongly inhibits growth (bacteriostatic effect), while the MBC indicates the lowest level of the antimicrobial agent that results in microbial death (bactericidal effect). In the case of the olive GTE, the MIC values are relatively reduced since even the lowest concentration at 10% could exert a bacteriostatic effect (see Tables 5 and 7). Interestingly, there was some evidence of a bacteriostatic effect on all the microorganisms tested, with *B. cereus* being the most sensitive and *E. coli*, together with *S. cerevisiae* being the most resistant. Regarding the MBC, in the case of *E. faecalis*, the 50% extract concentration induced bacterial death, while no bactericidal effect was detected in the case of *B. cereus*, *P. vulgaris* and *P. aeruginosa*. In the research conducted by Sudjana and colab. (2009), the MIC and MBC concentration of Australian olive leaf extracts ranged from 12.5% to 50% for *Bacillus cereus*, *E. faecalis*, *E. coli*, *L. monocytogenes*, *P. aeruginosa* and *S. enterica* [62]. In another study, the MIC value of a Turkish olive leaf extract was 32 mg/mL for *B. cereus*, *S. aureus*, *E. faecalis*, *P. vulgaris* and *E. coli*, while *L. monocytogenes*, *E. coli* O157 and *P. aeruginosa* showed 64 mg/mL [58]. The above MIC and MBC values and those reported by others do not appear to differ significantly from our data, suggesting that olive GTE and leaf extracts have similar antimicrobial activities.

Table 7. Antimicrobial features of the GTEs as revealed by different methods on the studied microorganisms.

Extract	Method	Microorganism								
		B. cereus	*S. aureus*	*E. faecalis*	*L. monocytogenes*	*P. vulgaris*	*P. aeruginosa*	*E. coli*	*S. enterica*	*S. cerevisiae*
OGTE	ADM	+++	+++	+	+	+++	nd	nd	nd	nd
	MIC	+++	+++	+++	+++	+++	++	++	+++	++
	MBC	nd	++	++	+	nd	nd	+	+	+
	MIC/MBC									
AGTE	ADM	+	nd	+++	nd	+++	nd	nd	nd	++
	MIC	+++	++	++	++	+++	++	+	++	+
	MBC	nd	nd	+	++	nd	+	nd	nd	nd
BMGTE	ADM	++	nd	nd	nd	++	nd	nd	nd	nd
	MIC	+++	+++	++	+++	+++	++	++	++	++
	MBC	nd	+	+	++	nd	nd	nd	+	+
WGTE	ADM	+++	nd	++	+++	+	nd	nd	nd	nd
	MIC	+++	+++	++	+++	+++	++	++	++	++
	MBC	nd	nd	+	+	nd	nd	nd	+	nd
BBGTE	ADM	++	nd	++	nd	+++	nd	nd	nd	+
	MIC	+++	+++	+++	+++	+++	++	++	++	++
	MBC	nd	+	+++	++	nd	+	nd	+	+
BkBGTE	ADM	nd	+++	nd	+++	+	nd	nd	nd	+
	MIC	+++	++	++	++	+++	++	++	++	++
	MBC	nd	++	+	++	nd	nd	nd	nd	+
BCGTE	ADM	nd	nd	nd	+	nd	nd	nd	nd	+
	MIC	+	+	nd	+	+++	++	+	+	+
	MBC	nd	nd	nd	nd	nd	nd	nd	nd	nd

(ADM)—agar diffusion method; (MIC)—minimal inhibition concentration; (MBC)—minimal bactericidal concentration; (+)—reduced but detectable effect on studied microorganisms at high 70–100% GTE concentrations; (++)—medium size effect on the studied microorganisms at 40–60% GTE concentration range; (+++)—significant effect on studied microorganisms for the lowest 10–30% GTE concentration interval; (nd)—not detected (had absolutely no effect on the studied microorganisms even at 100% concentrated GTE).

3.2. Blackberry GTE Is Effective against L. monocytogenes, S. aureus and P. vulgaris

The blackberry (*Rubus fruticosus* L.) GTE was found to be effective, with inhibition observed in eight of the fourteen microorganisms, as shown by the agar diffusion method (see Tables 2 and 7). The most sensitive microbe proved to be *L. monocytogenes*; the 100% concentrated blackberry GTE resulted in an inhibition zone of 19.20 ± 0.87 mm (Figure 1c) and even the 20% extract generated an inhibitory diameter of 13.4 ± 0.53 mm. In addition, significant zones of inhibition were visible for *S. aureus*, and a less pronounced inhibition was observed for *P. vulgaris* and *S. cerevisiae*. Moreover, no real inhibition was observed in the case of moulds, as colonies appeared in the inhibition zones produced, but it should be stressed that the GTE was able to produce some kind of inhibition, which represents a newly discovered effect. Weli and colab. (2020) investigated the antimicrobial effect of the Omani blackberry leaf extracts and found that the extract exerted an inhibitory effect on *E. coli*, *Haemophilus influenza*, *E. faecalis* and *S. aureus* bacteria [63]. Riaz and colab. (2011) examined the different plant parts of Pakistani blackberry, and based on their results, 100 μg of the stem extract as disks were effective against *E. coli*, *S. typhi*, *S. aureus*, *Proteus mirabilis*, *Micrococcus luteus*, *Citrobacter*, *B. subtilis* and *P. aeruginosa* bacteria [64]. Pavlović and colab. (2016) investigated the phenolic composition of different Serbian *Rubus* species and found that ellagic acid was the main phenolic acid in the leaf extract, and the largest amount was found in the blackberry leaf extract [65]. Also present in the leaf were the hydroxycinnamic acids, aesculin, catechin, myricetin, rutin, quercetin and kaempferol, the constituents of which can contribute to antimicrobial effects. It should also be noted that the presence of the above-mentioned phytonutrients was also confirmed in our HPLC-ESI-MS study. Some novel compounds, such as amino acids (4-hydroxyisoleucine and tryptophan), were also confirmed.

In the broth dilution analysis, the bacteriostatic effect of blackberry GTE was observed. *P. vulgaris* proved to be the most sensitive (MIC = 10%), while *S. aureus*, *E. faecalis*, *S. enterica* and *S. cerevisiae* were the least sensitive (MIC = 60%) (see Tables 5 and 7). Furthermore, when the MBC was analysed, it was observed that *L. monocytogenes* was the most efficient (40%), while *S. aureus* and *E. faecalis* showed a bactericidal effect at 60% and 70% GTE concentrations (see Table 6). The MBC value specific to *S. cerevisiae* was equivalent to 100% of the extract. Gil-Martínez and colab. (2023) investigated the antimicrobial effect of Spanish blackberry fruit and found that the MBC was 25 mg/mL for *L. monocytogenes* and *S. aureus*, 12.5 mg/mL for *E. faecalis*, *B. cereus*, *E. coli* and *S enterica*, and 100 mg/mL for *P. aeruginosa* [66]. Concerning the bactericidal effect and comparing their data with ours, it seems reasonable to predict that the extract from the blackberry fruit appears to be more effective than our GTE.

3.3. The Bilberry GTE Is a Relatively Effective Antimicrobial Agent against P. vulgaris, E. faecalis and L. monocytogenes

The agar diffusion method revealed the bilberry (*Vaccinium myrtillus* L.) GTE is the most effective in the case of *P. vulgaris* bacteria, as the 100% extract produced an inhibition zone of 12.76 ± 0.80 mm (Figure 1b), and then all the decreasing concentrations reaching even the 30% extract had inhibitory effects (10.15 ± 0.45 mm inhibition diameter), (see Tables 2 and 7).

For the other microbes, inhibition zones were detected for *B. cereus*, *E. faecalis* and *S. cerevisiae*. Based on the data in Table 2, there was no significant difference (p = 0.182) between the inhibition zones produced by the 90–50% GTE concentrations in the case of *E. faecalis* bacteria, meaning that these dilutions had an identical effect. In young bilberry shoots and leaves, including the GTE, the main phenolic classes are hydroxycinnamic acids, flavonols and proanthocyanidines, meaning that similar antimicrobial effects are expected to emerge [40,67].

The most sensitive bacteria to the bilberry GTE in the broth MIC assay method were *B. cereus* and *P. vulgaris* with a 10% extract concentration, which was shortly followed by *S. aureus*, *E. faecalis* and *L. monocytogenes* at the 20% concentration. The *S. cerevisiae* proved to be the least sensitive (see Tables 5 and 7). The MBC-generated bactericidal effect was detectable at a 30% GTE concentration for *E. faecalis*, whereas *L. monocytogenes* showed a 60% concentration value. Miljković and colab. (2018) investigated the antimicrobial properties of Serbian bilberry fruit, and their methanolic extract was effective against a significant number of Gram-positive and Gram-negative microbes, including *S. aureus* (MIC, MBC = 63 mg/mL), *E. faecalis* (MIC = 63 mg/mL, MBC = 126 mg/mL), *E. coli* and *P. aeruginosa* (MIC = 31.5 mg/mL, MBC = 126 mg/mL), [68]. Our observations corroborate their findings with the exception of *E. coli* bacteria. However, in the case of *S. cerevisiae*, 100% GTE-specific MBC data are a further novelty.

3.4. The Almond GTE Is Effective in Inhibiting *E. faecalis, P. vulgaris* and *L. monocytogenes*

The almond GTE has been shown to feature an impressive phytonutrient profile containing a high number of polyphenols (flavonoids and non-flavonoids), amino acids, carboxylic acids and fatty acids. Among the non-flavonoids, there are hydroxycinnamic acids, like chlorogenic acids, caffeic acids, coumaric acids and ferulic acids. The quantitative polyphenol profile showed that the almond GTE contained a high amount of rutoside, hyperoside and chlorogenic acid, and it is likely that these constituents confer some antimicrobial properties [51].

Performing the agar diffusion method, it turned out that the almond GTE proved its effectiveness against *E. faecalis* (10.11 ± 0.51 mm inhibition zone) at a 30% concentration and *P. vulgaris* (10.91 ± 0.76 mm inhibition zone) at 40% (see Tables 2, 3 and 7). The almond GTE showed antimicrobial activity for *S. cerevisiae* between 60 and 100% of the GTE concentration. There is no significant difference ($p = 0.084$) between the tested concentrations and the resulting inhibition zones for *B. cereus*, meaning that the 70–80–90–100% concentration solutions could have a greatly similar inhibitory effect. Another study conducted by Ibibia (2013) showed that different concentrations of the extract from Nigerian almond leaves proved effective against *E. coli, S. aureus, B. subtilis, P. aeruginosa* and *B. cereus* [25]. In a different study on the fresh Indian almond leaf alcoholic extract, it showed inhibition for *E. coli* (11 ± 1 mm) and *S. aureus* (17 ± 1) [69]. The antimicrobial properties in terms of microbial specificity are evident when comparing the almond GTE and the leaf extract.

For this extract, *B. cereus* and *P. vulgaris* proved to be the most sensitive in terms of MIC; even a 10% extract concentration exerted a bacteriostatic effect, while the least sensitive was *S. cerevisiae*. The bacterial growth inhibition was detected in the case of *E. faecalis, L. monocytogenes, P. aeruginosa, E. coli* and *S. enterica*.

Musarra-Pizzo and colab. (2019) investigated the antimicrobial effect of almond peel extract on the hospital strains of *S. aureus*, and in their research, the MIC values ranged from 0.31 to 1.25 mg/mL, while the MBC values were greater than 1.25 mg/mL [70]. Another study examined Italian almond peel; in this case, the MICs were 125 µg/mL for *L. monocytogenes*, 15.62–32.25 µg/mL for *S. aureus*, 500 µg/mL for *E. coli* and 250–500 µg/mL for *P. aeruginosa* while the MBC was greater than 1 mg/mL in all cases [71]. In the case of almond GTE, the most effective bactericidal outcome was seen for *L. monocytogenes* and *E. faecalis*. Our data suggest that the almond GTE and peel extracts have relatively different antimicrobial properties.

3.5. Walnut GTE Shows Broader Antimicrobial Specificity, Excelling against *L. monocytogenes* and *B. cereus*

Prior to our research, the antimicrobial properties of various parts of the walnut (*Juglans regia* L.) were investigated by others. Farooqui and colab. (2015) tested the Pakistani walnut bark extract against various antibiotic-resistant microbes, which proved to be effective for the following microbes: methicillin-resistant *S. aureus, B. subtilis, E. coli*, multidrug-resistant *Salmonella enterica* serovar Typhi, *P. aeruginosa, Streptococcus pyogenes, Streptococcus pneumoniae, Enterobacter cloacae, Pasteurella multocida, Helicobacter pylori, Campylobacter jejuni, Shigella species* and *Micrococcus* [5]. In another study conducted by Muzzaffer and Paul (2018), the Indian male *Juglans regia* flower extract was effective against *S. aureus, B. subtilis, E. coli, P. vulgaris, Candida albicans* and *Candida glabrata* microbes [72].

By means of the agar diffusion method, it was revealed that *L. monocytogenes, B. cereus, E. faecalis* and *P. vulgaris* were sensitive to different concentrations of walnut GTE (see

Tables 2, 3 and 7). It proved most effective against *L. monocytogenes*, where the 100% extract produced an inhibition zone of 21.98 ± 1.13 mm (Figure 1a), and even the 20% concentration had an inhibitory effect showing an inhibition diameter of 13.4 ± 0.53 mm.

The *B. cereus* was the most sensitive in the case of the MIC assay (MIC = 20%) when the walnut GTE was used, while *S. cerevisiae* was the least sensitive (MIC = 70%) (see Table 5). Furthermore, bacteriostatic effects were also observed for *S. aureus* (MIC = 30%), *L. monocytogenes* (MIC = 30%), *P. vulgaris* (MIC = 30%), *P. aeruginosa* and *E. faecalis*, both with a MIC of 40%, *S. enterica* (MIC = 50%) and *E. coli* (MIC = 50%). The bactericidal effect of the walnut GTE was observed only in the case of *L. monocytogenes* (MBC = 50%), *E. faecalis* (MBC = 90%) and *S. enterica* (MBC = 100%) (see Table 6). Interestingly, a study performed by Vieira and colab. (2019) exhibited that the Portuguese walnut leaf extract was effective against *E. coli* (MIC = 20 mg/mL, MBC > 20 mg/mL), *P. aeruginosa* (MIC and MBC > 20 mg/mL), *E. faecalis* and *L. monocytogenes* (MIC = 2.5 mg/mL, MBC > 20 mg/mL) bacteria [73]. The comparison of walnut GTE and leaf extract bactericidal activity showed a great level of similarity for *L. monocytogenes* and *E. faecalis*.

3.6. Black Mulberry GTE Predominantly Inhibits the Growth of B. cereus and P. vulgaris, While Exerting Moderate Bactericidal Activity against L. monocytogenes

Based on the research conducted by Aleya and colab. (2023), it has been shown that the black mulberry GTE contains mostly flavonoids and polyphenols, followed by amino acids and carboxylic acids [51]. Among the 29 non-flavonoid polyphenols, there were hydroxycinnamic acids (chlorogenic, caffeic, coumaric, ferulic) and hydroxybenzoic acids and stilbenes (such as resveratrol). All of these may be contributors to antimicrobial effects, and we used the agar diffusion method to investigate this prospect. Interestingly, only *B. cereus* and *P. vulgaris* bacteria were slightly sensitive to the black mulberry GTE (see Tables 2, 3 and 7). The 100% concentrated GTE resulted in an inhibition zone of 9.96 ± 0.55 mm for *B. cereus* and 10.40 ± 0.37 mm for *P. vulgaris*. Based on the data shown in Table 2, there were no significant differences ($p = 0.320$) between the inhibition zones obtained throughout the 70–100% concentration range in the case of *B. cereus* or the inhibition zones specific for *P. vulgaris* at the 90–100% concentration interval. Amazingly, besides *B. cereus*, it was shown that the Brazilian black mulberry leaf extract was effective against many other microbial species like *E. faecalis*, *E. coli*, *Klebsiella pneumoniae*, *Salmonella choleraesuis*, *Serratia marcescens*, *Shigella flexneri* and *Staphylococcus aureus* [74]. In another study, the Turkish black mulberry fruit extract was effective against *E. coli* and *S. aureus*, while the leaf extract was effective against *Enterobacter aerogenes*, *E. coli*, *Proteus miribalis*, *P. aeruginosa* and *S. aureus* [75]. It seems clear that the black mulberry GTE generates much different antimicrobial spectra then fruit or leaf extracts.

Regarding the MIC concentrations, *B. cereus*, followed by *P. vulgaris*, *L. monocytogenes* and *S. aureus*, proved to be the most sensitive, while *E. faecalis*, *E. coli* and *S. enterica* were the least sensitive. The minimal bactericidal effect of different concentrations was demonstrated for *S. aureus* (MBC = 80%GTE), *E. faecalis* (MBC = 70%GTE), *L. monocytogenes* (MBC = 50%GTE), *S. enterica* (MBC = 100%GTE) and *S. cerevisiae* (MBC = 100%GTE). In the literature, very diverse MIC and MBC values were reported for some leaf extracts; for example, in the case of *S. aureus*, the MIC values varied between 0.156 and 12.5 mg/mL [74,75].

3.7. The Blackcurrant GTE Is Less Effective as a Microbial Growth Inhibitor and Bactericide

The agar diffusion method has revealed that the studied blackcurrant GTE does not show any significant antimicrobial effect, having only an effect on *L. monocytogenes* and *S. cerevisiae* (see Tables 2 and 3). Interestingly, Raiciu and colab. (2010), studying a Romanian blackcurrant GTE showed an inhibitory effect against *S. aureus*, *P. aeruginosa*, *E. coli*, *A. niger* and *Candida albicans* microorganisms [18]. These apparently contradicting data could be explained by the different places of cultivation or the different types of extract production. Our blackcurrant GTE was alcoholic, whereas Raiciu and colab.

analysed an aqueous GTE. It has also been shown that the geographical location of the growing area can influence the phytonutrient profile of different plant species; for example, berries from Romania were found to be richer in antioxidant compounds than those from Russia [76]. Similarly, the antioxidant capacity of blackcurrant was found to vary depending on the season and cultivar [46]. In blackcurrant buds, the most common phenolic compounds are gallic acid, hydroxycinnamic acid derivatives, several flavonols (glycoside-alcoolics of quercetin, myricetin, kaempferol and isorhamnetin) and dihydroquercetin derivatives [20,48]. According to another study, the most common flavonols in blackcurrant buds are rutin, isoquercetin and astragalin [46,65]. It is predictable that all these compounds could be responsible for the antimicrobial effects. Bendokas and colabs. (2018) investigated the antimicrobial effect of different Lithuanian blackcurrant fruits and found that a 1% concentration had an inhibitory effect on *Rhodotorula rubra*, *Lactococcus lactis*, *Micrococcus luteus*, *S. aureus*, *L. monocytogenes*, *B. cereus*, *Salmonella typhimurium* and *E. coli* microbes [77]. Such a finding suggests that the blackcurrant fruit extract has a much broader antimicrobial spectrum than the GTE.

In the case of blackcurrant, the most sensitive bacteria revealed using the broth MIC assay was *P. vulgaris*, where the 20%GTE showed a bacteriostatic effect, while the least sensitive were *E. faecalis* (no inhibition at all) and *S. enterica* (inhibited only by the 100% extract), (see Table 5). The extract had no bactericidal effect on any of the tested microorganisms (see Table 6). In the research conducted by Paunović and colab. (2022) reported that the MIC values of Serbian blackcurrant fruit and the leaf extracts for *S. aureus*, *E. coli* and *P. vulgaris* varied between 55.82 and 199.21 mg/mL [78]. Also, in a study conducted by Trajković et al. (2023), the MIC of blackcurrant-lyophilised juice was 100 mg/mL for *S. aureus*, *E. faecalis*, *B. cereus*, *L. monocytogenes*, *E. coli* and *P. aeruginosa*, while the MBC was greater than 100 mg/mL [79]. These previously published studies strongly support the fact that blackcurrant fruit and GTE have reduced antimicrobial activity.

3.8. Comparative Evaluation of GTEs Revealing Variable Antimicrobial Activity Strength Levels

Based on obtained data, it was concluded that many of the studied GTEs showed a different kind of antimicrobial effectiveness (see also Table 7). The agar diffusion method (ADM) used is an excellent tool for the initial stage of the antimicrobial screening of GTEs, although it does not provide insight into the antimicrobial mechanism of action. Based on the ADM, the olive GTE showed 5 inhibitory microbial effects, while the almond, bilberry and blackberry GTEs featured 4, followed by walnut with 3, and the black mulberry and blackcurrant with 2 inhibitory microbial effects regarding the tested microbial strains. It was also interesting to note that when the antimicrobial effects of different GTE mixtures were assessed using ADM, the combination of individual olive, walnut and almond GTEs with others could produce synergistic interactions (see Table 4). This is a novel feature of such extracts and one that merits further analysis.

Bacteriostatic and bactericidal effects are considered to be two distinct types of antimicrobial properties based on different mechanisms. Bacteriostatic antibiotics inhibit the reproduction of microorganisms (they are kept in a stationary growth phase), and the latter is removed by the host's immune system, while bactericidal antibiotics kill the microorganisms. MICs provide a clearer indication of the microbial susceptibility, including resistance and the bacteriostatic efficacy of an antimicrobial, while the MBC indicates the direct lethal effect of the antimicrobial. Bacteriostatic antimicrobials are expected to inhibit bacterial protein synthesis, but this could affect transmembrane potential or interfere with antimicrobial resistance [80]. The MIC assay revealed the olive GTE to be the most bacteriostatic-effective (6 inhibited strains), followed by the blackberry, walnut and bilberry GTEs (with 4 restricted strains), then almond and blackberry GTEs (with 2 strains). Regarding the microbial spectrum's wideness, the less effective bacteriostatic result was specific to the blackcurrant GTE (limiting only one strain), while all these effects were generated at the lowest 10–30% GTE concentrations. Walnut and almond GTEs proved less effective in the case of the ADM method but presented a better outcome in the MIC assay.

These extracts showed lower bactericidal effectiveness, with 6 microorganisms on which no effect could be measured. The black mulberry and blackcurrant GTEs performed worse in the ADM assay but displayed higher effectiveness in the MIC assay.

In the MBC assay, bactericidal effects were relevant for the olive, bilberry and blackberry GTEs, but the almond and black mulberry GTEs also induced some lethality, while the blackcurrant extract GTE showed no life-limiting detrimental effect.

The observed results also provide a broader perspective on the antimicrobial applicability of the GTEs analysed. In fact, although some are more effective than others, all GTEs are able to inhibit the growth of the microbial species studied, but their effect is concentration-dependent (see Table 7).

The olive GTE emerged as an efficient antimicrobial with a remarkable bacteriostatic effect for *B. cereus*, followed by *S. aureus* and *E. faecalis*, while the most relevant bactericidal property was seen in the case of *S. aureus* and *E. faecalis*. The growth inhibition of *S. enterica* was also evident. Our study corroborates the recently published findings of Popović et al. [16] and extends our knowledge with respect to species like *P. vulgaris*, *P. aeruginosa*, *S. enterica* and *S. cerevisiae*. The *S. aureus* is an opportunistic pathogen that can lead to different acute or chronic diseases and difficult-to-treat infections in hospitals and other community locations. The *E. faecalis* has been seen in most healthy individuals but could also cause endocarditis, urinary tract infections, meningitis and eventually sepsis. The *S. enterica* has many serovars that might bring about gastrointestinal diseases.

The walnut GTE showed a significant sensitivity and prominent bacteriostatic effect towards *B. cereus* and *L. monocytogenes*, while the bactericidal property was almost absent (Table 7). This suggests the possible use of the walnut GTE as an enhancer for classical antibiotic treatments to increase efficacy.

The bilberry GTE featured significant bacteriostatic properties, but a substantial bactericidal effect was displayed mostly for *E. faecalis* and *L. monocytogenes*. The *L. monocytogenes* is considered a virulent foodborne pathogen-inducing neuro- or pregnancy-related listeriosis leading to meningitis [81]. It is also important to mention that the bilberry GTE displayed some specificity towards *P. vulgaris*, which is an opportunistic pathogen of humans causing resistant hospital infections.

The blackberry GTE proved itself as a potent antimicrobial with a broad bacteriostatic but a more specific bactericidal effect on *L. monocytogenes* and *S. aureus*. Our observations suggest the putative suitability of bilberry and blackberry GTEs for the treatment of listeriosis, although the bilberry–blackberry GTE mixture did not show any interacting property.

The almond and black mulberry GTEs emerged as more bacteriostatic than bactericide (see Table 6), displaying some kind of specificity towards *L. monocytogenes*, and noticeably, their mixture does not reveal any interacting features.

Among the most interesting observations reported in this study are the mixtures of some GTEs that showed synergistic antimicrobial interactions. Mixtures such as blueberry–almond, walnut–black mulberry and walnut–blackcurrant are combinations of GTEs that showed effective antimicrobial activity against *S. aureus*. It is noteworthy that the individual GTEs mentioned above did not inhibit the growth of *S. aureus*, while the mixture of two GTEs resulted in the formation of some kinds of molecular hybrids that could gain antimicrobial properties and might be used for the development of novel hybrid antibiotics [82,83].

Taken together, comparing the ADM with the MIC and MBC broth assays, it could be seen that the studied microorganisms were much more sensitive to being suspended in broth. The analysis of MIC and MBC facilitated the comparison of bacteriostatic and bactericidal effects. It has been suggested that bactericidal activity at lower concentrations, as with olive, bilberry, or blackberry GTEs, is beneficial for a new antibacterial factor, inhibiting the emergence of resistance by preventing bacterial regrowth [84]. Furthermore, in clinical practice, the categorisation of antibiotics into bacteriostatic and bactericidal is debatable in situations concerning abdominal, skin and soft tissue infections and pneumonia [85]. In the case of pneumonia, it was demonstrated that bactericidal effects are not statistically different compared with bacteriostatic antibiotics in clinical cure rates, treatment failure, or relapse rates [86]. This could imply that an important element of personalised antimicrobial treatment should be the application of a decision regarding the possible superiority of bacteriostatic over bactericidal antibiotics or vice versa. In case the bacteriostatic effect is more favoured over the bactericidal property, the olive, bilberry, black mulberry, walnut and blackcurrant GTEs should be further studied in the context of enteritis. The olive, black mulberry, blackcurrant and blueberry GTEs have been shown to contain many phytonutrients with expected or proven anti-inflammatory properties, so they can have a synergistic healing effect by limiting microbial growth and overcoming inflammation. The quest for new antimicrobials continues, and as the scientific considerations become more diverse, looking for natural solutions seems to be an endless source of inspiration.

4. Materials and Methods

4.1. The Gemmotherapy Extracts

The reported research is based on seven different GTEs that correspond to species like *Olea europaea*, *Prunus amygdalus*, *Morus nigra*, *Juglans regia*, *Rubus fruticosus*, *Ribes nigrum* and *Vaccinium myrtillus*. The buds and young shoots were collected from different places at different times. *Olea europaea* young shoots and *Prunus amygdalus* buds were harvested from a plantation in Calabria, Italy, in June and April 2022, respectively; *Morus nigra*, *Juglans regia* and *Ribes nigrum* buds were obtained from the organic plantations of the PlantExtrakt company, collected in March–April 2022; *Rubus fruticosus* and *Vaccinium myrtillus* young shoots were collected from wild flora in the Mărișel area, Cluj county, Romania, in June 2022. The fresh vegetal material was processed at a maximum of 6 h from collection or stored in the refrigerator at 4 °C for a maximum of 24 h until manufacturing.

4.2. Sample Preparation and Extraction

The extraction method is based on the method written in European Pharmacopoeia, monograph 07/2022:2371, method 2.1.3. The extracts were prepared from freshly harvested vegetal materials that were preserved in a 1:1 mixture of 96% (v/v) ethanol and glycerol, with a plant-to-solvent ratio of 1:2. A moisture content analysis was performed on the fresh samples. Based on the determined moisture content, the solvent quantity was calculated to achieve a ratio of dry plant-to-solvent at 1:20. The solvent was a 1:1 mixture of 96% (v/v) ethanol and glycerol. The obtained plant–solvent mixture was mixed periodically for 20 days, 2×20 min/day. For the next step, the solid and the liquid parts of the mixture were separated, and the extracted solid plant material was further pressed to increase the yield of extraction. The two extracted solutions (separated from the solid part and those obtained after the pressing of the solid part) were mixed, forming the concentrated extracts that were used in further studies.

4.3. Studied Microorganisms

The reference bacterial and microscopic fungi strains used in this study were obtained from the National Collection of Agricultural and Industrial Microorganisms (NCAIM). The determination of antimicrobial activity of different GTEs was carried out on the following eight bacteria strains: *Escherichia coli* B.00200, *Pseudomonas aeruginosa* B.01064, *Salmonella enterica* subsp. *enterica* B.00834, *Proteus vulgaris* B.00642 (Gram-negative bacteria); *Bacillus cereus* B.00076, *Staphylococcus aureus* B.01055 and *Enterococcus faecalis* B.01054 (Gram-positive bacteria). It was also carried out on five mycotoxigenic fungi, including *Aspergillus flavus* F.00048, *A. niger* F.00071, *A. ochraceus* F.00850, *Penicillium citrinum* F.00815, *P. expansum* F.00601 and one yeast strain *Saccharomyces cerevisiae* Y.00481. Bacterial strains were cultivated on nutrient agar (peptone 10 g, meat extract 10 g, NaCl 5 g, agar 18 g, distilled water 1000 mL) at 37 °C for 24 h, moulds and yeast were cultivated on a complex medium (peptone 10 g, yeast extract 10 g, glucose 40 g, agar 20 g, distilled water 1000 mL) at 28 °C for 72 h, obtained from VWR International L.L.C. (Debrecen, Hungary).

4.4. Antimicrobial Activity Assessment

The GTE-specific antimicrobial effects were studied using the agar-well diffusion method. Prior to analysis, ethanol was removed from the extracts using a rotavapor, operated at a maximum of 40 °C degrees and at 200 mbar, avoiding in these conditions the degradation and loss of the bioactive compounds. The removed ethanol was replaced immediately after evaporation with purified water. The obtained samples were stored in the refrigerator at 4 °C degrees until the study was performed.

A set of GTE concentrations from 0 to 100% (*v*/*v*) was obtained, where 100% corresponded to the concentrated GTE, and the rest were diluted with sterile distilled water. The concentrations of the diluted GTE/set were as follows: 100%–50 mg/mL, 90%–45 mg/mL, 80%–40 mg/mL, 70%–35 mg/mL, 60%–30 mg/mL, 50%–25 mg/mL, 40%–20 mg/mL, 30%–15 mg/mL, 20%–10 mg/mL, 10%–5 mg/mL. Based on their effects on a given microorganism, a few of the concentrated solutions were also mixed together in a 1:1 ratio and tested as a GTE mixture combination for effectiveness.

The bacterial and fungal suspension of 1 OD (optical density) was prepared in a turbidity tube, from which 0.1 mL of microbial suspension (10^8 CFU/mL) was inoculated on the surface of the nutrient medium. After this, an 8 mm diameter hole was cut in the centre of the medium, into which 0.1 mL of the extract was pipetted into different concentrations. After incubation for 24 h at 37 °C for *Bacillus cereus*, *Escherichia coli*, *Pseudomonas aeruginosa*, *Salmonella enterica* subsp. *enterica*, *Proteus vulgaris*, *Staphylococcus aureus*, *Enterococcus faecalis* and *Listeria monocytogenes*, the diameter of the inhibition zones (together with the hole) was measured using a digital calliper [87]. To accurately evaluate the obtained results, the average of three parallel measurements was calculated. The same method was used for yeast and moulds (*Saccharomyces cerevisiae*, *Aspergillus niger*, *Aspergillus flavus*, *Aspergillus ochraceus*, *Penicillium citrinum*, *Penicillium expansum*), except that the medium was a complex medium and the incubation was performed at 28 °C for 48 h.

4.5. Broth Microdilution Method

The antimicrobial assay was performed using the broth microdilution method with 96 well plates. Each of the stock-concentrated GTE samples was diluted serially in the microplate wells to obtain 100 µL of the mixed solution using nutrient broth as the medium for dilution. A concentration range between 10 and 100% (concentrations in mg/mL are mentioned above) was achieved as a result.

4.6. Minimum Inhibitory Concentration Assay (MIC)

The MICs were determined according to a method described by Agbeby et al. (2022) [88] and El Baabouaa et al. (2022) [49]. The overnight culture of the tested microorganism was diluted to 1 OD, which is equivalent to an inoculum size of 1.0×10^8 CFU/mL. Each well of the microtiter plate contained 100 µL of various concentrations of the GTEs (as explained above), and 20 µL of the tested microorganisms (eight bacteria and one yeast) were inoculated into them. The bacteria-containing microplates were incubated at 37 °C, while the yeast-containing microplates were incubated at 28 °C for 24 h. After incubation, 10 µL of 0.01 mg/mL resazurin was added to each well and incubated for another 2 h and microbial growth was revealed by a change in colouration from purple to pink. The lowest concentration of each extract with no visible growth was recorded as the minimum inhibitory concentration (MIC) against the respective microbial isolates. As a verifying method, samples were inoculated on a nutrient medium from several wells, and the colonies formed were counted to determine the authenticity of the colour change.

4.7. Minimum Bactericidal Concentration Assay (MBC)

The MBC was determined using the microtiter plate method used in the MIC determination. The nutrient broth in the wells of the microtiter plate, which did not show any growth after incubation during the MIC assays was diluted and spread separately on nutrient agar and incubated in an inverted position at 37 °C for 24 h (bacteria) and at 28 °C for 48 h (yeast). The MBC was regarded as the lowest concentration of the extract, which did not produce any growth on the nutrient agar after 24–48 h of incubation.

4.8. The Phytochemical Analysis

The LC/MS method was performed on a Shimadzu Nexera I LC/MS—8045 (Kyoto, Japan) UHPLC system equipped with a quaternary pump and autosampler, an ESI probe and quadrupole rod mass spectrometer, respectively [51].

The separation was carried out on a Luna C18-reversed phase column (150 mm × 4.6 mm × 3 mm, 100 Å) from Phenomenex (Torrance, CA, USA). The column was maintained at 40 °C degrees during the analyses.

The mobile phase (see Figure 5) was a gradient made from methanol (Merck, Darmstadt, Germany) and ultra-purified water prepared using the Simplicity Ultra-Pure Water Purification System (Merck Millipore, Billerica, MA, USA). As an organic modifier, formic acid (Merck, Darmstadt, Germany), in the form of a 2% solution in ultra-purified water, methanol and formic acid was of the LC/MS grade. The used flow rate was of 0.5 mL/minute. The total time of the analysis was 35 min.

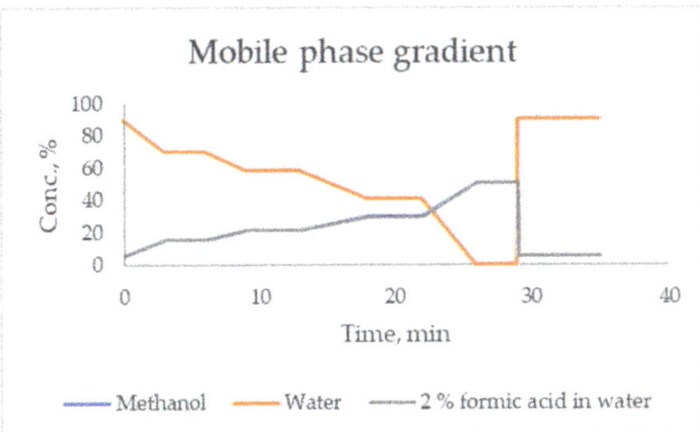

Figure 5. The mobile phase gradient.

The detection was performed on a quadrupole rod mass spectrometer operated with electrospray ionisation (ESI), both in the negative and positive MRM (multiple reaction monitoring) ion mode (see Table 8). The interface temperature was set at 300 °C degrees. For vaporisation, drying gas nitrogen was used at 35 psi and 10 mL/min, respectively. The capillary potential was set at +3000 V.

Table 8. The main MS transitions of the standards.

Name of Standard	Retention Time, min	*m*/*z*, and Main Transition	MRM
Caffeic acid	13.8	179.0 > 135.0	Negative
Chlorogenic acid	11.9	353.0 > 191.0	Negative
Ferulic acid	18.4	193.0 > 134.0	Negative
Gallic acid	7.0	168.9 > 125.0	Negative
Salicylic acid	23.5	137.0 > 93.0	Negative
Apigenina	28.1	269.0 > 117.0	Negative
Catechin	10.3	289.0 > 202.9	Negative
Chrysin	29.7	253.0 > 143.0	Negative
Hyperoside	20.3	463.1 > 300.0	Negative
Kaempferol	27.9	285.0 > 187.0	Negative
Luteolin	26.8	287.0 > 153.0	Positive
Luteolin-7-*O*-glucosid	19.9	447.0 > 284.9	Negative
Naringenin	26.2	271.0 > 119.0	Negative
Quercetin	25.4	300.9 > 151.0	Negative
Rutoside	20.2	609.0 > 300.0	Negative

The substances from Table 9 were used as the standards. From each standard at each concentration, 1 µL was injected. The identification was performed by a comparison of MS spectra and their transitions between the separated compounds and standards (see Table 8). The identification and quantification were made basely on the main transition from the MS spectra of the substance. For the purpose of quantification, the calibration curves were determined (the equations for which are given in Table 9).

Table 9. The standards used for LC/MS analysis.

Name of Standard	Origin	Concentration Range, mg/mL	Calibration Curve Equation	Correlation Factor	Detection Limit, µg/mL	Quantification Limit, µg/mL
Caffeic acid	Phytolab, Vestenbergs-greuth, Germany	0.11–1.10	Area = 4 × 10^7 × conc[mg/mL] − 319,689	0.9998	3.20	4.80
Chlorogenic acid		0.13–1.30	Area = 2 × 10^8 × conc[mg/mL] − 269,699	0.9997	5.00	8.00
Ferulic acid		0.100–1.000	Area = 5 × 10^6 × conc[mg/mL] − 50,000	0.9992	4.00	6.00
Gallic acid		0.107–1.070	Area = 8 × 10^6 × conc[mg/mL] − 37,131	0.9999	1.90	2.80
Apigenina		0.10–0.98	Area = 2 × 10^8 × conc[mg/mL] + 15,916	0.9999	0.20	0.30
Hyperoside		0.012–0.107	Area = 4 × 10^8 × conc[mg/mL] − 567,182	0.9986	0.60	0.90
Kaempferol		0.10–1.00	Area = 10^7 × conc[mg/mL] − 20,574	0.9996	0.80	1.20
Luteolin		0.01–0.10	Area = 2 × 10^8 × conc[mg/mL] − 2295.4	0.9977	0.05	0.07
Luteolin-7-*O*-glucosid		0.07–0.70	Area = 1 × 10^9 × conc[mg/mL] − 700,317	0.9990	3.00	4.00
Naringenin		0.16–1.60	Area = 3 × 10^8 × conc[mg/mL] − 43,443	0.9999	0.60	0.90
Quercetin		0.09–0.91	Area = 5 × 10^7 × conc[mg/mL] − 9556	0.9964	0.80	1.10
Rutoside		0.17–1.70	Area = 2 × 10^8 × conc[mg/mL] − 191,937	0.9996	4.00	6.00
Salicylic acid	Merck, Darmstadt, Germany	0.16–1.60	Area = 4 × 10^7 × conc[mg/mL] + 44,120	0.9997	1.50	2.00
Catechin		0.10–1.01	Area = 5 × 10^6 × conc[mg/mL] − 1706	0.9984	1.00	2.00
Chrysin		0.10–1.00	Area = 1 × 10^8 × conc[mg/mL] − 82,818	0.9997	3.00	5.00

4.9. Statistical Analysis

All analyses were performed in triplicate, and data were then expressed as the mean ± standard deviation (SD). The statistical analysis of the data was performed using IBM SPSS Statistics 26. For antimicrobial activity, the data were subjected to the statistical analysis of variance (ANOVA-1) followed by Tukey's HSD test to evaluate the significant differences between various concentrations and extracts. The difference was regarded as significant when $p < 0.05$.

5. Conclusions

The current study aims to elucidate the antimicrobial properties of seven GTEs, and for five of them, the reported phytonutrient profiles suggest putative antidiabetic, anti-inflammatory and antimicrobial implications. The comparative nature of this study permits us to directly compare GTEs and even draw conclusions about their relative antimicrobial strength. Interestingly, the agar diffusion method revealed the blackberry (*R. fruticosus*) GTE to inhibit the growth of eight microbial species among the tested ones and, quite remarkably, included the mould and yeast strains. The blackberry GTE emerges as a potent antimicrobial that inhibits the growth of many microorganisms, while the microbial death-inducing effect is more relevant for *S. aureus* and *L. monocytogenes*. Furthermore, the olive (*O. europaea* L.) GTE appeared to feature the strongest bacteriostatic and bactericidal effects with increased specificity for *S. aureus*, *E. faecalis* and *L. monocytogenes*. Next to olive, the bilberry (*V. myrtillus*) GTE showed increased bacteriostatic but diminished bactericidal properties with some specificity towards *E. faecalis* and *L. monocytogenes*. Walnut (*J. regia*) and black mulberry (*M. nigra*) GTEs featured similar bacteriostatic and bactericidal strengths, while the walnut GTE looked more specifically towards *E. faecalis* and *L. monocytogenes* which were shortly followed by *B. cereus* and *P. vulgaris*. The black mulberry (*M. nigra*) GTE presented further bacteriostatic specificity towards *L. monocytogenes* and then *B. cereus* and *P. vulgaris*, on which the GTE did not induce any bactericide effect. The almond (*P. amygdalus*) GTE brought about a weaker bacterial growth inhibition that was completed by a slight death induction for *E. faecalis*. Finally, the blackcurrant (*R. nigrum*) GTE had very little effect on bacterial growth or death, indicating that this GTE had no significant antimicrobial activity. Taken together, with the exception of blackcurrant, all the other GTEs have a more significant inhibition of bacterial growth than the induction of microbial death, which is a feature that suggests their applicability to enhance the antimicrobial effects of other antibiotics under less stringent conditions.

Author Contributions: Conceptualisation, É.G., N.K.O. and E.M. (Endre Máthé); methodology, M.H., E.M. (Emőke Mihok), A.A. and M.J.; software, M.H. and N.M.; validation, M.H., E.M. (Emőke Mihok), A.A. and N.M.; formal analysis, É.G., N.K.O., V.T. and E.M. (Endre Máthé); investigation, M.H., E.M. (Emőke Mihok), A.A., M.J. and N.M.; resources, É.G., V.T., N.K.O. and E.M. (Endre Máthé); data curation, M.H., E.M. (Emőke Mihok), A.A. and M.J.; writing—original draft preparation, M.H., É.G. and E.M. (Endre Máthé); writing—review and editing, É.G., V.T., N.K.O. and E.M. (Endre Máthé); visualisation, M.H., É.G. and E.M. (Emőke Mihok); supervision, É.G., V.T., N.K.O. and E.M. (Endre Máthé); project administration, É.G., N.K.O. and E.M. (Endre Máthé); funding acquisition, N.K.O. and E.M. (Endre Máthé). All authors have read and agreed to the published version of the manuscript.

Funding: M.H. has been partly funded by the ÚNKP-23-3 new national excellence program of the Ministry for Culture and Innovation Hungary from the source of the National Research, Development and Innovation Fund.

Institutional Review Board Statement: Not applicable.

Informed Consent Statement: Not applicable.

Data Availability Statement: Data can be made available by the corresponding author on request.

Acknowledgments: The authors would like to thank György Tankó, Bence Pecsenye and Judit Szepesi for their helpful comments on this manuscript.

Conflicts of Interest: Author Neli Kinga Oláh was employed by the company PlantExtrakt Ltd. All authors declare that the research was conducted in the absence of any commercial or financial relationships that could be construed as a potential conflict of interest.

References

1. Dadgostar, P. Antimicrobial Resistance: Implications and Costs. *Infect. Drug Resist.* **2019**, *12*, 3903–3910. [CrossRef]
2. Qadri, H.; Haseeb Shah, A.; Mudasir Ahmad, S.; Alshehri, B.; Almilaibary, A.; Ahmad Mir, M. Natural Products and Their Semi-Synthetic Derivatives against Antimicrobial-Resistant Human Pathogenic Bacteria and Fungi. *Saudi J. Biol. Sci.* **2022**, *29*, 103376. [CrossRef] [PubMed]
3. Brown, E.D.; Wright, G.D. Antibacterial Drug Discovery in the Resistance Era. *Nature* **2016**, *529*, 336–343. [CrossRef] [PubMed]
4. Mascarello, A.; Orbem Menegatti, A.C.; Calcaterra, A.; Martins, P.G.A.; Chiaradia-Delatorre, L.D.; D'Acquarica, I.; Ferrari, F.; Pau, V.; Sanna, A.; De Logu, A.; et al. Naturally Occurring Diels-Alder-Type Adducts from *Morus nigra* as Potent Inhibitors of Mycobacterium Tuberculosis Protein Tyrosine Phosphatase B. *Eur. J. Med. Chem.* **2018**, *144*, 277–288. [CrossRef]
5. Farooqui, A.; Khan, A.; Borghetto, I.; Kazmi, S.U.; Rubino, S.; Paglietti, B. Synergistic Antimicrobial Activity of *Camellia sinensis* and *Juglans regia* against Multidrug-Resistant Bacteria. *PLoS ONE* **2015**, *10*, e0118431. [CrossRef] [PubMed]

6. Moori Bakhtiari, N.; Jamshidian, J.; Khalafi, E. Effect of *Juglans regia* Li. Stem Bark Hydroalcoholic Extract on Methicillin Resistant *Staphylococcus aureus*. *Jundishapur. J. Nat. Pharm. Prod.* **2016**, *11*, e29095. [CrossRef]
7. Dolatabadi, S.; Moghadam, H.N.; Mahdavi-Ourtakand, M. Evaluating the Anti-Biofilm and Antibacterial Effects of *Juglans regia* L. Extracts against Clinical Isolates of *Pseudomonas aeruginosa*. *Microb. Pathog.* **2018**, *118*, 285–289. [CrossRef]
8. Ildiz, N.; Korkmaz, F.; Yusufbeyoglu, S.; Baldemir Kilic, A.; Ocsoy, I. Silver Nanoparticles Biosynthesized from *Vaccinium myrtillus* L. against Multiple Antibiotic Resistance and Biofilm Forming *Escherichia coli* and *Pseudomonas aeruginosa*. *Indian J. Pharm. Educ. Res.* **2021**, *55*, s220–s224. [CrossRef]
9. Christenhusz, M.J.M.; Byng, J.W. The Number of Known Plants Species in the World and Its Annual Increase. *Phytotaxa* **2016**, *261*, 201. [CrossRef]
10. Borges, A.; Abreu, A.; Dias, C.; Saavedra, M.; Borges, F.; Simões, M. New Perspectives on the Use of Phytochemicals as an Emergent Strategy to Control Bacterial Infections Including Biofilms. *Molecules* **2016**, *21*, 877. [CrossRef]
11. Khameneh, B.; Iranshahy, M.; Soheili, V.; Fazly Bazzaz, B.S. Review on Plant Antimicrobials: A Mechanistic Viewpoint. *Antimicrob. Resist. Infect. Control* **2019**, *8*, 118. [CrossRef]
12. Lai, P.; Roy, J. Antimicrobial and Chemopreventive Properties of Herbs and Spices. *Curr. Med. Chem.* **2004**, *11*, 1451–1460. [CrossRef]
13. Lopes, G.; Pinto, E.; Salgueiro, L. Natural Products: An Alternative to Conventional Therapy for Dermatophytosis? *Mycopathologia* **2017**, *182*, 143–167. [CrossRef]
14. Ogbulie, J.N.; Ogueke, C.C.; Okoli, I.C.; Anyanwu, B.N. Antibacterial Activities and Toxicological Potentials of Crude Ethanolic Extracts of *Euphorbia hirta*. *Afr. J. Biotechnol.* **2007**, *6*, 1544–1548.
15. Mostafa, A.A.; Al-Askar, A.A.; Almaary, K.S.; Dawoud, T.M.; Sholkamy, E.N.; Bakri, M.M. Antimicrobial Activity of Some Plant Extracts against Bacterial Strains Causing Food Poisoning Diseases. *Saudi J. Biol. Sci.* **2018**, *25*, 361–366. [CrossRef]
16. Popović, M.; Burčul, F.; Veršić Bratinčević, M.; Režić Mužinić, N.; Skroza, D.; Frleta Matas, R.; Nazlić, M.; Ninčević Runjić, T.; Jukić Špika, M.; Bego, A.; et al. In the Beginning Was the Bud: Phytochemicals from Olive (*Olea europaea* L.) Vegetative Buds and Their Biological Properties. *Metabolites* **2023**, *13*, 237. [CrossRef] [PubMed]
17. Kovalikova, Z.; Lnenicka, J.; Andrys, R. The Influence of Locality on Phenolic Profile and Antioxidant Capacity of Bud Extracts. *Foods* **2021**, *10*, 1608. [CrossRef] [PubMed]
18. Raiciu, A.D.; Mihele, D.E.; Ioni, C.; Nistoric, V.; Manea, T. Antimicrobial Activity of *Ribes nigrum*, *Rosmarinus officinalis*, *Betula Pubescens Salix Alba*, *Vaccinium myrtillus* Gemoderivatives. *Farmacia* **2010**, *58*, 735–748.
19. Nicoletti, M.; Piterà di Clima, F. *Gemmotherapy, and the Scientific Foundations of a Modern Meristemotherapy*; Cambridge Scholars Publishing: Newcastle upon Tyne, UK, 2020.
20. Ieri, F.; Innocenti, M.; Possieri, L.; Gallori, S.; Mulinacci, N. Phenolic Composition of "Bud Extracts" of *Ribes nigrum* L., *Rosa canina* L. and *Tilia tomentosa* M. *J. Pharm. Biomed. Anal.* **2015**, *115*, 1–9. [CrossRef] [PubMed]
21. Donno, D.; Beccaro, G.L.; Cerutti, A.K.; Mellano, M.G.; Bounous, G. Bud Extracts as New Phytochemical Source for Herbal Preparations—Quality Control and Standardization by Analytical Fingerprint. In *Phytochemicals—Isolation, Characterisation and Role in Human Health*; Rao, A.V., Rao, L.G., Eds.; InTech: London, UK, 2015. [CrossRef]
22. Rocha, J.; Borges, N.; Pinho, O. Table Olives and Health: A Review. *J. Nutr. Sci.* **2020**, *9*, e57. [CrossRef] [PubMed]
23. Ben Attia, T.; Ben Ali, R.; Nahdi, A.; Galai, S.; Ghali, R.; Rammeh, S.; Véronique El May, M.; Mhamdi, A. *Olea europaea* L. Leaf Extract Mitigates Oxidative and Histological Damage in Rat Heart Tissue Exposed to Combined Noise and Toluene: An Experimental Study. *Saudi Pharm. J.* **2023**, *31*, 101683. [CrossRef] [PubMed]
24. Said Nasser Al-Owamri, F.; Saleh Abdullah Al Sibay, L.; Hemadri Reddy, S.; Althaf Hussain, S.; Subba Reddy Gangireddygari, V. Phytochemical, Antioxidant, Hair Growth and Wound Healing Property of Juniperus Excelsa, *Olea oleaster* and *Olea europaea*. *J. King Saud. Univ. Sci.* **2023**, *35*, 102446. [CrossRef]
25. Ibibia, E.-K.T. Determination of the Total Phenolic Contents, Antimicrobial and Antioxidant Effects in the Ethanolic Leaf Extract of *Prunus amgydalus*. *J. Appl. Pharm. Sci.* **2013**, *3*, 94–100.
26. Arangia, A.; Ragno, A.; Cordaro, M.; D'Amico, R.; Siracusa, R.; Fusco, R.; Marino Merlo, F.; Smeriglio, A.; Impellizzeri, D.; Cuzzocrea, S.; et al. Antioxidant Activity of a Sicilian Almond Skin Extract Using In Vitro and In Vivo Models. *Int. J. Mol. Sci.* **2023**, *24*, 12115. [CrossRef] [PubMed]
27. Ramachandran, S.; Nikitha, J.; Gopi, C.; Amala, M.; Dhanaraju, M.D. Effect of *Prunus dulcis* and *Salvia hispenica* in the Management of Polycystic Ovary Syndrome in Wistar Rats. *J. Taibah Univ. Med. Sci.* **2020**, *15*, 122–128. [CrossRef]
28. Kamiloglu, S.; Serali, O.; Unal, N.; Capanoglu, E. Antioxidant Activity and Polyphenol Composition of Black Mulberry (*Morus nigra* L.) Products. *J. Berry Res.* **2013**, *3*, 41–51. [CrossRef]
29. Thabti, I.; Elfalleh, W.; Tlili, N.; Ziadi, M.; Campos, M.G.; Ferchichi, A. Phenols, Flavonoids, and Antioxidant and Antibacterial Activity of Leaves and Stem Bark of *Morus* Species. *Int. J. Food Prop.* **2014**, *17*, 842–854. [CrossRef]
30. Pycia, K.; Kapusta, I.; Jaworska, G. Impact of the Degree of Maturity of Walnuts (*Juglans regia* L.) and Their Variety on the Antioxidant Potential and the Content of Tocopherols and Polyphenols. *Molecules* **2019**, *24*, 2936. [CrossRef]
31. Pycia, K.; Kapusta, I.; Jaworska, G.; Jankowska, A. Antioxidant Properties, Profile of Polyphenolic Compounds and Tocopherol Content in Various Walnut (*Juglans regia* L.) Varieties. *Eur. Food Res. Technol.* **2019**, *245*, 607–616. [CrossRef]
32. Oliveira, I.; Sousa, A.; Ferreira, I.C.F.R.; Bento, A.; Estevinho, L.; Pereira, J.A. Total Phenols, Antioxidant Potential and Antimicrobial Activity of Walnut (*Juglans regia* L.) Green Husks. *Food Chem. Toxicol.* **2008**, *46*, 2326–2331. [CrossRef]

33. Pereira, J.A.; Oliveira, I.; Sousa, A.; Ferreira, I.C.F.R.; Bento, A.; Estevinho, L. Bioactive Properties and Chemical Composition of Six Walnut (*Juglans regia* L.) Cultivars. *Food Chem. Toxicol.* **2008**, *46*, 2103–2111. [CrossRef]
34. Cintesun, S.; Ozman, Z.; Kocyigit, A.; Mansuroglu, B.; Kocacaliskan, I. Effects of Walnut (*Juglans regia* L.) Kernel Extract and Juglone on Dopamine Levels and Oxidative Stress in Rats. *Food Biosci.* **2023**, *51*, 102327. [CrossRef]
35. Pires, T.C.S.P.; Caleja, C.; Santos-Buelga, C.; Barros, L.; Ferreira, I.C.F.R. *Vaccinium myrtillus* L. Fruits as a Novel Source of Phenolic Compounds with Health Benefits and Industrial Applications—A Review. *Curr. Pharm. Des.* **2020**, *26*, 1917–1928. [CrossRef]
36. Satoh, Y.; Ishihara, K. Investigation of the Antimicrobial Activity of Bilberry (*Vaccinium myrtillus* L.) Extract against Periodontopathic Bacteria. *J. Oral Biosci.* **2020**, *62*, 169–174. [CrossRef] [PubMed]
37. Dragana, M.V.; Miroslav, R.P.; Branka, B.R.G.; Olgica, D.S.; Sava, M.V.; Ljiljana, R.Č. Antibacterial and Antioxidant Activities of Bilberry (*Vaccinium myrtillus* L.) in Vitro. *Afr. J. Microbiol. Res.* **2013**, *7*, 5130–5136. [CrossRef]
38. Elkiran, O.; Avşar, C. Chemical Composition and Biological Activities of the Essential Oil from the Leaves of *Vaccinium myrtillus* L. *Bangladesh J. Bot.* **2020**, *49*, 91–96. [CrossRef]
39. Klavins, L.; Mezulis, M.; Nikolajeva, V.; Klavins, M. Composition, Sun Protective and Antimicrobial Activity of Lipophilic Bilberry (*Vaccinium myrtillus* L.) and Lingonberry (*Vaccinium vitis-idaea* L.) Extract Fractions. *LWT* **2021**, *138*, 110784. [CrossRef]
40. Neamtu, A.A.; Szoke-Kovacs, R.; Mihok, E.; Georgescu, C.; Turcus, V.; Olah, N.K.; Frum, A.; Tita, O.; Neamtu, C.; Szoke-Kovacs, Z.; et al. Bilberry (*Vaccinium myrtillus* L.) Extracts Comparative Analysis Regarding Their Phytonutrient Profiles, Antioxidant Capacity along with the In Vivo Rescue Effects Tested on a Drosophila melanogaster High-Sugar Diet Model. *Antioxidants* **2020**, *9*, 1067. [CrossRef] [PubMed]
41. Habanova, M.; Saraiva, J.A.; Haban, M.; Schwarzova, M.; Chlebo, P.; Predna, L.; Gažo, J.; Wyka, J. Intake of Bilberries (*Vaccinium myrtillus* L.) Reduced Risk Factors for Cardiovascular Disease by Inducing Favorable Changes in Lipoprotein Profiles. *Nutr. Res.* **2016**, *36*, 1415–1422. [CrossRef] [PubMed]
42. Kaume, L.; Howard, L.R.; Devareddy, L. The Blackberry Fruit: A Review on Its Composition and Chemistry, Metabolism and Bioavailability, and Health Benefits. *J. Agric. Food Chem.* **2012**, *60*, 5716–5727. [CrossRef]
43. Bushway, L.J.; Pritts, M.P.; Handley, D.T. (Eds.) *Raspberry & Blackberry Production Guide for the Northeast, Midwest, and Eastern Canada*; NRAES; Natural Resource, Agriculture, and Engineering Service, Cooperative Extension: Ithaca, NY, USA, 2008.
44. Gopalan, A.; Reuben, S.C.; Ahmed, S.; Darvesh, A.S.; Hohmann, J.; Bishayee, A. The Health Benefits of Blackcurrants. *Food Funct.* **2012**, *3*, 795. [CrossRef] [PubMed]
45. Tabart, J.; Kevers, C.; Evers, D.; Dommes, J. Ascorbic Acid, Phenolic Acid, Flavonoid, and Carotenoid Profiles of Selected Extracts from *Ribes nigrum*. *J. Agric. Food Chem.* **2011**, *59*, 4763–4770. [CrossRef] [PubMed]
46. Tabart, J.; Kevers, C.; Pincemail, J.; Defraigne, J.-O.; Dommes, J. Antioxidant Capacity of Black Currant Varies with Organ, Season, and Cultivar. *J. Agric. Food Chem.* **2006**, *54*, 6271–6276. [CrossRef]
47. Kendir, G.; Süntar, I.; Çeribaşı, A.O.; Köroğlu, A. Activity Evaluation on *Ribes* Species, Traditionally Used to Speed up Healing of Wounds: With Special Focus on Ribes Nigrum. *J. Ethnopharmacol.* **2019**, *237*, 141–148. [CrossRef]
48. Téglás, T.; Mihok, E.; Cziáky, Z.; Oláh, N.-K.; Nyakas, C.; Máthé, E. The Flavonoid Rich Black Currant (*Ribes nigrum*) Ethanolic Gemmotherapy Extract Elicits Neuroprotective Effect by Preventing Microglial Body Swelling in Hippocampus and Reduces Serum TNF-α Level: Pilot Study. *Molecules* **2023**, *28*, 3571. [CrossRef] [PubMed]
49. El Baaboua, A.; El Maadoudi, M.; Bouyahya, A.; Belmehdi, O.; Kounnoun, A.; Cheyadmi, S.; Ouzakar, S.; Senhaji, N.S.; Abrini, J. Evaluation of the Combined Effect of Antibiotics and Essential Oils against *Campylobacter* Multidrug Resistant Strains and Their Biofilm Formation. *S. Afr. J. Bot.* **2022**, *150*, 451–465. [CrossRef]
50. Pisoschi, A.M.; Pop, A.; Georgescu, C.; Turcuş, V.; Olah, N.K.; Mathe, E. An overview of natural antimicrobials role in food. *Eur. J. Med. Chem.* **2018**, *143*, 922–935. [CrossRef] [PubMed]
51. Aleya, A.; Mihok, E.; Pecsenye, B.; Jolji, M.; Kertész, A.; Bársony, P.; Vígh, S.; Cziaky, Z.; Máthé, A.-B.; Burtescu, R.F.; et al. Phytoconstituent Profiles Associated with Relevant Antioxidant Potential and Variable Nutritive Effects of the Olive, Sweet Almond, and Black Mulberry Gemmotherapy Extracts. *Antioxidants* **2023**, *12*, 1717. [CrossRef]
52. Dengyu, Y.; Tiancheng, W.; Miao, L.; Peng, L. Quercetin: Its Main Pharmacological Activity and Potential Application in Clinical Medicine. *Oxid. Med. Cell Longev.* **2020**, *2020*, 8825387.
53. Kępa, M.; Miklasińska-Majdanik, M.; Wojtyczka, R.D.; Idzik, D.; Korzeniowski, K.; Smoleń-Dzirba, J.; Wąsik, T.J. Antimicrobial Potential of Caffeic Acid against *Staphylococcus aureus* Clinical Strains. *BioMed Res. Int.* **2018**, *2018*, 7413504. [CrossRef]
54. Aliabadi, M.A.; Darsanaki, R.K.; Rokhi, M.L.; Raeisi, G. Antimicrobial Activity of Olive Leaf Aqueous Extract. *Ann. Biol. Res.* **2012**, *3*, 4189–4191.
55. Himour, S.; Yahia, A.; Belattar, H. Oleuropein and Antibacterial Activities of *Olea europaea* L. Leaf Extract. *Eur. Sci. J.* **2017**, *13*, 342. [CrossRef]
56. Nora, N.B.; Hamid, K.; Snouci, M.; Boumedien, M.; Abdellah, M. Antibacterial Activity and Phytochemical Screening of *Olea europaea* Leaves from Algeria. *TOPROCJ* **2012**, *3*, 66–69. [CrossRef]
57. Borges, A.; José, H.; Homem, V.; Simões, M. Comparison of Techniques and Solvents on the Antimicrobial and Antioxidant Potential of Extracts from *Acacia dealbata* and *Olea europaea*. *Antibiotics* **2020**, *9*, 48. [CrossRef]
58. Gökmen, M.; Kara, R.; Akkaya, L.; Torlak, E.; Önen, A. Evaluation of Antimicrobial Activity in Olive (*Olea europaea* L.) Leaf Extract. *Am. J. Microbiol.* **2014**, *5*, 37–40. [CrossRef]

59. Dobrinčić, A.; Repajić, M.; Garofulić, I.E.; Tuđen, L.; Dragović-Uzelac, V.; Levaj, B. Comparison of Different Extraction Methods for the Recovery of Olive Leaves Polyphenols. *Processes* **2020**, *8*, 1008. [CrossRef]
60. Bisignano, G.; Tomaino, A.; Cascio, R.L.; Crisafi, G.; Uccella, N.; Saija, A. On the In-Vitro Antimicrobial Activity of Oleuropein and Hydroxytyrosol. *J. Pharm. Pharmacol.* **1999**, *51*, 971–974. [CrossRef]
61. Thielmann, J.; Kohnen, S.; Hauser, C. Antimicrobial Activity of *Olea europaea* Linné Extracts and Their Applicability as Natural Food Preservative Agents. *Int. J. Food Microbiol.* **2017**, *251*, 48–66. [CrossRef] [PubMed]
62. Sudjana, A.N.; D'Orazio, C.; Ryan, V.; Rasool, N.; Ng, J.; Islam, N.; Riley, T.V.; Hammer, K.A. Antimicrobial Activity of Commercial *Olea europaea* (Olive) Leaf Extract. *Int. J. Antimicrob. Agents* **2009**, *33*, 461–463. [CrossRef] [PubMed]
63. Weli, A.M.; Al-Saadi, H.S.; Al-Fudhaili, R.S.; Hossain, A.; Putit, Z.B.; Jasim, M.K. Cytotoxic and Antimicrobial Potential of Different Leaves Extracts of *R. fruticosus* Used Traditionally to Treat Diabetes. *Toxicol. Rep.* **2020**, *7*, 183–187. [CrossRef] [PubMed]
64. Riaz, M.; Ahmad, M.; Rahman, N. Antimicrobial Screening of Fruit, Leaves, Root and Stem of *Rubus fruticosus*. *J. Med. Plants Res.* **2011**, *5*, 5920–5924.
65. Pavlović, A.V.; Papetti, A.; Zagorac, D.Č.D.; Gašić, U.M.; Mišić, D.M.; Tešić, Ž.L.; Natić, M.M. Phenolics Composition of Leaf Extracts of Raspberry and Blackberry Cultivars Grown in Serbia. *Ind. Crops Prod.* **2016**, *87*, 304–314. [CrossRef]
66. Gil-Martínez, L.; Mut-Salud, N.; Ruiz-García, J.A.; Falcón-Piñeiro, A.; Maijó-Ferré, M.; Baños, A.; De La Torre-Ramírez, J.M.; Guillamón, E.; Verardo, V.; Gómez-Caravaca, A.M. Phytochemicals Determination, and Antioxidant, Antimicrobial, Anti-Inflammatory and Anticancer Activities of Blackberry Fruits. *Foods* **2023**, *12*, 1505. [CrossRef]
67. Ieri, F.; Martini, S.; Innocenti, M.; Mulinacci, N. Phenolic distribution in liquid preparations of *Vaccinium myrtillus* L. and *Vaccinium vitis idaea* L. *Phytochem. Anal.* **2013**, *24*, 467–475. [CrossRef] [PubMed]
68. Miljković, V.M.; Nikolić, G.S.; Zvezdanović, J.; Mihajlov-Krstev, T.; Arsić, B.B.; Miljković, M.N. Phenolic Profile, Mineral Content and Antibacterial Activity of the Methanol Extract of *Vaccinium myrtillus* L. *Not. Bot. Horti Agrobo.* **2018**, *46*, 122–127. [CrossRef]
69. Tiwari, U.; Dubey, N.; Kaushik, S. Antibacterial and Antioxidant Efficacy Analysis of Leaves Extracts of *Prunus amygdalus* (Badam) in Different Solvents. *Int. J. Curr. Microbiol. Appl. Sci.* **2015**, *4*, 728–736.
70. Musarra-Pizzo, M.; Ginestra, G.; Smeriglio, A.; Pennisi, R.; Sciortino, M.T.; Mandalari, G. The Antimicrobial and Antiviral Activity of Polyphenols from Almond (*Prunus dulcis* L.) Skin. *Nutrients* **2019**, *11*, 2355. [CrossRef] [PubMed]
71. Smeriglio, A.; Mandalari, G.; Bisignano, C.; Filocamo, A.; Barreca, D.; Bellocco, E.; Trombetta, D. Polyphenolic Content and Biological Properties of Avola Almond (*Prunus dulcis* Mill. D.A. Webb) Skin and Its Industrial Byproducts. *Ind. Crops Prod.* **2016**, *83*, 283–293. [CrossRef]
72. Muzaffer, U.; Paul, V.I. Phytochemical Analysis, in Vitro Antioxidant and Antimicrobial Activities of Male Flower of *Juglans regia* L. *Int. J. Food Prop.* **2018**, *21*, 345–356. [CrossRef]
73. Vieira, V.; Pereira, C.; Pires, T.C.S.P.; Calhelha, R.C.; Alves, M.J.; Ferreira, O.; Barros, L.; Ferreira, I.C.F.R. Phenolic Profile, Antioxidant and Antibacterial Properties of *Juglans regia* L. (Walnut) Leaves from the Northeast of Portugal. *Ind. Crops Prod.* **2019**, *134*, 347–355. [CrossRef]
74. Souza, G.R.; Oliveira-Junior, R.G.; Diniz, T.C.; Branco, A.; Lima-Saraiva, S.R.G.; Guimarães, A.L.; Oliveira, A.P.; Pacheco, A.G.M.; Silva, M.G.; Moraes-Filho, M.O.; et al. Assessment of the Antibacterial, Cytotoxic and Antioxidant Activities of *Morus nigra* L. (Moraceae). *Braz. J. Biol.* **2018**, *78*, 248–254. [CrossRef] [PubMed]
75. Yiğit, D.; Yiğit, N. Antibacterial Activity of Black Mulberry (*Morus nigra*) Fruits and Leaves. *Erzincan Univ. J. Sci. Technol.* **2008**, *1*, 39–48.
76. Georgescu, C.; Frum, A.; Virchea, L.-I.; Sumacheva, A.; Shamtsyan, M.; Gligor, F.-G.; Olah, N.K.; Mathe, E.; Mironescu, M. Geographic Variability of Berry Phytochemicals with Antioxidant and Antimicrobial Properties. *Molecules* **2022**, *27*, 4986. [CrossRef] [PubMed]
77. Bendokas, V.; Šarkinas, A.; Jasinauskienë, D.; Anisimovienë, N.; Morkûnaitë-Haimi, Š.; Stanys, V.; Šikšnianas, T. Antimicrobial Activity of Berries Extracts of Four *Ribes* Species, Their Phenolic Content and Anthocyanin Composition. *Folia Hortic.* **2018**, *30*, 249–257. [CrossRef]
78. Paunović, S.; Mašković, P.; Milinković, M. Phytochemical and Antimicrobial Profile of Black Currant Berries and Leaves. *Acta Agric. Serbica* **2022**, *27*, 25–29. [CrossRef]
79. Trajković, M.; Kitić, D.; Mihajilov-Krstev, T.; Šavikin, K.; Ranđelović, M.; Milutinović, M.; Branković, S.; Kitić, N.; Miladinović, B. Antimicrobial Activity Evaluation of Black Currant (*Ribes nigrum* L.) Variety Čačanska Crna Juice and Extract. *Acta Fac. Med. Naissensis* **2023**, *40*, 208–216. [CrossRef]
80. Zhang, F.; Cheng, W. The Mechanism of Bacterial Resistance and Potential Bacteriostatic Strategies. *Antibiotics* **2022**, *11*, 1215. [CrossRef]
81. Koopmans, M.M.; Brouwer, M.C.; Vázquez-Boland, J.A.; van de Beek, D. Human Listeriosis. *Clin. Microbiol. Rev.* **2023**, *36*, e0006019. [CrossRef]
82. Sbaraglini, M.L.; Talevi, A. Hybrid Compounds as Anti-infective Agents. *Curr. Top. Med. Chem.* **2017**, *17*, 1080–1095. [CrossRef]
83. Kuppusamy, R.; Browne, K.; Suresh, D.; Rosario, R.M.D.; Chakraborty, S.; Yang, S.; Willcox, M.D.; Black, D.S.; Chen, R.; Kumar, N. Transition Towards Antibiotic Hybrid Vehicles: The Next Generation Antibacterials. *Curr. Med. Chem.* **2022**, *30*, 104–125. [CrossRef]

84. Thwaites, M.; Hall, D.; Shinabarger, D.; Serio, A.W.; Krause, K.M.; Marra, A.; Pillar, C. Evaluation of the Bactericidal Activity of Plazomicin and Comparators against Multidrug-Resistant Enterobacteriaceae. *Antimicrob. Agents Chemother.* **2018**, *62*, e00236-18. [CrossRef] [PubMed]
85. Nemeth, J.; Oesch, G.; Kuster, S.P. Bacteriostatic versus bactericidal antibiotics for patients with serious bacterial infections: Systematic review and meta-analysis. *J. Antimicrob. Chemother.* **2015**, *70*, 382–395. [CrossRef] [PubMed]
86. Saleem, N.; Ryckaert, F.; Snow, T.A.C.; Satta, G.; Singer, M.; Arulkumaran, N. Mortality and clinical cure rates for pneumonia: A systematic review, meta-analysis, and trial sequential analysis of randomized control trials comparing bactericidal and bacteriostatic antibiotic treatments. *Clin. Microbiol. Infect.* **2022**, *28*, 936–945. [CrossRef]
87. Bauer, A.W.; Kirby, W.M.M.; Sherris, J.C.; Turck, M. Antibiotic Susceptibility Testing by a Standardized Single Disk Method. *Am. J. Clin. Pathol.* **1966**, *45*, 493–496. [CrossRef]
88. Agbebi, E.A.; Alabi, O.S.; Nkrumah, A.O.; Ogbole, O.O. Evaluation of the Antibacterial and Antifungal Potentials of Peptide-Rich Extracts from Selected Nigerian Plants. *Eur. J. Integr. Med.* **2022**, *54*, 102163. [CrossRef]

antibiotics

MDPI

Article

Combinations of *Terminalia bellirica* (Gaertn.) Roxb. and *Terminalia chebula* Retz. Extracts with Selected Antibiotics Against Antibiotic-Resistant Bacteria: Bioactivity and Phytochemistry

Gagan Tiwana [1], Ian Edwin Cock [2] and Matthew James Cheesman [1,*]

1 School of Pharmacy and Medical Sciences, Gold Coast Campus, Griffith University, Gold Coast 4222, Australia; g.tiwana@griffith.edu.au

2 School of Environment and Science, Nathan Campus, Griffith University, Brisbane 4111, Australia; i.cock@griffith.edu.au

* Correspondence: m.cheesman@griffith.edu.au; Tel.: +61-7-55529230

Abstract: Antimicrobial resistance (AMR) has arisen due to antibiotic overuse and misuse. Antibiotic resistance renders standard treatments less effective, making it difficult to control some infections, thereby increasing morbidity and mortality. Medicinal plants are attracting increased interest as antibiotics lose efficacy. This study evaluates the antibacterial activity of solvent extracts prepared using *Terminalia bellirica* and *Terminalia chebula* fruit against six bacterial pathogens using disc diffusion and broth microdilution assays. The aqueous and methanol extracts of *T. bellirica* and *T. chebula* showed substantial zones of inhibition (ZOIs) against *Staphylococcus aureus* and methicillin-resistant *S. aureus* (MRSA). The activity against those bacteria was strong, with minimum inhibitory concentrations (MIC) ranging from 94 μg/mL to 392 μg/mL. Additionally, the *T. bellirica* methanolic extract showed noteworthy antibacterial activity against *Escherichia coli* and an extended spectrum β-lactamase (ESBL) *E. coli* strain (MIC values of 755 μg/mL for both). The aqueous *T. bellirica* and *T. chebula* extracts also inhibited *Klebsiella pneumoniae* growth (MIC values of 784 μg/mL and 556 μg/mL, respectively). The corresponding methanolic extracts also inhibited ESBL *K. pneumoniae* growth (MIC values of 755 μg/mL and 1509 μg/mL, respectively). Eighteen additive interactions were observed when extracts were combined with reference antibiotics. Strong antagonism occurred when any of the extracts were mixed with polymyxin B. Liquid chromatography-mass spectroscopy (LC-MS) analysis of the extracts revealed several interesting flavonoids and tannins, including 6-galloylglucose, 1,2,6-trigalloyl-β-D-glucopyranose, 6-O-[(2E)-3-phenyl-2-propenoyl]-1-O-(3,4,5-trihydroxybenzoyl)-β-D-glucopyranose, propyl gallate, methyl gallate, sanguiin H4, hamamelitannin, pyrogallol, gallic acid, ellagic acid, chebulic acid, and chebuloside II. All extracts were nontoxic in brine shrimp assays. This lack of toxicity, combined with their antibacterial activities, suggests that these plant species may be promising sources of antibacterial compound(s) that warrant further study.

Keywords: MRSA; ESBL; plant extracts; natural therapies; combinational therapies; metabolomics

1. Introduction

Antimicrobial resistance (AMR) is one of the most concerning public health issues of the 21st century. The development of AMR mechanisms in bacterial pathogens leads to lower efficacies for standard antimicrobial therapies, which in turn promotes the transmission of these infections. The World Health Organization (WHO) has highlighted antimicrobial resistance (AMR) as a major danger to global health, food security, and future development, with far-reaching effects on human health and economic stability [1].

Antibiotic-resistant bacterial strains have rapidly arisen due to antibiotic misuse and overuse in humans and animals, as well as in agriculture. Antibiotic misuse includes excessive antibiotic prescriptions, poor treatment compliance, and the widespread use of antibiotics in livestock for growth promotion and disease prevention. This results in longer illness durations, higher mortality rates, and elevated healthcare costs [1]. AMR mortality and morbidity are concerning. AMR caused 1.27 million deaths worldwide in 2019, and current trends indicate that this number will climb dramatically [1]. Infections caused by antibiotic-resistant bacteria, such as methicillin-resistant *Staphylococcus aureus* (MRSA) and multidrug-resistant *Escherichia coli*, are particularly concerning due to their high resistance rates and severe clinical outcomes [2]. The costs associated with AMR are multifaceted, encompassing direct medical costs such as longer hospital stays and more intensive care, as well as indirect costs such as lost productivity and long-term disability. According to the World Bank, by 2050, AMR is likely to cause a loss of global economic output amounting to USD 1 trillion annually, with healthcare costs also projected to increase significantly [3].

The 2022 Global Antimicrobial Resistance and Use Surveillance System (GLASS) report underscores the significant concern regarding the alarming resistance rates of third-generation cephalosporin-resistant *E. coli* and MRSA in 76 countries [1,4]. That report also found a significant rise in *E. coli* infections resistant to ampicillin, co-trimoxazole, and fluoroquinolones. The common intestinal bacterium *Klebsiella pneumoniae* has also shown increased resistance to penicillins, cephalosporins and fluoroquinolones. These elevated levels of antibiotic resistance may lead to an increase in the use of last-resort medications, such as carbapenems [1,4]. The rise of antibiotic-resistant bacteria has outpaced drug development. The high expenditures and limited financial returns of antibiotic research and development have caused a sharp fall in the number of novel antibiotics approved for clinical use [5]. According to the WHO, there is a concerning lack of new antibacterials in the pipeline due to the lengthy research and development processes, and the high probability of failure during clinical testing [6]. Thirteen new antibiotics have received therapeutic authorization since July 2017. However, only two of these antibiotics constitute a new chemical class and are considered innovative [6]. This highlights the significant scientific and technical difficulties in finding new antibacterials that are both effective against bacteria and safe for human use.

Exploring the potential of medicinal plants in the development of antimicrobial drugs presents numerous benefits compared to conventional antibiotics. Traditional medicinal plants offer an accessible and cost-effective alternative, requiring fewer resources and less time for production [7]. They often interact with the body in a safe manner, causing minimal side effects, and often have complementary effects that enhance overall well-being. However, medicinal plants can also cause toxicity if misused. Therefore, careful dosing, accurate identification, and monitoring are essential to avoid adverse effects. Phytochemicals in medicinal plants may work together to boost antibacterial efficacy, potentiating the treatment's efficacy [7,8]. Medicinal plants possess a variety of mechanisms of action, which holds great promise in combating antibiotic-resistant bacteria [8]. The combination of plant extracts/compounds with conventional antibiotics is a strategy that can be utilized in the development of new antimicrobial therapies [9]. Phytochemicals may enhance antibiotic efficacies through synergistic and additive interactions, potentially overcoming resistance issues. This approach offers a promising solution for developing effective treatments against antibiotic-resistant bacterial strains. For example, propolis ethanolic extract potentiates the efficacy of ampicillin and vancomycin against the methicillin-resistant *S. aureus* (MRSA) [10].

The current study focuses on the antibacterial activity, phytochemistry, and toxicity of fruit extracts (aqueous, methanol, and ethyl acetate) derived from *Terminalia bellirica* (Gaertn.) Roxb. and *Terminalia chebula* Retz. Antibiotic-sensitive and antibiotic-resistant bacterial pairs of *S. aureus*, *E. coli*, and *K. pneumoniae* were examined for their growth in the presence of the extracts, as well as a panel of reference antibiotics. Our previous work revealed enhancements of *E. coli* antibacterial activity when *T. bellirica* and *T. chebula* fruit extracts were combined [11]. However, antibiotic-resistant bacterial species were not tested in that study, nor were combinational interactions between pure antibiotics and the plant extracts examined. Thakur et al. (2024) recently identified good antibacterial activities of the *T. bellirica* aqueous fruit extract against *S. aureus*, *E. coli*, and *E. coli* 385 (an antibiotic-resistant strain), with minimum inhibitory concentrations (MICs) of 312 μg/mL, 1250 μg/mL and 625 μg/mL against these species, respectively [12]. Phytochemical analysis was conducted by liquid chromatography–mass spectrometry (LC-MS), which identified a single polyphenol compound, bergenin [12]. Interestingly, flavonoids, tannins and terpenoids were not identified in the *T. bellirica* fruit extracts in that study. Furthermore, combinational interactions between reference antibiotics and the extracts were not explored. In addition, prior studies have demonstrated that fruit extracts of *T. bellirica* exhibit antibacterial activity against *S. aureus*, *E. coli*, and *K. pneumoniae* [13–15]. However, those investigations did not include combinational studies of extracts with antibiotics and testing of antibiotic-resistant bacterial strains. Other investigations reported inconsistent results for *T. chebula* fruit extracts (aqueous, ethanol, and dimethylformamide) against *S. aureus* and *K. pneumoniae*, with ZOIs of 15–18 mm on agar, using 500 μg extract per disc [16]. Furthermore, low-to-inactive antibacterial activities of *T. chebula fruit* extracts were observed against antibiotic-sensitive and antibiotic-resistant strains of *S. aureus* and *E. coli* [17,18].

In order to address the discrepancies in the previous studies regarding the activities of *T. bellirica* and *T. chebula*, and the absence of thorough phytochemical analyses of the extracts, we investigated the antibacterial properties of aqueous, methanolic, and ethyl acetate fruit extracts obtained from *T. bellirica* and *T. chebula*. Our study focused on selected bacterial pathogens, but included resistant strains of *S. aureus*, *E. coli*, and *K. pneumoniae*. We conducted disc diffusion and liquid microdilution assays to assess their effectiveness. Additionally, LC-MS was utilized to examine the phytochemical composition of *T. bellirica* and *T. chebula* and to identify specific flavonoid, phenolic acid, terpenoid, and tannin molecules. In addition, our study investigated the interactions between active plant extracts and a panel of reference antibiotics when tested as extract–antibiotic combinations in MIC assays. Finally, the toxicities of the extracts were assessed using *Artemia franciscana* Kellogg nauplii lethality assays to provide initial insights into the safety of the extracts for possible clinical use.

2. Results

2.1. Antimicrobial Susceptibility Assays

Individual 1 g masses of *T. bellirica* and *T. chebula* fruit powder was extracted separately using sterile deionized water, methanol, or ethyl acetate. The extracts were subsequently dried and resuspended in 10 mL of 1% DMSO. The extract concentrations for the two plants were generally similar, where the highest yields were obtained using methanol as a solvent, whilst ethyl acetate produced very low yields for each plant. Specifically, *T. bellirica* extract yields for water, methanol and ethyl acetate solvent extractants were 50.2, 48.3, and 3.6 mg/mL, respectively, whilst for *T. chebula* they were 35.6, 48.3, and 4.9 mg/mL.

The antibacterial efficacies of all extracts and reference antibiotics were evaluated using agar disc diffusion assays and broth microdilution assays. The aqueous and methanolic extracts of both plants exhibited activities varying from low to high against the six bacterial pathogens tested in the disc diffusion and broth dilution assays (Figure 1 and Table 1, respectively). The broth microdilution assays were used to quantify MIC values of the extracts and reference antibiotics (Table 1). The differences between the antibiotic-sensitive and antibiotic-resistant strains of the pathogens can be readily observed by the generally higher MIC values for many of the antibiotics against the resistant bacteria compared to their sensitive counterparts, as well as the lower ZOIs resulting from agar disc diffusion assays. This demonstrates that the antibiotic-resistant strains are much less sensitive to many of the antibiotics tested in this study.

When aqueous and methanol extracts of *T. bellirica* were evaluated against *S. aureus* and MRSA, they exhibited MIC values ranging from 94 and 392 μg/mL, respectively. The *T. bellirica* ethyl acetate extract also inhibited *S. aureus* and MRSA growth, albeit with a higher MIC value of 900 µg/mL. In contrast, all *T. chebula* extracts exhibited good antibacterial activity against *S. aureus* and MRSA, with MIC values ranging from 139 µg/mL to 306 µg/mL. Concordant findings were obtained for both plant extracts against *S. aureus* and MRSA in agar disc diffusion assays, where only small but detectable ZOIs were observed for the *T. bellirica* ethyl acetate extracts against the two *Staphylococcus* species, although much larger ZOIs of 9–15 mm were produced by all other extracts against *S. aureus* and MRSA (Figure 1).

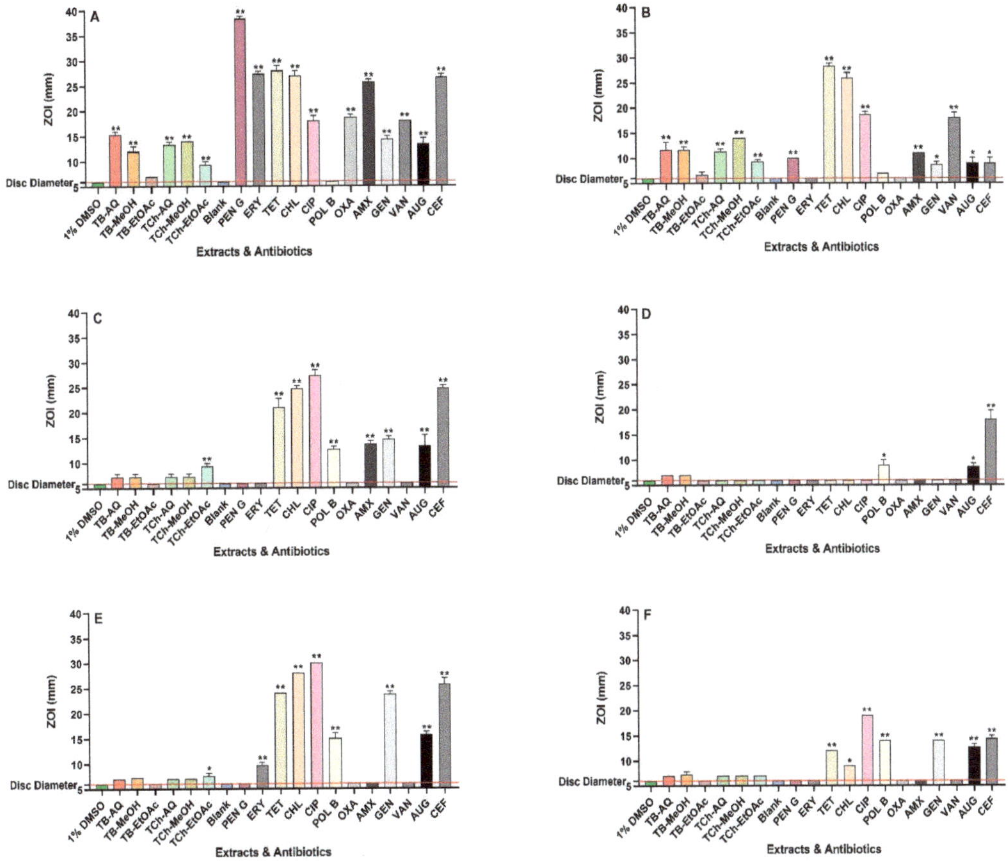

Figure 1. Antimicrobial activities of *T. bellirica* and *T. chebula* fruit extracts in agar disc diffusion assays against (**A**) *S. aureus*, (**B**) MRSA, (**C**) *E. coli*, (**D**) ESBL *E. coli*, (**E**) *K. pneumoniae*, and (**F**) ESBL *K. pneumoniae*. TB-AQ = *T. bellirica* aqueous; TB-MeOH = *T. bellirica* methanol; and TB-EtOAc = *T. bellirica* ethyl acetate. TCh-AQ = *T. chebula* aqueous; TCh-MeOH = *T. chebula* methanol; and TCh-EtOAc = *T. chebula* ethyl acetate. Negative controls = 1% DMSO and Blank = sterile water. Reference antibiotics: PEN G = penicillin G (10 IU), ERY = erythromycin (10 µg), TET = tetracycline (30 µg), CHL = chloramphenicol (30 µg), CIP = ciprofloxacin (1 µg), POL B = polymyxin B (300IU), OXA = oxacillin (1 µg), AMX = amoxycillin (10 µL of 0.01 mg/mL stock solution), GEN = gentamicin (10 µg), VAN = vancomycin (30 µg), AUG = Augmentin® (15 µg), and CEF = cefoxitin (30 µg). Horizontal red lines on the *y*-axis at 6 mm indicates the disc diameter used in the assay. Mean values (±SEM) are reported from three independent studies. *p*-values < 0.01 are represented with a single asterisk symbol (*), while *p*-values < 0.001 are represented with a double asterisk symbol (**).

Similarly, the extracts were also screened against *E. coli* and *K. pneumoniae*, as well as their antibiotic-resistant ESBL counterparts. The agar disc diffusion experiments showed limited growth inhibition for most of the extracts when tested against *E. coli*, ESBL *E. coli*, *K. pneumoniae*, and ESBL *K. pneumoniae*. However, these results cannot be considered as zones of inhibition (ZOIs) because complete inhibition surrounding the disc is necessary. Interestingly, the *T. chebula* ethyl acetate extract produced a small but distinct ZOI against *E. coli* and *K. pneumoniae* on agar (7–9 mm) in the disc diffusion assay (Figure 1). Furthermore, relatively high MIC values were determined for the *T. bellirica* aqueous extracts and the *T. chebula* aqueous and methanol extracts against *E. coli* and ESBL *E. coli* (MIC = 1509 µg/mL to 3138 µg/mL). Notably, an MIC value of 755 µg/mL was obtained for the *T. bellirica* methanolic extract against these two species. The aqueous *T. bellirica* and *T. chebula* extracts also exhibited noteworthy antibacterial activity against *K. pneumoniae*, with MIC values of 784 µg/mL and 556 µg/mL, respectively. Moderate activities towards this bacterium were found when the *T. bellirica* and *T. chebula* methanolic extracts were tested (MIC = 1509 µg/mL), as well as the ethyl acetate *T. chebula* extract (MIC = 1225 µg/mL). Additionally, the ESBL *K. pneumoniae* was inhibited in broth assays by the methanolic *T. bellirica* and *T. chebula* extracts (MIC values of 755 µg/mL and 1509 µg/mL, respectively). However, the aqueous extracts yielded low activities (relatively high MIC values) against ESBL *K. pneumoniae* (MIC values of 3138 µg/mL and 2225 µg/mL, respectively).

Table 1. MIC values (µg/mL) for aqueous, methanol, and ethyl acetate of *T. bellirica* and *T. chebula* extracts, and the reference (positive control) antibiotics against the six bacterial strains.

Extract Type or Antibiotic	**Bacterial Species and MIC (µg/mL)**					
	S. aureus	**MRSA**	***E. coli***	**ESBL *E. coli***	***K. pneumoniae***	**ESBL *K. pneumoniae***
TB-AQ	392	196	**3138**	1569	784	**3138**
TB-MeOH	94	189	755	755	1509	755
TB-EtOAc	900	900	Inactive	Inactive	Inactive	Inactive
TCh-AQ	139	139	**2225**	**2225**	556	**2225**
TCh-MeOH	189	189	**3019**	1509	1509	1509
TCh-EtOAc	306	306	Inactive	Inactive	1225	Inactive
PENG	**1.25**	>2.5	>2.5	>2.5	>2.5	>2.5
ERY	**0.31**	>2.5	>2.5	>2.5	>2.5	>2.5
TET	**0.16**	**0.04**	**0.31**	>2.5	**0.625**	>2.5
CHL	>2.5	>2.5	**2.5**	>2.5	**2.5**	>2.5
CIP	**0.16**	**0.625**	**0.02**	>2.5	**0.02**	**0.16**
POLB	>2.5	>2.5	**0.02**	**0.02**	**0.02**	**0.04**
OXA	**0.16**	>2.5	>2.5	>2.5	>2.5	>2.5
AMX	**0.625**	>2.5	>2.5	>2.5	>2.5	>2.5
GEN	>2.5	>2.5	**0.625**	>2.5	**0.625**	>2.5

MIC values for extracts with no antibacterial activity (Inactive; MIC > 10,000 µg/mL), low activity (2000–5000 µg/mL; shown in bold), moderate activity (1000–2000 µg/mL; shown in blue), noteworthy activity (400–1000 µg/mL; shown in red), or good activity (100–400 µg/mL; shown in green). Reference antibiotics: PENG = penicillin G, ERY = erythromycin, TET = tetracycline, CHL = chloramphenicol, CIP = ciprofloxacin, POLB = polymyxin B, OXA = oxacillin, AMX = amoxycillin, GEN = gentamicin, and VAN = vancomycin. Active antibiotics are shown in bold, while lack of antibiotic activity was observed when MIC values > 2.5 µg/mL.

2.2. Combination Assays: Sum of Fractional Inhibitory Concentration (ΣFIC) Determinations

Combinations of the *T. bellirica* and *T. chebula* extracts with conventional antibiotics were tested to detect any possible interactions between the two components against the antibiotic-sensitive and antibiotic-resistant bacterial strains (Table 2). For these assays to be conducted, both the extract and the antibiotic must demonstrate efficacy against the bacterial species under examination, as MIC values for both components are required to determine ΣFIC values. No synergistic interactions were observed for any of the combinations. Eighteen combinations caused additive effects, and eighty combinations were indifferent. Additionally, nineteen combinations had antagonistic effects.

Table 2. ∑FIC values calculated for combinations of T. bellirica and T. chebula extracts and conventional antibiotics.

Bacteria	Extracts	PENG	ERY	TET	CHL	CIP	POLB	OXA	AMX	GEN	VAN
S. aureus	TB-AQ	0.53	1.26	1.50	-	1.50	-	1.25	0.56	-	1.06
	TB-MeOH	1.02	2.13	1.13	-	2.25	-	1.25	1.03	-	2.03
	TB-EtOAc	0.75	1.13	1.06	-	2.06	-	2.13	1.25	-	1.50
	TChAQ	1.06	1.25	0.75	-	1.50	-	1.50	1.13	-	1.06
	TCh-MeOH	1.03	1.13	1.25	-	1.25	-	1.25	1.06	-	1.03
	TCh-EtOH	0.75	0.75	1.25	-	2.50	-	2.50	1.00	-	1.50
MRSA	TB-AQ	-	-	1.00	-	1.06	-	-	-	-	1.03
	TB-MeOH	-	-	1.50	-	1.03	-	-	-	-	1.02
	TB-EtOAc	-	-	1.02	-	0.63	-	-	-	-	1.50
	TCh-AQ	-	-	1.00	-	2.13	-	-	-	-	2.06
	TCh-MeOH	-	-	1.00	-	1.06	-	-	-	-	1.03
	TCh-EtOAc	-	-	1.06	-	1.00	-	-	-	-	1.50
E. coli	TB-AQ	-	-	1.50	1.25	2.25	64.50	-	-	2.00	-
	TB-MeOH	-	-	1.52	1.06	4.00	17.50	-	-	1.25	-
	TCh-AQ	-	-	1.50	1.25	2.25	64.50	-	-	2.00	-
	TCh-MeOH	-	-	0.76	1.25	2.25	32.25	-	-	2.00	-
ESBL *E. coli*	TB-AQ	-	-	-	-	-	16.50	-	-	-	-
	TB-MeOH	-	-	-	-	-	5.00	-	-	-	-
	TCh-AQ	-	-	-	-	-	32.50	-	-	-	-
	TCh-MeOH	-	-	-	-	-	16.50	-	-	-	
K. pneumoniae	TB-AQ	-	-	1.25	1.06	2.00	9.00	-	-	1.25	-
	TB-MeOH	-	-	1.50	1.12	3.00	16.50	-	-	1.50	-
	TB-EtOAc	-	-	-	-	-	-	-	-	-	-
	TCh-AQ	-	-	1.25	1.06	4.00	9.00	-	-	1.25	-
	TCh-MeOH	-	-	0.75	0.56	3.00	16.50	-	-	1.50	-
	TCh-EtOAc	-	-	0.63	1.00	2.12	63.00	-	-	4.00	-
ESBL *K. pneumoniae*	TB-AQ	-	-	-	-	1.25	8.25	-	-	-	-
	TB-MeOH	-	-	-	-	1.00	2.50	-	-	-	-
	TCh-AQ	-	-	-	-	2.50	16.60	-	-	-	-
	TCh-MeOH	-	-	-	-	1.50	8.75	-	-	-	-

∑ FIC values of aqueous (TB-AQ, TCh-AQ), methanolic (TB-MeOH, TCh-MeOH) and ethyl acetate (TB-EtOAc, TCh-EtOAc) extracts of *T. bellirica* and *T. chebula*, respectively, in combination with reference antibiotics against antibiotic-sensitive and antibiotic-resistant strains of *S. aureus*, MRSA, *E. coli*, ESBL *E. coli*, *K. pneumoniae*, and ESBL *K. pneumoniae*. Additive interaction: >0.5 ≤ 1.00 and are in blue color, indifferent interaction: >1.01–≤4.00, antagonistic interaction: >4.0 and are in red color.—indicates the extract and/or the antibiotic was inactive against the bacteria being tested. Reference antibiotics: PENG = penicillin G, ERY = erythromycin, TET = tetracycline, CHL = chloramphenicol, CIP = ciprofloxacin, POL B = polymyxin B, OXA = oxacillin, AMX = amoxycillin, GEN = gentamicin, and VAN = vancomycin.

2.3. *Compound Identification by LC-MS Metabolomics Fingerprinting*

LC-MS fingerprinting analysis was employed to investigate the metabolomic fingerprints of all extracts, with particular focus on the flavonoid, tannin, and terpenoid compounds. Most of the extract compounds eluted in the gradient stage of the chromatogram from 30% to 90% acetonitrile (Supplementary Materials Figures S1 and S2), suggesting that most of the extract components were of relatively high polarity [19]. Organic acids and amines are more likely to elute in polar environments and therefore do so early in the chromatogram. Conversely, lipophilic substances and hydrocarbons, which exhibit a stronger interaction with the non-polar stationary phase, elute later as the gradient persists. Only compounds that were completely matched in any of the databases (and were not present in the blank controls) were chosen to create a potential inventory of all the identified compounds (Supplementary Materials: Tables S1 and S2). In this study, we have focused on the flavonoid, tannin, terpenoid and phenolic acid compounds (Table 3).

Table 3. LC-MS putative identification and % relative abundance of phytochemicals identified in the fruit extracts of *T. bellirica* (TB) and *T. chebula* (TCh).

Retention Time (min)	Molecular Weight	Empirical Formula	Putative Compounds	% Relative Abundance (TB)			% Relative Abundance (TCh)		
				AQ	MeOH	EtOAc	AQ	MeOH	EtOAc
1.496	192.06305	$C_7H_{12}O_6$	Quinic acid	3.13%	0.33%	0.19%	0.39%	-	1.53%
1.573	344.07409	$C_{14}H_{16}O_{10}$	Theogallin	-	3.47%	-	-	0.03%	0.02%
1.784	302.06328	$C_{12}H_{14}O_9$	Pyrogallol-2-O-glucuronide	-	0.21%	-	0.07%	-	-
1.793	244.0581	$C_{10}H_{12}O_7$	1-O-Galloylglycerol	-	-	0.02%	-	-	-
1.905	236.0684	$C_{12}H_{12}O_5$	Dillapional	0.01%	-	-	-	T	0.01%
1.923	316.0793	$C_{13}H_{16}O_9$	Ginnalin B	0.01%	-	-	-	-	-
1.975	149.08397	$C_9H_{11}NO$	Venoterpine	-	-	0.05%	0.04%	-	-
2.045	294.03749	$C_{13}H_{10}O_8$	Banksiamarin B	-	-	0.15%	0.17%	0.05%	0.13%
2.058	174.05268	$C_7H_{10}O_5$	Shikimic acid	-	0.41%	0.67%	2.64%	3.14%	4.80%
2.237	154.02646	$C_7H_6O_4$	Gentisic acid	0.02%	0.05%	-	0.01%	-	0.09%
2.296	448.15769	$C_{19}H_{28}O_{12}$	8-O-Acetyl shanzhiside methyl ester	-	-	-	0.19%	0.18%	-
2.356	332.07411	$C_{13}H_{16}O_{10}$	6-Galloylglucose	6.06%	3.97%	3.39%	3.74%	0.68%	-
2.444	448.06386	$C_{20}H_{16}O_{12}$	Ellagic acid 2-rhamnoside	0.11%	1.44%	0.69%	0.01%	0.21%	0.33%
2.51	292.02177	$C_{13}H_8O_8$	Brevifolincarboxylic acid	0.09%	-	-	0.11%	0.03%	0.61%
2.56	288.0844	$C_{12}H_{16}O_8$	Phlorin	-	0.02%	-	0.03%	0.02%	-
3.11	484.0848	$C_{20}H_{20}O_{14}$	Gallic acid 3-O-(6-galloylglucoside)	0.74%	-	-	-	-	-
3.158	212.06824	$C_{10}H_{12}O_5$	Propyl gallate	-	-	-	0.30%	0.35%	0.12%
4.4	277.05821	$C_{13}H_{11}NO_6$	Salfredin C1	-	-	-	0.14%	-	0.03%
4.847	184.03703	$C_8H_8O_5$	Methyl gallate	0.25%	11.39%	-	0.04%	1.05%	-
5.638	444.19969	$C_{21}H_{32}O_{10}$	Cynaroside A	-	-	-	0.02%	0.02%	-
8.848	636.09627	$C_{27}H_{24}O_{18}$	1,3,4-Trigalloyl-β-D-glucopyranose	-	-	-	-	0.07%	0.25%
8.44	484.0855	$C_{20}H_{20}O_{14}$	1,6-Bis-O-(3,4,5-trihydroxybenzoyl) hexopyranose	5.13%	5.19%	2.52%	6.52%	2.16%	3.78%

Table 3. *Cont.*

Retention Time (min)	Molecular Weight	Empirical Formula	Putative Compounds	% Relative Abundance (TB)			% Relative Abundance (TCh)		
				AQ	MeOH	EtOAc	AQ	MeOH	EtOAc
8.961	478.07436	$C_{21}H_{18}O_{13}$	Quercetin 7-glucuronide	-	-	-	-	-	0.49%
8.985	478.0743	$C_{21}H_{18}O_{13}$	Quercetin 3-O-glucuronide	-	0.08%	-	-	-	-
9.316	470.01176	$C_{21}H_{10}O_{13}$	Sanguisorbic acid dilactone	-	0.08%	-	0.56%	0.61%	0.19%
9.567	634.08082	$C_{27}H_{22}O_{18}$	Sanguiin H4	0.84%	-	0.07%	-	5.63%	0.54%
9.811	478.07452	$C_{21}H_{18}O_{13}$	Miquelianin	0.04%	0.42%	-	0.37%	0.60%	0.39%
9.902	152.04703	$C_8H_8O_3$	Vanillin	-	-	-	0.16%	0.17%	0.17%
9.921	126.03146	$C_6H_6O_3$	Phloroglucinol	0.10%	1.93%	-	0.07%	0.24%	0.27%
10.043	636.09614	$C_{27}H_{24}O_{18}$	1,2,6-Trigalloyl-β-D-glucopyranose	0.09%	5.44%	2.85%	0.11%	1.42%	2.22%
10.158	634.08037	$C_{27}H_{22}O_{18}$	Corilagin	-	-	-	-	0.15%	-
10.357	524.1533	$C_{24}H_{28}O_{13}$	Barbatoflavan	0.01%	-	-	-	-	-
10.419	484.08522	$C_{20}H_{20}O_{14}$	Hamamelitannin	2.10%	0.02%	0.62%	0.02%	0.11%	-
10.421	126.0316	$C_6H_6O_3$	Pyrogallol	6.28%	5.28%	2.19%	6.29%	3.82%	4.87%
10.422	296.05248	$C_{13}H_{12}O_8$	cis-Coutaric acid	0.33%	0.86%	0.19%	0.31%	0.93%	1.05%
10.476	636.09612	$C_{27}H_{24}O_{18}$	1,4,6-Trigalloyl-β-D-glucopyranose	-	-	-	-	-	0.63%
10.55	601.99658	$C_{28}H_{10}O_{16}$	Diellagilactone	-	-	-	1.13%	0.60%	-
10.703	372.1055	$C_{16}H_{20}O_{10}$	Veranisatin C	0.02%	0.04%	-	-	-	-
10.754	636.09608	$C_{27}H_{24}O_{18}$	1,3,6-Tri-O-galloyl-β-D-glucose	-	0.25%	0.93%	0.64%	-	-
11.305	170.02138	$C_7H_6O_5$	Phloroglucinic acid	0.98%	2.80%	4.33%	0.98%	0.83%	1.24%
11.091	610.1535	$C_{27}H_{30}O_{16}$	Rutin	-	0.14%	0.10%	-	0.03%	0.08%
11.176	432.10539	$C_{21}H_{20}O_{10}$	Vitexin	-	-	-	-	0.05%	-
11.257	304.0579	$C_{15}H_{12}O_7$	Nigrescin	T	0.02%	-	-	-	-
11.272	610.1527	$C_{27}H_{30}O_{16}$	Quercetin 3-O-rhamnoside-7-O-glucoside	0.05%	-	-	-	-	-
11.448	302.04213	$C_{15}H_{10}O_7$	Quercetin	0.11%	0.33%	0.17%	0.02%	-	-
11.473	464.0951	$C_{21}H_{20}O_{12}$	Myricitrin	0.05%	0.13%	0.19%	-	-	-
11.529	422.0846	$C_{19}H_{18}O_{11}$	1,5,8-Trihydroxy-9-oxo-9H-xanthen-3-yl β-D-glucopyranoside	0.02%	0.05%	-	-	-	-
11.589	170.02147	$C_7H_6O_5$	Gallic acid	26.23%	8.64%	2.60%	23.90%	1.90%	1.56%
11.756	216.0994	$C_{10}H_{16}O_5$	(4S,5S,8S,10R)-4,5,8-trihydroxy-10-methyl-3,4,5,8,9,10-hexahydro-2H-oxecin-2-one	0.05%	-	-	0.06%	-	1.23%
11.822	462.07961	$C_{21}H_{18}O_{12}$	Aureusidin 6-glucuronide	-	-	2.52%	-	-	0.04%
11.905	286.04729	$C_{15}H_{10}O_6$	Maritimetin	-	-	-	T	0.01%	0.01%
11.906	594.15829	$C_{27}H_{30}O_{15}$	Palasitrin	-	-	-	0.01%	-	0.03%

Table 3. *Cont.*

Retention Time (min)	Molecular Weight	Empirical Formula	Putative Compounds	% Relative Abundance (TB)			% Relative Abundance (TCh)		
				AQ	MeOH	EtOAc	AQ	MeOH	EtOAc
11.938	176.04708	$C_{10}H_8O_3$	4-Methylumbelliferone hydrate	-	-	-	0.03%	0.03%	-
11.953	310.10477	$C_{15}H_{18}O_7$	(E)-1-O-Cinnamoyl-β-D-glucose	-	-	-	-	-	1.67%
12.141	584.1169	$C_{28}H_{24}O_{14}$	2′′-O-Galloylisovitexin	-	-	-	-	-	0.01%
12.183	448.0996	$C_{21}H_{20}O_{11}$	Maritimein	-	0.01%	0.02%	-	-	-
12.185	302.00627	$C_{14}H_6O_8$	Ellagic acid	2.45%	10.74%	33.49%	8.39%	10.46%	11.96%
12.201	220.07336	$C_{12}H_{12}O_4$	Eugenitin	-	-	-	-	-	0.04%
12.233	262.0476	$C_{13}H_{10}O_6$	Maclurin	-	0.02%	-	0.04%	-	-
12.254	148.05223	$C_9H_8O_2$	trans-Cinnamic acid	-	-	-	0.76%	0.96%	0.87%
12.38	334.0325	$C_{15}H_{10}O_9$	3,5,6,7,2′,3′,4′-Heptahydroxyflavone	-	0.20%	-	-	-	-
12.503	192.07847	$C_{11}H_{12}O_3$	(R)-Shinanolone	-	-	-	0.04%	0.03%	0.05%
12.504	310.10483	$C_{15}H_{18}O_7$	(2S,3R,4S,5S,6R)-3,4,5-trihydroxy-6-(hydroxymethyl) oxan-2-yl (2E)-3-phenylprop-2-enoate	-	-	-	2.25%	-	-
12.509	610.1894	$C_{28}H_{34}O_{15}$	Neohesperidin	-	-	0.16%	-	-	-
12.584	498.1741	$C_{23}H_{30}O_{12}$	Eucaglobulin	-	0.02%	-	-	-	-
12.593	436.13688	$C_{21}H_{24}O_{10}$	Nothofagin	-	-	-	-	-	0.12%
12.721	680.37692	$C_{36}H_{56}O_{12}$	Tenuifolin	-	-	-	-	0.11%	0.37%
12.8	486.33397	$C_{30}H_{46}O_5$	Bassic acid	-	-	-	-	-	0.05%
12.844	518.1785	$C_{26}H_{30}O_{11}$	Phellodensin E	-	-	0.05%	-	-	-
12.889	346.1052	$C_{18}H_{18}O_7$	Hamilcone	-	-	-	0.02%	-	0.01%
12.914	190.13544	$C_{13}H_{18}O$	β-Damascenone	-	-	-	-	0.02%	0.06%
12.915	666.39739	$C_{36}H_{58}O_{11}$	Chebuloside II	-	-	-	-	3.85%	-
12.924	302.1152	$C_{17}H_{18}O_5$	Lusianin	0.01%	-	-	-	-	-
12.929	356.03763	$C_{14}H_{12}O_{11}$	(+)-Chebulic acid	0.54%	-	-	3.98%	1.40%	2.88%
12.967	330.14651	$C_{19}H_{22}O_5$	Hericenone A	-	-	-	-	0.03%	-
12.969	504.34417	$C_{30}H_{48}O_6$	Madecassic acid	-	-	-	-	-	1.42%
12.971	202.13522	$C_{14}H_{18}O$	(±)-Anisoxide	-	-	-	-	-	0.05%
12.973	244.14583	$C_{16}H_{20}O_2$	Lahorenoic acid C	-	-	-	-	-	0.02%
13.208	288.06318	$C_{15}H_{12}O_6$	Eriodictyol	-	-	-	-	-	0.27%
13.354	314.1154	$C_{18}H_{18}O_5$	Crotaoprostrin	-	-	-	-	-	0.01%
13.428	442.1992	$C_{25}H_{30}O_7$	Exiguaflavanone M	-	-	0.13%	-	-	-
13.443	460.13716	$C_{23}H_{24}O_{10}$	7-Hydroxy-5,6-dimethoxyflavone 7-glucoside	-	-	-	-	0.01%	-
13.451	274.08371	$C_{15}H_{14}O_5$	Phloretin	-	-	-	0.01%	0.02%	0.01%
13.536	462.11641	$C_{22}H_{22}O_{11}$	Leptosin	-	0.01%	-	0.01%	0.06%	-
13.59	302.04255	$C_{15}H_{10}O_7$	Bracteatin	-	-	-	0.01%	0.01%	-

Table 3. *Cont.*

Retention Time (min)	Molecular Weight	Empirical Formula	Putative Compounds	% Relative Abundance (TB)			% Relative Abundance (TCh)		
				AQ	MeOH	EtOAc	AQ	MeOH	EtOAc
13.592	450.07961	$C_{20}H_{18}O_{12}$	Quercetin 4′-galactoside	-	-	-	0.01%	-	-
13.593	502.1836	$C_{26}H_{30}O_{10}$	Flavaprin	-	-	0.07%	-	-	-
13.642	514.18403	$C_{27}H_{30}O_{10}$	Baohuoside 1	-	-	-	T	0.01%	-
13.678	568.12178	$C_{28}H_{24}O_{13}$	Isoorientin 2″-p-hydroxybenzoate	-	-	-	-	-	0.04%
13.703	280.13067	$C_{15}H_{20}O_{5}$	Artabsinolide A	-	-	-	-	-	0.02%
13.725	330.0374	$C_{16}H_{10}O_{8}$	Blighinone	0.12%	-	-	-	-	-
13.805	444.10499	$C_{22}H_{20}O_{10}$	3′-O-Methylderhamnosylmaysin	-	-	-	0.04%	0.12%	0.08%
13.805	292.09447	$C_{15}H_{16}O_{6}$	(S)-Angelicain	-	-	-	0.05%	-	-
13.806	462.11629	$C_{22}H_{22}O_{11}$	6-O-[(2E)-3-Phenyl-2-propenoyl]-1-O-(3,4,5-trihydroxybenzoyl)-β-D-glucopyranose	-	-	-	0.08%	1.02%	0.18%
14.024	500.1674	$C_{26}H_{28}O_{10}$	Ikarisoside A	-	-	0.03%	-	-	-
14.078	534.28285	$C_{29}H_{42}O_{9}$	Corchoroside A	-	-	-	-	-	0.02%
14.358	272.06832	$C_{15}H_{12}O_{5}$	Naringenin	-	-	-	-	-	0.18%
14.367	470.33907	$C_{30}H_{46}O_{4}$	Glycyrrhetinic acid	-	-	-	-	0.08%	0.01%
14.561	226.1203	$C_{12}H_{18}O_{4}$	Allixin	-	-	0.03%	-	-	-
14.783	234.16167	$C_{15}H_{22}O_{2}$	Valerenic acid	-	-	-	-	-	0.13%
14.928	202.17175	$C_{15}H_{22}$	Rulepidadiene B	-	-	-	-	-	0.08%
14.93	222.16153	$C_{14}H_{22}O_{2}$	Rishitin	-	-	-	-	-	0.04%
15.046	426.09477	$C_{22}H_{18}O_{9}$	Epiafzelechin 3-O-gallate	-	-	-	-	-	0.01%
15.454	650.4026	$C_{36}H_{58}O_{10}$	Pedunculoside	-	-	-	-	1.18%	2.61%
16.257	738.41926	$C_{39}H_{62}O_{13}$	Isonuatigenin 3-[rhamnosyl-(1->2)-glucoside]	-	-	-	-	0.04%	0.12%
16.301	470.1941	$C_{26}H_{30}O_{8}$	Limonin	-	-	0.14%	-	-	-
16.478	540.1663	$C_{25}H_{32}O_{11}S$	Sumalarin B	-	-	0.02%	-	-	-
16.532	316.1308	$C_{18}H_{20}O_{5}$	Methylodoratol	-	-	0.02%	-	-	-
16.787	472.2097	$C_{26}H_{32}O_{8}$	Kushenol H	-	-	0.07%	-	-	-
16.844	344.0532	$C_{17}H_{12}O_{8}$	3,4,3′-Tri-O-methylellagic acid	-	-	0.01%	-	-	-
16.876	252.20856	$C_{16}H_{28}O_{2}$	Isoambrettolide	-	-	-	-	-	0.32%
16.889	300.1361	$C_{18}H_{20}O_{4}$	Angoletin	-	-	T	-	-	-
17.064	440.1828	$C_{25}H_{28}O_{7}$	Lonchocarpol E	-	-	0.15%	-	-	-
17.209	544.2668	$C_{30}H_{40}O_{9}$	Physagulin F	-	-	0.10%	-	-	-
17.275	342.14638	$C_{20}H_{22}O_{5}$	Brosimacutin C	-	-	-	-	T	-
17.276	180.11471	$C_{11}H_{16}O_{2}$	Jasmolone	-	0.61%	1.48%	0.05%	-	-
17.31	504.34409	$C_{30}H_{48}O_{6}$	Protobassic acid	-	-	-	1.26%	0.02%	0.01%
17.33	468.32326	$C_{30}H_{44}O_{4}$	Glabrolide	-	-	-	0.87%	-	3.19%

Table 3. *Cont.*

Retention Time (min)	Molecular Weight	Empirical Formula	Putative Compounds	% Relative Abundance (TB)			% Relative Abundance (TCh)		
				AQ	MeOH	EtOAc	AQ	MeOH	EtOAc
17.33	502.32964	$C_{30}H_{46}O_6$	Medicagenic acid	-	-	-	-	T	0.07%
17.331	200.15605	$C_{15}H_{20}$	(S)-gamma-Calacorene	-	-	-	0.02%	-	0.29%
17.363	696.40877	$C_{37}H_{60}O_{12}$	Momordicoside E	-	-	-	-	0.01%	0.04%
17.626	286.08357	$C_{16}H_{14}O_5$	Homobutein	-	T	0.01%	-	-	0.01%
17.635	282.12541	$C_{18}H_{18}O_3$	Ohobanin	0.01%	T	0.09%	T	-	0.06%
17.671	652.27302	$C_{32}H_{44}O_{14}$	Dicrocin	-	-	-	-	-	0.03%
17.902	424.1881	$C_{25}H_{28}O_6$	Paratocarpin G	T	-	-	-	-	-
17.949	456.2144	$C_{26}H_{32}O_7$	Antiarone J	-	0.54%	-	-	-	-
18.124	372.2509	$C_{20}H_{36}O_6$	Sterebin Q4	-	-	0.01%	-	-	-
18.164	328.1309	$C_{19}H_{20}O_5$	2′,3′,4′,6′-Tetrameth oxychalcone	-	-	0.05%	-	-	-
18.237	428.1831	$C_{24}H_{28}O_7$	Heteroflavanone B	-	-	0.05%	-	-	-
18.237	312.13615	$C_{19}H_{20}O_4$	Desmosdumotin C	T	-	0.02%	T	-	0.02%
18.292	546.35535	$C_{32}H_{50}O_7$	Hovenidulcigenin B	-	-	-	0.04%	-	-
18.339	236.1776	$C_{15}H_{24}O_2$	Capsidiol	-	-	-	-	-	0.02%
18.346	268.13069	$C_{14}H_{20}O_5$	Kamahine C	0.02%	0.01%	-	-	0.01%	0.15%
18.363	336.0994	$C_{20}H_{16}O_5$	Ciliatin A	-	-	-	-	0.01%	-
18.47	466.1989	$C_{27}H_{30}O_7$	Eriotriochin	-	0.50%	-	-	-	-
18.498	340.09447	$C_{19}H_{16}O_6$	Ambanol	-	-	-	-	0.01%	-
18.507	484.31803	$C_{30}H_{44}O_5$	Liquoric acid	-	-	-	T	0.01%	0.04%
18.623	488.35017	$C_{30}H_{48}O_5$	Pitheduloside I	-	-	-	T	0.06%	0.11%
19.641	226.09903	$C_{15}H_{14}O_2$	7-Hydroxyflavan	-	0.84%	-	0.03%	-	0.05%
18.748	208.1096	$C_{12}H_{16}O_3$	Isoelemicin	0.01%	-	0.19%	-	-	-
18.767	526.2565	$C_{30}H_{38}O_8$	Kosamol A	-	0.52%	-	-	-	-
18.824	300.0997	$C_{17}H_{16}O_5$	2′,4′-Dihydroxy-3,4-dimethoxychalcone	-	-	0.07%	-	-	-
18.987	372.1208	$C_{20}H_{20}O_7$	Tangeretin	-	-	0.03%	-	-	-

Compounds identified in both plant extracts are in black; compounds identified only in *T. bellirica* (TB) extracts are in red; compounds identified only in *T. chebula* (TCh) extracts are in green; and compounds less than 0.01% of the total area were considered as trace amounts and are denoted as T.

2.4. Toxicity Quantification

The plant extracts were evaluated for toxicity in triplicate assays conducted on 48-well plates using *Artemia franciscana* Kellogg nauplii lethality assays (ALA). The toxicity level was determined, and plant extracts were classified as toxic if their LC_{50} values were less than 1000 µg/mL following 24 h exposure [11]. More than half of the nauplii evaluated in this study remained alive for all extracts after their 24 h duration of incubation. Consequently, all plant extracts tested were classified as nontoxic. Indeed, the outcomes of all extracts were comparable to those of the negative control (artificial seawater).

3. Discussion

Our study tested *T. bellirica* and *T. chebula* fruit extracts against a group of bacterial pathogens that are significant for human health, including strains that are resistant to antibiotics. Significantly, the aqueous and methanolic extracts effectively suppressed the growth of the six bacterial pathogens examined in this study, underscoring their potential as targets for plant-based antibiotics development. The methanolic extracts exhibited the highest antibacterial efficacy in both the disc diffusion and liquid microdilution experiments against all pathogens. The ethyl acetate *T. bellirica* and *T. chebula* extracts also exhibited good antibacterial activities against *S. aureus* and MRSA in the disc diffusion and broth microdilution assays. In addition, the *T. chebula* ethyl acetate extract showed moderate antibacterial efficacy against *K. pneumoniae*. The differences in net yields and the populations of phytochemicals extracted by different solvents may account for these variances in potency. Methanol and water have a higher polarity compared to ethyl acetate, which results in the extraction of a larger quantity of phytochemicals with high-to-mid polarity. In contrast, ethyl acetate extracts a smaller number of compounds with mid-to-lower polarity [20]. The differences in phytochemical contents among the extracts may potentially contribute to the varied antibacterial growth inhibition effects observed in the disc diffusion and liquid dilution investigations. Phytochemicals that have lower polarity or are larger in size diffuse less rapidly through solid agar, resulting in a decrease in their apparent antibacterial effectiveness in disc diffusion assays [21]. The solubility of these phytochemicals in broth is also influenced by their polarity [22], which in turn impacts their ability to dissolve and may lead to inaccurate MIC values. Prior research has demonstrated that the depth of agar in petri dishes, as well as the regularity of the agar, may impact the extent of zones of inhibition (ZOIs) in agar diffusion studies [23]. Whilst we followed manufacturers' instructions to create agar of uniform consistency and poured it at a consistent depth of 4 mm, repeating the disc diffusion experiments at varying agar depths may be useful to confirm the ZOIs of all the extracts and antibiotics. In this investigation, we noticed that the borders of the zone of inhibition (ZOI) were clearly visible for *S. aureus* and MRSA, although they were less clear (regarded as no ZOI) for the other bacterial pathogens studied. It is important to note that in future research, the use of methylene blue or crystal violet to stain the plates may enhance the visibility of ZOIs if there is low clarity [24].

Notably, the MRSA strain tested herein showed resistance to many commonly used antibiotics, such as β-lactams (penicillin G, oxacillin, amoxicillin), and macrolides (erythromycin). Nevertheless, the emergence of extended spectrum β-lactamase enzymes has made these medications less effective against some bacterial strains. Likewise, macrolide antibiotics such as erythromycin are commonly employed because they have the ability to impede protein synthesis in bacteria [25]. The existence of MRSA resistance to macrolides complicates the availability of treatment options, highlighting the need for new therapeutic drugs and procedures. Hence, it is imperative to identify innovative compounds that can elude or surmount these resistance mechanisms. The antibacterial activities observed with *T. bellirica* and *T. chebula* extracts against *S. aureus* and MRSA produced similar MIC values ranging from 94 μg/mL to 900 μg/mL. These findings indicate that the resistance mechanisms observed in the MRSA strain have little influence on the active compounds of the extracts. Thus, the extract compounds either function through different mechanisms, or they may inhibit the bacterial antibiotic-resistance pathways.

The *mecA* gene plays a crucial role in the resistance of MRSA [26]. This gene codes for a new penicillin-binding protein (PBP2a) that has a reduced ability to bind to β-lactam antibiotics. This protein provides the bacteria with resistance against many β-lactam antibiotics by enabling them to produce cell walls, even in the presence of these medications. Hence, the mechanisms by which the phytochemicals in the extract function may vary from those of β-lactam antibiotics, even in bacteria that are resistant to β-lactam antibiotics. Alternatively, these extracts may contain phytochemicals that disrupt the bacterial strains' defense mechanisms against these medicines, thereby allowing them to function at higher potency [26]. This outcome is promising because, when compared to the susceptible strain, the MRSA strain in our study exhibited significantly diminished susceptibilities/increased resistance to a range of antibiotics from the β-lactams, macrolides and fluoroquinolones classes.

Aqueous and methanol *T. bellirica* and *T. chebula* extracts exhibited antibacterial activity against *E. coli* and its antibiotic-resistant counterpart, ESBL *E. coli*. The methanolic *T. bellirica* extract showed noteworthy antibacterial activity against both bacterial pathogens, with identical MIC values. Similarly, the methanolic *T. bellirica* and *T. chebula* extracts also inhibited the growth of *K. pneumoniae* and ESBL *K. pneumoniae*, with similar MIC values. These results suggest that the methanolic extracts of both plants may contain compounds that have a broad efficacy against strains of *E. coli* and *K. pneumoniae*, including those that produce ESBL enzymes. Their efficacy might be linked to a distinct mechanism of action that contrasts those of β-lactam antibiotics. For example, the plant extracts may affect how bacteria form their cell walls, how well their membrane's function, or they may affect other essential processes independent of the β-lactam antibiotic mechanism [27]. In addition, it is possible that the methanolic extracts of both plants are exerting antibacterial effects through mechanisms that do not directly interfere with or inhibit the ESBL enzymes. Additional research is necessary to ascertain whether the plant extracts specifically hinder the resistance mechanisms of ESBL bacterial pathogens, or if they function via independent antibiotic pathways. This may require assessment of the effects of the extract/isolated components on β-lactamase inhibition, or by investigating the impact of the extract on the production of resistance genes in ESBL strains.

We also examined the use of *T. bellirica* and *T. chebula* extracts in combinations with conventional antibiotics. This method holds great promise for developing novel antibiotic chemotherapies, as many bacteria have developed resistance to conventional antibiotics, and plant compounds may provide ways of inhibiting/blocking these resistance mechanisms [4]. Our goal was to enhance the efficacy of antibiotics and possibly negate the bacterial resistance mechanisms by mixing them with extracts from plants. Augmentin®, a combination of amoxicillin and clavulanic acid, is a well-known example of how combining medications can improve treatment outcomes [28] since clavulanic acid inhibits β-lactamase enzymes present in resistant bacteria. This enables amoxicillin to specifically target and eliminate the bacteria with greater efficiency, even in β-lactam-resistant bacterial strains. Clavulanic acid acts as a β-lactamase inhibitor by binding permanently to the active site of the enzyme, therefore inhibiting the breakdown of the antibiotic.

Our investigation found that penicillin G, amoxicillin, in combination with the plant extracts, have additive effects against *S. aureus*, which may be due to the presence of phytochemicals that possess anti-β-lactamase activities [29]. These phytochemicals can hinder the activity of β-lactamase enzymes, thereby contributing to antibiotic resistance by breaking down the β-lactam ring found in β-lactam antibiotics, such as penicillin and amoxicillin [30]. In addition, phytochemicals found in the plant extracts may interact with β-lactamase enzymes in a way that is comparable to clavulanic acid, although this requires confirmation. Regardless of the mechanism, this interaction helps protect the antibiotics from being broken down by bacterial enzymes and improves their ability to fight against bacterial pathogens. Plant extracts may possess the capacity to function as an alternative treatment method and could be a safe and less detrimental option for addressing antibiotic resistance [9]. In comparison to synthetic antibiotics, natural compounds found in plants frequently exhibit fewer adverse effects and a lower likelihood of generating resistance [8]. Moreover, the likelihood of further antibiotic-resistance development may be reduced by the variety of phytochemicals present in plant extracts, which may act on multiple bacterial pathways.

The ethyl acetate *T. chebula* extract exhibited additive effects against *S. aureus* in combination with erythromycin. It is possible that the extract and erythromycin may target distinct bacterial processes. Erythromycin inhibits protein synthesis by binding to the 50S ribosomal subunit [31], whereas the plant extract may impact other bacterial targets, including cell wall synthesis, membrane integrity, or metabolic processes [30]. Further studies are required to determine which of these mechanisms are affected by the extracts. Notably, this complementary targeting has the potential to improve the overall antibacterial effect. Furthermore, the plant extract may also influence other mechanisms associated with bacterial resistance, such as the disruption of efflux pumps or the modification of cell wall structures [30], which could render bacteria more susceptible to erythromycin. The extract may also disrupt bacterial protective barriers, which could facilitate the improved penetration of erythromycin into the cell. Additionally, the plant extract may contain a variety of bioactive compounds [8] that work in conjunction to enhance the efficacy of erythromycin. Alternatively, the extract may exhibit broad-spectrum antimicrobial activity that complements the specific effects of erythromycin. Similarly, the methanolic and ethyl acetate extracts of *T. chebula* exhibited additional antibacterial effects against *K. pneumoniae* when combined with chloramphenicol. This antibiotic binds to the 23S rRNA component of the 50S ribosomal subunit of the bacterial ribosome [32]. This binding suppresses peptidyl transferase activity, a crucial process for the creation of peptide bonds during protein synthesis. Chloramphenicol inhibits bacterial protein production by blocking the formation of peptide bonds.

Our research determined that when tetracycline is combined with *T. chebula* extracts, the combination exhibited additive interactions against *S. aureus*, MRSA, *E. coli* and *K. pneumoniae,* suggesting enhanced antibacterial efficacy. However, the aqueous *T. bellirica* extract only showed an additive interaction against MRSA. Tetracycline resistance is mostly commonly attributed to tetracycline-specific efflux pumps [33]. Hence, the observed additive effect indicates that the *T. bellirica* and *T. chebula* extracts might have hindered the functioning of these efflux pumps. By inhibiting efflux pumps, tetracycline is allowed to remain inside cells for a longer period, which increases its effectiveness. Whilst ribosomal changes may also contribute to tetracycline resistance, this pathway is substantially less common [33]. Our research findings suggest that a broad range of phytochemicals found in the extracts of *T. bellirica* and *T. chebula* may have antibacterial action against several different bacteria. Similarly, plant extracts prepared from *Phyllanthus niruri* L., *Berberis vulgaris* L., and *Piper nigrum* L. exhibit additive interactions in combination with tetracycline, and can inhibit tetracycline efflux pumps [34,35].

Interestingly, the *T. bellirica* and *T. chebula* ethyl acetate extracts exhibited additive interactions in combination with ciprofloxacin against MRSA. This indicates that ethyl acetate extracts contain phytochemicals that may target different bacterial processes such as cell membrane disruption, inhibition of cell wall synthesis, or interference with metabolic pathways [30]. The plant extract's unique mechanisms may enhance the effectiveness of ciprofloxacin's DNA-targeting action, resulting in a more comprehensive treatment [8]. The plant extract may also enhance the cellular absorption of ciprofloxacin (thereby increasing its intracellular concentration) or it may block/inhibit MRSA's antibiotic-resistance mechanisms [35].

Notably, polymyxin B and *T. bellirica*, and *T. chebula* extracts combinations exhibited substantial antagonistic interactions. The antagonistic interaction between polymyxin B and the plant extracts may be affected by variations in pH levels in the broth. Polymyxin B, which breaks bacterial cell membranes by binding to lipopolysaccharides, is pH sensitive, with substantially reduced potency under acidic or alkaline circumstances [36]. The inclusion of plant extracts may cause a change in the pH of the broth, which could affect the efficacy of both polymyxin B and the plant chemicals, potentially resulting in a decrease in overall antibacterial activity, although this remains to be confirmed in future studies. Changes in pH may also impact bacterial physiology, thereby reducing the vulnerability of bacteria to the combined actions of the two substances. Polymyxin B and the components of plant extracts may also have chemical interactions that are regulated by pH [36], which may further contribute to the antagonistic effects of the combination. Moreover, the antagonistic interactions between the extracts and polymyxin B can be ascribed to the binding of bioactive phytochemicals with polymyxin B, which impedes its absorption and efficacy in targeting bacterial cells [37]. Hence, understanding these dynamics is critical for optimizing combination medicines and assuring antimicrobial efficacy. Future studies are planned to examine these effects.

LC-MS metabolomics analysis of the *T. bellirica* and *T. chebula* fruit extracts highlighted the presence of flavonoids, tannins, terpenoids and phenolic acid compounds (Table 3). Complete, comprehensive lists of phytochemicals present in the individual plant extracts are available as the Supplementary Files (Supplementary Materials: Tables S1 and S2). Notable phytochemicals identified in both plant extracts include quinic acid (Figure 2A), shikimic acid (Figure 2B), aureusidin 6-glucuronide (Figure 2C), madecassic acid (Figure 2D), pedunculoside (Figure 2E), 6-galloylglucose (Figure 2F), 1,2,6-trigalloyl-β-D-glucopyranose (Figure 2G), propyl gallate (Figure 2H), methyl gallate (Figure 2I), theogallin (Figure 2J), gallic acid (Figure 2K), ellagic acid (Figure 2L), sanguiin H4 (Figure 2M), hamamelitannin (Figure 2N), pyrogallol (Figure 2O), chebulic acid (Figure 2P), chebuloside II (Figure 2Q), and 1,6-bis-O-(3,4,5-trihydroxybenzoyl) hexopyranose (Figure 2R). The scientific literature has documented the presence of gallic acid, ellagic acid, chebulic acid, chebuloside II, methyl gallate, propyl gallate, ethyl gallate, phloroglucinol, pyrogallol, quercetin, kaempferol, and various others compound in the fruit extracts of *T. bellirica* and *T. chebula* [38–40]. In our previous study, we conducted qualitative GC-MS headspace analysis on aqueous, methanol and ethyl acetate fruit extracts of *T. bellirica* and *T. chebula*. Our analysis revealed the presence of several notable volatile terpenoids, including eucalyptol, linalool, methoxycitronellal, terpinene-4-ol, camphor, pinocarveol, carvone, endo borneol, L-fenchone, hyscylene, patchoulane, p-cumic aldehyde, and phenylbutanal [11].

Notably, Embaby et al. (2019) showed synergistic antibacterial activity of quinic acid-rich acetone bark extract of *Ficus macrocarpa* var. nitida. with tetracycline against *E. coli* and *S. aureus* [41]. Furthermore, an in-silico molecular docking study revealed that 5-caffeol quinic acid (and other phenolic compounds) may have antibacterial activity due to their efflux pump inhibitory effect. However, the study did not investigate the interactions between the plant extracts and conventional antibiotics. Another study reported the antibacterial activity of quinic acid against *E. coli* and *S. aureus*, with an MIC of 500 μg/mL to 1000 μg/mL, respectively [42]. Additionally, Zhang et al. (2024) reported synergistic antibacterial effects for shikimic acid (625 μg/mL) in combination with penicillin, ampicillin, amoxicillin, and ceftiofur against MRSA, and significantly reduced MIC values reported for the combinations (4 to 16-fold decreases) [43]. Similarly, other investigations have shown that phloroglucinol derivatives exhibited synergistic antibacterial activity against MRSA in combination with vancomycin, penicillin and doxycycline [44–46], despite phloroglucinol itself lacking antibacterial activity against MRSA, yielding a high MIC of over 10,000 μg/mL [45].

We identified the flavonoid glucuronide, aureusidin 6-glucuronide in the ethyl acetate extracts of *T. bellirica* and *T. chebula*. Notably, studies evaluating the antibacterial activity of this compound are lacking in the literature, as are studies evaluating its effects in combination with conventional antibiotics. In addition, madecassic acid, a pentacyclic triterpenoid has been identified in the *T. chebula* ethyl acetate extracts in our study. Previous studies have reported noteworthy antibacterial activity of madecassic acid against *S. aureus*, MRSA, and *E. coli*, with MIC values of 31.25 (61.9 μM), 62.5 (124 μM), 250 μg/mL (495 μM), respectively [47]. These findings indicate that the madecassic acid exhibits more efficacy against Gram-positive bacteria, including *S. aureus* and MRSA, compared to Gram-negative bacteria such as *E. coli*. This discrepancy in effectiveness may be attributed to variations in cell wall structures and methods of action. These values aid in determining the most effective dosage levels and emphasize the potential of madecassic acid as a specific treatment for antibiotic-resistant bacteria, such as MRSA. Moreover, these findings establish a basis for future investigations, such as carrying out studies with different antibiotics to improve effectiveness. Antibacterial mechanism-focused experiments showed that madecassic acid destroys cell wall integrity, inhibiting the synthesis of soluble proteins and DNA topoisomerase I and II [47]. Pedunculoside, a triterpene saponin has been identified in the methanol and ethyl acetate *T. chebula* extracts. Interestingly, an older study reported the antibacterial effects of pedunculoside against *S. aureus* and *E. coli*, with MIC values of 200 μg/mL [48]. However, there is a shortage of literature on the combined effects of pedunculoside and antibiotics.

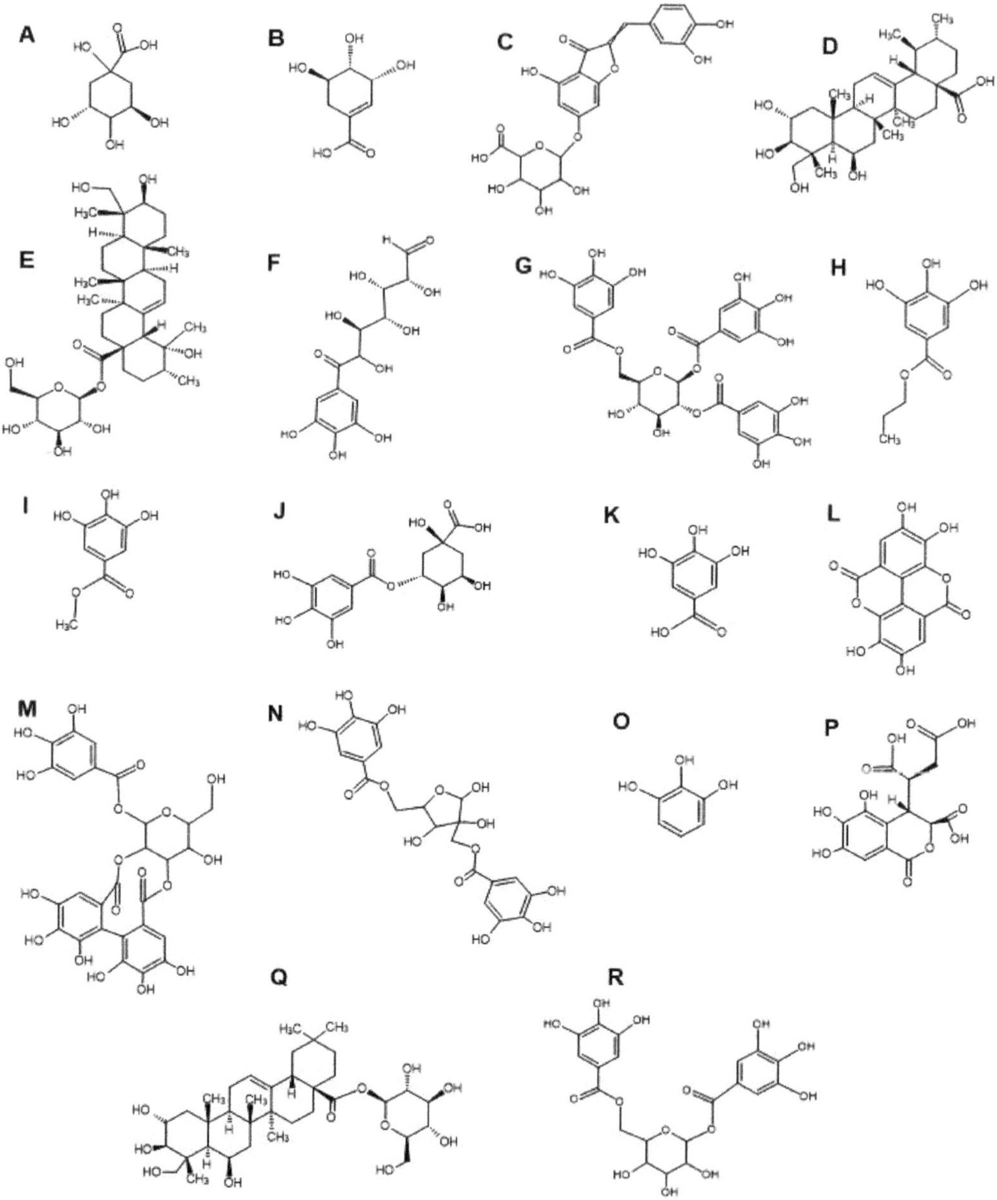

Figure 2. Structures of noteworthy compounds identified in the fruit extracts of *T. bellirica* and *T. chebula*. Quinic acid (**A**), shikimic acid (**B**), aureusidin 6-glucuronide (**C**), madecassic acid (**D**), pedunculoside (**E**), 6-galloylglucose (**F**), 1,2,6-trigalloyl-β-D-glucopyranose (**G**), propyl gallate (**H**), methyl gallate (**I**), theogallin (**J**), gallic acid (**K**), ellagic acid (**L**), sanguiin H4 (**M**), hamamelitannin (**N**), pyrogallol (**O**), chebulic acid (**P**), chebuloside II (**Q**), and 1,6-bis-O-(3,4,5-trihydroxybenzoyl) hexopyranose (**R**).

Previous work has documented the antibacterial activity of penta-galloyl-glucose against *S. aureus* and *E. coli*, with an MIC of 250 μg/mL (266 μM) against both bacteria [49]. The postulated mechanism of antibacterial activity is related to the suppression of the bacterial type II fatty acid production pathway. Another study reported broad-spectrum antibacterial activity of penta-galloyl-glucose against both methicillin-resistant *S. aureus* and quinolone-resistant *S. aureus* and *E. coli*, with MIC values ranging from 64 to 128 μg/mL (68 μM and 136 μM, respectively) [50]. The antibacterial activities of four derivatives of galloyl-β-D-glucose have also been investigated against multidrug-resistant *E. coli* and *K. pneumoniae* strains, with MIC values from 32 μg/mL to 128 μg/mL, respectively (26–136 μM) [51]. However, combinational interactions of galloyl-β-D-glucose derivatives with reference antibiotics have not been conducted to date.

Our LC/MS experiments also identified the galloyl-glucose derivatives 1,2,6-trigalloyl-β-D-glucopyranose, 1,6-bis-O-(3,4,5-trihydroxybenzoyl) hexopyranose, and 6-O-[(2E)-3-phenyl-2-propenoyl]-1-O-(3,4,5-trihydroxybenzoyl)-β-D-glucopyranose in both *T. bellirica* and *T. chebula* extracts. Previous studies have reported that relatively high levels of gallotannins are present in *T. bellirica* and *T. chebula* extracts [40,52–54]. Notably, efflux pump inhibitory activity has previously been demonstrated for 1,2,6-tri-*O*-galloyl-β-D-glucopyranose against multidrug-resistant (MDR) uropathogenic *E. coli* [55]. Additionally, 1,2,6-tri-*O*-galloyl-β-D-glucopyranose exhibits synergistic antibacterial activity in combination with gentamicin and trimethoprim against *E. coli* [56]. Synthetic gallotannins also exhibit antibiofilm and antimicrobial activity against *S. aureus* and MRSA strains [57].

Synergistic interactions between orbifloxacin and propyl gallate against the *E. coli*-resistant strain KVCC 1423 have previously been reported, with MIC values of the combination being reduced from 125 μg/mL (316 μM, orbifloxacin only) to 7.8 μg/mL (19.7 μM), and 312.5 μg/mL (1472 μM, propyl gallate only) to 78 μg/mL (367 μM), respectively [58]. In the present study, through LC-MS analysis, propyl gallate was identified only in the *T. chebula* extracts, although methyl gallate was identified in both *Terminalia* species. Tamang et al. (2022) investigated the antibacterial activities of erythromycin, ampicillin, gentamicin, kanamycin, and ciprofloxacin in combination with gallic acid, methyl gallate, ethyl gallate, propyl gallate, butyl gallate, octyl gallate, dodecyl gallate, and stearyl gallate against MRSA [59]. It was noted in that study that octyl gallate (4 μg/mL) exhibited significant antimicrobial synergy against MRSA in combination with penicillin, ampicillin, cephalothin, gentamicin, tetracycline, erythromycin and lincomycin, reducing their MIC values from 64 μg/mL to 0.25–16 μg/mL.

A recent study reviewed the antimicrobial characteristics of sanguiins, highlighting their capacity to inhibit bacterial growth and the production of biofilms [60]. The antibacterial activity of sanguiin H6, a closely related compound to sanguiin H4, was demonstrated against *S. aureus* and MRSA, with an MIC value of 250 μg/mL [60,61]. Sanguiin H4 has been identified in the polyphenolic extract of *Sanguisorba officinalis* L., which exhibited antibacterial activity against *S. aureus* and *E. coli* [62]. However, data are not available for the combinatorial interactions of sanguiins with antibiotics to combat AMR. The combination of gallic acid and thiamphenicol, and the combination of hamamelitannin with thiamphenicol or erythromycin, exhibited synergistic antibacterial effects against *E. coli*. (ATCC 25922) [63]. Furthermore, a study detected additional antibacterial interactions against *E. coli* when combining gallic acid with ampicillin, or cefotaxime, and/or marbofloxacin, as well as when combining hamamelitannin with amoxicillin or marbofloxacin. Interestingly, gallic acid and hamamelitannin each have moderate antibacterial activity against *E. coli*, with MIC values of 1024 μg/mL (6024 μM) and 2048 μg/mL (4230 μM), respectively [63]. Bassyouni et al. (2015) noted that hamamelitannin (20 μg/mL) reduces the MIC of vancomycin (4 μg/mL), and clindamycin (32 μg/mL) to 0.25 μg/mL against MRSA strains [64]. Furthermore, hamamelitannin in combination with vancomycin and clindamycin effectively inhibits the biofilm formation in MRSA strains.

Our present study identified chebulic acid, a gallotannin compound in the aqueous extract of *T. bellirica* and all extracts of *T. chebula*. Chebulic acid has demonstrated numerous biological activities including anti-tumor activity, anti-atherogenic, anti-fibrotic, anti-ulcer, and antioxidant effects [65]. Yang et al. (2020) identified and isolated twenty chebulic acid and brevifolincarboxylic acid derivatives from an ethanolic extract prepared from the arial parts of *Euphorbia hirta* L. [66]. All of those compounds exhibited significant free radical scavenging activities, although antibacterial activity was not investigated in that study. Both ethyl gallate and tri-n-butyl chebulate have been isolated from the aqueous *T. chebula* fruit extract [67]. Both compounds inhibit *K. pneumoniae* growth, with MIC values of 156 μg/mL (787 μM) and 1250 μg/mL, respectively. However, combinational interactions with antibiotics were not investigated in that study. In the present study, chebuloside II was only identified in the methanolic *T. chebula* fruit extract. In contrast, several earlier studies reported the presence of chebuloside II in both *T. bellirica* and *T. chebula* extracts [40,53,54,68]. Chebuloside II-rich *T. chebula* extracts exhibit hepatoprotective effects and prevent liver toxicity in animal models [68], although there is a lack of studies examining the antibacterial activity and combinational interactions of chebuloside II with conventional antibiotics.

In the present study, the extracts were found to be rich in gallic acid, ellagic acid and pyrogallol. Previous studies showed that gallic acid acts synergistically in combination with norfloxacin against *S. aureus* [69]. This combination decreases the MIC of norfloxacin from 156 μg/mL to 49 μg/mL. In addition, gallic acid lowered the MIC of gentamicin against *S. aureus* from 49 μg/mL to 2.5 μg/mL. Similarly, ellagic acid lowered the MIC of tetracycline, chloramphenicol, and tobramycin against a multidrug resistant isolate of *E. coli* [70]. Quave et al. (2012) showed that ellagic acid and its derivatives isolated from the roots of *Rubus ulmifolius* Schott. inhibited *S. aureus* growth by inhibiting biofilm formation [71]. Pyrogallol exhibited antibacterial activity against *S. aureus* and reduced the MIC of norfloxacin from 156 μg/mL to 78 μg/mL, and gentamicin from 49 μg/mL to 2.5 μg/mL [69]. In addition, pyrogallol exhibited broad-spectrum antibacterial activities against methicillin-susceptible *S. aureus*, MRSA, *E. coli* (ATCC 25922), colistin-resistant *E. coli*, and colistin-resistant *K. pneumoniae* [72].

We were unable to detect synergistic enhancement of antibacterial activity between *T. bellirica* and *T. chebula* extracts and any of the antibiotics we selected against the bacterial pathogens investigated. However, additive interactions of extracts were noted in some combinations containing penicillin G, amoxicillin, erythromycin, chloramphenicol, tetracycline and ciprofloxacin against *S. aureus*, MRSA, *E. coli*, and ESBL *K. pneumoniae*. This indicates that the phytochemicals present in the *T. bellirica* and *T. chebula* extracts may possess β-lactamase and/or efflux pump inhibitory properties. Further research is required to investigate the effects of these extracts against those resistance mechanisms.

The toxicity assays using *Artemia* nauplii revealed that all *T. bellirica* and *T. chebula* extracts are nontoxic, thereby indicating their safety as an antimicrobial agent. To determine whether these extracts are suitable for use in medicine, additional testing should be conducted utilizing a panel of mammalian cell lines. Taken together, the findings of our study indicate that *T. bellirica* and *T. chebula* fruit extracts may be a valuable source of antimicrobial compounds for future research and development in the fight against bacterial infections.

4. Materials and Methods

4.1. Plant Origins

Terminalia bellirica fruit powder (batch no: BNFP/01) was produced by Organic Prime and was purchased online from Navafresh Australia. *Terminalia chebula* fruit powder (batch no: HRP1020) developed by Aarshaveda was obtained online from Sattvic Australia. The traditional Ayurvedic names of *T. bellirica* (Bhitaki, Baheda) and *T. chebula* (Haritaki, Harad) were used to search for the plant herb on the supplier's website. The provider verified the authenticity and quality of the plant materials. The plant samples were labelled, and voucher specimens NBG-TB0220GU and NBG-TC0220GU for *T. bellirica* and *T. chebula*, respectively, were kept at Griffith University's Gold Coast campus in the School of Pharmacy and Medical Sciences.

4.2. Extract Preparation

After weighing individual 1 g masses of *T. bellirica* and *T. chebula* fruit powders into three separate 50 mL tubes, sterile deionized water, methanol (AR grade), or ethyl acetate

(AR grade) were added individually to achieve a total volume of 50 mL [11,34]. The organic solvents (methanol and ethyl acetate) were provided by ChemSupply (Gillman, Australia). Samples were mixed at room temperature for 24 h and then filtered through Whatman No. 54 filter paper (Sigma-Aldrich, Melbourne, Australia) into pre-weighed 50 mL tubes under vacuum pressure. The aqueous samples were lyophilized in an Alpha 1–4 LSC plus benchtop freeze dryer (Martin Christ, Osterode am Harz, Germany) for 72 h to dry the aqueous extracts. The organic solvent samples were subjected to evaporation at a temperature of 40 °C until the evaporation process was fully completed. To calculate the final yields, all dried extracts were weighed, and the mass of extract was determined. The crude extracts were resuspended in 10 mL of 1% dimethyl sulfoxide (DMSO; Merck, Macquarie Park, Australia) and sterilized by passage through 0.22 µm syringe-driven filters (Sarstedt, Mawson Lakes, Australia) and stored at −20 °C until use.

4.3. Antibiotics and Bacterial Strains

Powdered antibiotics were purchased from Sigma-Aldrich (Melbourne, Australia), which included penicillin G (potency of 1440–1680 µg/mg), erythromycin (potency ≥850 µg/mg), tetracycline (≥95% purity by HPLC), chloramphenicol (≥98% purity by HPLC), ciprofloxacin (≥98% purity by HPLC), polymyxin B (purity >90%), oxacillin (≥95% purity by TLC), amoxycillin (potency of 900 µg/mg), gentamicin (≥98% purity by HPLC), and vancomycin (potency of ≥900 µg per mg). Antibiotic stock solutions (1 mg/mL) were prepared for broth microdilution assays and stored at −20 °C until required. Oxoid Ltd. (Thebarton, Australia) supplied preloaded standard discs that contained penicillin G (10 IU), erythromycin (10 µg), tetracycline (30 µg), chloramphenicol (30 µg), ciprofloxacin (1 µg), polymyxin B (300IU), oxacillin (1 µg), gentamicin (10 µg), vancomycin (30 µg), Augmentin® (15 µg) and cefoxitin (30 µg). A 10 µL volume of amoxicillin stock solution (0.01 mg/mL) was infused into sterile filter paper discs, which were subsequently placed on Mueller–Hinton (MH) agar and used immediately for disc diffusion assays. Broth microdilution assays were conducted with all reference antibiotics, except for Augmentin® and cefoxitin.

The American Type Culture Collection (ATCC, Manassas, VA, USA) provided the reference strains of *Escherichia coli* (ATCC 25922), *Staphylococcus aureus* (ATCC 25923), MRSA (ATCC 43300), *Klebsiella pneumoniae* (ATCC 13883), and ESBL *Klebsiella pneumoniae* (ATCC 700603). A clinical isolate strain of ESBL *Escherichia coli* was obtained from the Gold Coast University Hospital in Southport, QLD, Australia and its resistance profile has been previously confirmed by our group [34]. Mueller–Hinton (MH) agar and broth (Oxoid Ltd., Australia) were utilized to cultivate all bacterial strains. The resistance phenotype of the MRSA strain was preserved by culture at 35 °C [73], whilst all other bacterial strains were cultured at 37 °C for 18–24 h. All MH agar plates were prepared in accordance with the instructions provided by the manufacturer and with an agar depth of 4 millimeters.

4.4. Antibacterial Susceptibility Screening

The antibacterial activity of all plant extracts in MH agar was investigated using a modified Kirby–Bauer disc diffusion method [34]. In summary, individual colonies isolated from MH agar plates were inoculated in 40 mL MH broth and grown at 37 °C for 18–24 h, except for MRSA, which was grown at 35 °C. The individual bacterial cultures were used to make 0.5 McFarland standards for each strain. Volumes of 100 µL of the 0.5 McFarland standards were spread on fresh MH agar plates. Using sterile forceps, Whatman sterile filter paper discs (6 mm in diameter) were affixed to MH agar, and 10 µL of all extracts resuspended in 1% DMSO was infused into them. Reference antibiotic discs were also tested in this way. The plates were incubated at 37 °C for 18–24 h, except for MRSA, which was incubated at 35 °C. All samples were examined in triplicate.

The zones of inhibition (ZOIs) were reported as the diameter of the inhibition zones around each disc, which was measured to the nearest whole millimeter (mm) to assess the bacterial growth inhibition. Samples with no visible inhibition were reported to have ZOIs of 6 mm (the diameter of the discs). The ZOI data are presented in the form of bar graphs as the average ± SEM (standard error of mean) of a minimum of three independent studies. One-way analysis of variance (ANOVA) was employed to analyze the differences between the treatment groups and the negative controls. p-values of less than 0.01 and 0.001 were deemed to be statistically highly significant and very highly significant, respectively.

4.5. Minimum Inhibitory Concentration Determinations

The minimum inhibitory concentration (MIC) values for all extracts and reference antibiotics were determined using a standard 96-well microtiter plate broth microdilution assay [11,34]. A 100 µL volume of the individual extracts and reference antibiotics were added to the top row of the plates. The dilutions were then made down each column of the plates using doubling dilutions. After adding a volume of 100 µL of a 1:100 dilution of 0.5 McFarland cell suspension to every well (except from the sterile controls), the wells were incubated for 20–24 h at 37 °C. After the initial incubation period, a solution (0.4 mg/mL) of p-iodonitrotetrazolium violet (INTZ; Sigma Aldrich, Australia) dye was added to each well on the plate. The plate was then incubated for an additional 2–4 h at room temperature. For determining the MIC values, the lowest concentration of plant extracts or antibiotics that effectively prevented bacterial growth was determined by visual inspection and was indicated by the absence of a red-pink color change. The experiments were conducted in duplicate. MIC values greater than 10,000 µg/mL were classified as inactive, while values between 2000 and 10,000 µg/mL were considered to have low activity. Moderate activity was assigned to MIC values between 1000 and 2000 µg/mL, noteworthy activity to values between 400 and 1000 µg/mL, and good activity to values between 100 and 400 µg/mL. MIC values below 100 µg/mL were regarded as having high activity.

4.6. Fractional Inhibitory Concentration Evaluation

Plant extracts and antibiotics that showed antibacterial activity at minimum inhibitory concentrations (MICs) $\leq$ 3000 µg/mL and $\leq$2.5 µg/mL, respectively, were selected for combination studies. These were combined in equal proportions (50:50) to study their interactions with susceptible bacterial pathogens. The study examined the interactions between the extracts and antibiotics by calculating the sum of the fractional inhibitory concentrations (ΣFIC) for each combination using the following equations (a = extracts; b = antibiotics):

FIC(a) = MIC (a in combination with b)/MIC (a independently)

FIC(b) = MIC (b in combination with a)/MIC (b independently).

The sum of the fractional inhibitory concentrations (∑FIC) was determined by applying the formula ∑FIC = FIC(a) + FIC(b).

The interactions were classified as synergistic (∑FIC $\leq$ 0.5), additive (∑FIC > 0.5–$\leq$ 1.0), indifferent (∑FIC > 1.0–$\leq$ 4.0), or antagonistic (∑FIC > 4.0) [74].

4.7. Toxicity Assays

The toxicity of the plant extracts and controls were assessed using standard *Artemia franciscana* Kellogg nauplii lethality assays (ALA) [11]. In summary, 400 µL of plant extracts (2 mg/mL concentration, diluted in artificial seawater) and 400 µL of artificial seawater with newly hatched (within 1 day) *A. franciscana* nauplii were added separately in each well of a 48-well plate. On all plates, a 400 µL volume of negative control (32 g/L artificial seawater; Red Sea) and positive control (1 mg/mL sodium azide) was added. The plates were then incubated at 25 °C ± 1 °C for 24 h, and the number of live shrimps was determined. Probit analysis was employed to determine the LC_{50} values, which represent the concentration of extract or control required to cause mortality in 50% of the *A. franciscana* nauplii in separate wells. The LC_{50} values were calculated graphically using the mean percentage of three repeated experiments, representing the concentration that resulted in 50% mortality.

4.8. Non-Targeted Headspace LC-MS for Quantitative Analysis

A Vanquish Ultra High-Performance Liquid Chromatography (UHPLC) system (Thermo Fisher Scientific, Waltham, MA, USA) was utilized to conduct a non-targeted headspace metabolic profile analysis on all samples [34]. The separation of compounds was achieved using an Accucore ™ RP-MS column (100 mm × 2.1 mm) with a particle size of 2.6 µm, which was linked to an Orbitrap Exploris 120 mass spectrometer (Thermo Fisher Scientific). The UHPLC system was fitted with a quaternary pump at a flow rate of 0.6 mL/min. The separation used the following mobile phases: (A) a solution of 0.1% v/v formic acid in ultrapure water and (B) acetonitrile (MeCN) solution containing 0.1% v/v formic acid. The Xcalibur acquisition software (version 2.0) was utilized to create a gradient flow for compound separation. The flow consisted of the following steps, with a total duration of 24 min: 5% B for 5 min, a linear increase from 5% to 30% B over 5 min, 30% B for 3 min, a linear increase from 30% to 90% B over 4 min, isocratic elution at 90% B for 4 min to flush the column, and a linear decrease from 90% to 5% B over 1 min. The column was re-equilibrated by running an isocratic separation at 5% B of the mobile phase for a duration of 2 min between each separation. To obtain chromatogram peaks of high quality, plant extract samples were analyzed at three distinct concentrations (0.25 mg/mL, 0.5 mg/mL, and 1 mg/mL) using the Vanquish HPLC system (Thermo Fisher Scientific, Waltham, MA, USA) linked to the same column as mentioned above. Plant samples exhibited enhanced chromatogram peaks of superior quality when used at a concentration of 1 mg/mL.

The mass spectra of the eluted compounds were examined using the Orbitrap Exploris 120 mass spectrometer in the information-dependent acquisition (IDA) mode. The Orbitrap system employed electrospray ionization (ESI) in the negative ionization mode, utilizing specified settings including a vaporizer temperature of 350 °C, sheath gas pressure of 60 psi, auxiliary gas pressure of 15 psi, sweep gas pressure of 2 psi, and a spray voltage ranging from 2.5 KV to 5 KV. The data were analyzed using Compound Discoverer^{TM} software 3.3. The identification of the unknown natural products utilized local database searches and online statistical analysis. To remove the background and differentiate individual components of the extract, the data files for each extract were analyzed individually and compared to the blank file. In the Compound Discoverer function, result filters were employed to utilize databases such as Mz cloud, ChemSpider, Predicted Compositions, and MassList to achieve either a partial or complete match of the compounds that were discovered. The Compound Discoverer software 3.3 was utilized to generate Excel files containing the discovered compounds from each extract. The files were subsequently analyzed to generate a catalogue containing potential putative compounds. Following the consolidation of duplicates by pivot table analysis in Microsoft Excel, the relative abundance was calculated as a percentage of the total area.

5. Conclusions

Due to increasing levels of antibiotic-resistant bacterial strains, there is a pressing demand for new antibacterial medications, which has generated interest in natural products as potential sources. The results of our study demonstrate that the active extracts derived from *Terminalia bellirica* and *Terminalia chebula* can effectively hinder the growth of both resistant and susceptible strains of bacteria. This suggests that the extracts possess unique antibacterial mechanisms that require further examination. In addition, all extracts enhanced the effectiveness of various conventional antibiotics, specifically β-lactam antibiotics and tetracycline. This may allow the reactivation of these antibiotics, even in bacterial strains that are otherwise resistant to their actions. The method of potentiation has not been discovered yet, although it is probable that the components of the extract may deactivate bacterial extended spectrum β-lactamase enzymes and efflux pumps, leading to an increase in the concentration of antibiotics inside the cells. Future studies are required to confirm these mechanisms, as well as to test other possible potentiation pathways. Several phytochemicals that were identified in the extracts may contribute to these actions, suggesting that they could be valuable targets for new antibacterial agent development, although further confirmation is required. Subsequent studies should prioritize the isolation of these compounds and examine their capacity to augment the effectiveness of existing antibiotics. Also, nuclear magnetic resonance (NMR) is essential for the conclusive structural identification of the components present in the extract.

Supplementary Materials: The following supporting information can be downloaded at: https://www.mdpi.com/article/10.3390/antibiotics13100994/s1, Figure S1: LC-MS total compound chromatograms of (**A**) TB-Aq (*Terminalia bellirica* aqueous extract), (**B**) TB-MeOH (*Terminalia bellirica* methanolic extract), and (**C**) TB-EtOAc (*Terminalia bellirica* ethyl acetate extract). Figure S2: LC-MS total compound chromatograms of (**A**) TCh-Aq (*Terminalia chebula* aqueous extract), (**B**) TB-MeOH (*Terminalia chebula* methanolic extract), and (**C**) TB-EtOAc (*Terminalia chebula* ethyl acetate extract). Table S1: LC-MS putative identification and % relative abundance of phytochemicals identified in the extracts of *Terminalia bellirica*. Compounds less than 0.01% of the total area were considered as trace amounts and denoted as T. Table S2: LC-MS putative identification and % relative abundance of phytochemicals identified in the extracts of *Terminalia chebula*. Compounds less than 0.01% of the total area were considered as trace amounts and denoted as T.

Author Contributions: Conceptualization, investigation, resources, M.J.C. and I.E.C.; methodology, G.T. and M.J.C.; validation, formal analysis, data curation, G.T.; writing—original draft preparation, G.T.; writing—review and editing, supervision, M.J.C. and I.E.C.; project administration and funding acquisition, I.E.C. and M.J.C. All authors have read and agreed to the published version of the manuscript.

Funding: Financial support for this work was provided by the Environmental Futures Research Institute, Griffith University, Australia.

Institutional Review Board Statement: Not applicable.

Informed Consent Statement: Not applicable.

Data Availability Statement: Data are either presented within the manuscript or are available from the corresponding author upon reasonable request.

Acknowledgments: The authors wish to thank Muhammad Jawad Zai for assistance with compound identification.

Conflicts of Interest: The authors declare no conflicts of interest.

References

1. WHO. *Antimicrobial Resistance*; World Health Organization: Geneva, Switzerland, 2023. Available online: https://www.who.int/news-room/fact-sheets/detail/antimicrobial-resistance (accessed on 26 July 2024).
2. Centers for Disease Control and Prevention (CDC). 2019 Antibiotic Resistance Threats Report. Available online: https://www.cdc.gov/antimicrobial-resistance/data-research/threats/ (accessed on 26 July 2024).
3. World Bank. Drug-Resistant Infections: A Threat to Our Economic Future. Available online: https://www.worldbank.org/en/topic/health/publication/drug-resistant-infections-a-threat-to-our-economic-future (accessed on 6 June 2024).
4. Ajulo, S.; Awosile, B. Global antimicrobial resistance and use surveillance system (GLASS 2022): Investigating the relationship between antimicrobial resistance and antimicrobial consumption data across the participating countries. *PLoS ONE* **2024**, *19*, e0297921. [CrossRef] [PubMed]
5. Renwick, M.J.; Brogan, D.M.; Mossialos, E. A systematic review and critical assessment of incentive strategies for discovery and development of novel antibiotics. *J. Antibiot.* **2016**, *69*, 73–88. [CrossRef] [PubMed]
6. World Health Organization. WHO Releases Report on State of Development of Antibacterials. 2024. Available online: https://www.who.int/news/item/14-06-2024-who-releases-report-on-state-of-development-of-antibacterials (accessed on 18 June 2024).
7. Abdallah, E.M.; Alhatlani, B.Y.; de Paula Menezes, R.; Martins, C.H.G. Back to nature: Medicinal plants as promising sources for antibacterial drugs in the post-antibiotic era. *Plants* **2023**, *12*, 3077. [CrossRef]
8. Tiwana, G.; Cock, I.E.; Cheesman, M.J. A review of Ayurvedic principles and the use of Ayurvedic plants to control diarrhoea and gastrointestinal infections. *Pharmacogn. Commun.* **2023**, *13*, 152–162. [CrossRef]
9. Cheesman, M.; Ilanko, A.; Blonk, B.; Cock, I. Developing new antimicrobial therapies: Are synergistic combinations of plant extracts/compounds with conventional antibiotics the solution? *Pharmacogn. Rev.* **2017**, *11*, 57. [CrossRef]
10. Belmehdi, O.; Bouyahya, A.; Jekő, J.; Cziáky, Z.; Zengin, G.; Sotkó, G.; El Baaboua, A.; Senhaji, N.S.; Abrini, J. Synergistic interaction between propolis extract, essential oils, and antibiotics against *Staphylococcus epidermidis* and methicillin-resistant *Staphylococcus aureus*. *Int. J. Sec. Metab.* **2021**, *8*, 195–213. [CrossRef]

11. Tiwana, G.; Cock, I.E.; White, A.; Cheesman, M.J. Use of specific combinations of the triphala plant component extracts to potentiate the inhibition of gastrointestinal bacterial growth. *J. Ethnopharmacol.* **2020**, *260*, 112937. [CrossRef]
12. Thakur, M.; Yadav, A.; Dubey, K.K.; Dakal, T.C.; Yadav, V. Antimicrobial activity against antibiotic-resistant pathogens and antioxidant activity and LCMS/MS phytochemical content analysis of selected medicinal plants. *J. Pure Appl. Microbiol.* **2024**, *18*, 722–738. [CrossRef]
13. Badoni, H.; Sharma, P.; Mohsin Waheed, S.; Singh, S. Phytochemical analyses and evaluation of antioxidant, antibacterial, and toxic properties of *Emblica officinalis* and *Terminalia bellirica* fruit extracts. *Asian J. Pharm. Clin. Res.* **2016**, *9*, 96–102. [CrossRef]
14. Mani, P.; Devi, P.N.; Kaleeswari, S.; Poonkothai, M. Antimicrobial activity and phytochemical analysis of fruit extracts of *Terminalia bellirica. Int. J. Pharm. Pharm. Sci.* **2014**, *43*, 364.
15. Sharma, R.; Raizada, S.; Gautam, A.; Bhatia, A.K. Phytochemical and antibacterial analysis of *Terminalia chebula* and *Terminalia bellirica*. In *Green Chemistry in Environmental Sustainability and Chemical Education*; Springer: Singapore, 2018; pp. 131–137. [CrossRef]
16. Parekh, J.; Chanda, S. Evaluation of antimicrobial activity of *Terminalia chebula* Retz. fruit in different solvents. *J. Herbs Spices Med. Plants* **2008**, *13*, 107–116. [CrossRef]
17. Bag, A.; Kumar Bhattacharyya, S.; Bharati, P.; Pal, N.K.; Chattopadhyay, R.R. Evaluation of antibacterial properties of Chebulic myrobalan (fruit of *Terminalia chebula* Retz.) extracts against methicillin-resistant *Staphylococcus aureus* and trimethoprim-sulphamethoxazole resistant uropathogenic *Escherichia coli. Afr. J. Plant Sci.* **2009**, *3*, 25–29.
18. Zearah, S.A. Antifungal and antibacterial activity of flavonoid extract from *Terminalia chebula* retz. fruits. *J. Basrah Res. (Sci.)* **2014**, *40*, 122–131.
19. Cajka, T.; Hricko, J.; Rudl Kulhava, L.; Paucova, M.; Novakova, M.; Kuda, O. Optimization of mobile phase modifiers for fast LC-MS-based untargeted metabolomics and lipidomics. *Int. J. Mol. Sci.* **2023**, *24*, 1987. [CrossRef]
20. Altemimi, A.; Lakhssassi, N.; Baharlouei, A.; Watson, D.G.; Lightfoot, D.A. Phytochemicals: Extraction, isolation, and identification of bioactive compounds from plant extracts. *Plants* **2017**, *6*, 42. [CrossRef]
21. Bonev, B.; Hooper, J.; Parisot, J. Principles of assessing bacterial susceptibility to antibiotics using the agar diffusion method. *J. Antimicrob. Chemother.* **2008**, *61*, 1295–1301. [CrossRef]
22. Jain, S.; Patel, N.; Lin, S. Solubility and dissolution enhancement strategies: Current understanding and recent trends. *Drug Dev. Ind. Pharm.* **2015**, *41*, 875–887. [CrossRef]
23. Flanagan, J.N.; Steck, T.R. The relationship between agar thickness and antimicrobial susceptibility testing. *Indian J. Microbiol.* **2017**, *57*, 503–506. [CrossRef]
24. Bhattacharjee, M.K. Better visualization and photodocumentation of zone of inhibition by staining cells and background agar differently. *J. Antibiot.* **2015**, *68*, 657–659. [CrossRef]
25. Livermore, D.M. Antibiotic resistance in staphylococci. *Int. J. Antimicrob. Agents* **2000**, *16*, 3–10. [CrossRef]
26. Kim, C.; Mwangi, M.; Chung, M.; Milheirço, C.; de Lencastre, H.; Tomasz, A. The mechanism of heterogeneous beta-lactam resistance in MRSA: Key role of the stringent stress response. *PLoS ONE* **2013**, *8*, e82814. [CrossRef] [PubMed]
27. Vaou, N.; Stavropoulou, E.; Voidarou, C.; Tsigalou, C.; Bezirtzoglou, E. Towards advances in medicinal plant antimicrobial activity: A review study on challenges and future perspectives. *Microorganisms* **2021**, *9*, 2041. [CrossRef] [PubMed]
28. Huttner, A.; Bielicki, J.; Clements, M.N.; Frimodt-Møller, N.; Muller, A.E.; Paccaud, J.P.; Mouton, J.W. Oral amoxicillin and amoxicillin–clavulanic acid: Properties, indications, and usage. *Clin. Microbiol. Infect.* **2020**, *26*, 871–879. [CrossRef]
29. Oelschlaeger, P. β-Lactamases: Sequence, structure, function, and inhibition. *Biomolecules* **2021**, *11*, 986. [CrossRef]
30. Khameneh, B.; Eskin, N.A.M.; Iranshahy, M.; Fazly Bazzaz, B.S. Phytochemicals: A promising weapon in the arsenal against antibiotic-resistant bacteria. *Antibiotics* **2021**, *10*, 1044. [CrossRef] [PubMed]
31. Platon, V.M.; Dragoi, B.; Marin, L. Erythromycin formulations—A journey to advanced drug delivery. *Pharmaceutics* **2022**, *14*, 2180. [CrossRef]
32. Kehrenberg, C.; Schwarz, S.; Jacobsen, L.; Hansen, L.H.; Vester, B. A new mechanism for chloramphenicol, florfenicol, and clindamycin resistance: Methylation of 23S ribosomal RNA at A2503. *Mol. Microbiol.* **2005**, *57*, 1064–1073. [CrossRef] [PubMed]
33. Sharma, A.; Gupta, V.K.; Pathania, R. Efflux pump inhibitors for bacterial pathogens: From bench to bedside. *Indian J. Med. Res.* **2019**, *149*, 129. [CrossRef]
34. Tiwana, G.; Cock, I.E.; Cheesman, M.J. *Phyllanthus niruri* Linn.: Antibacterial activity, phytochemistry, and enhanced antibiotic combinatorial strategies. *Antibiotics* **2024**, *13*, 654. [CrossRef]
35. Gibbons, S. Phytochemicals for bacterial resistance--strengths, weaknesses, and opportunities. *Planta Med.* **2008**, *74*, 594–602. [CrossRef]
36. Cai, X.; Javor, S.; Gan, B.H.; Köhler, T.; Reymond, J.L. The antibacterial activity of peptide dendrimers and polymyxin B increases sharply above pH 7.4. *Chem. Commun.* **2021**, *57*, 5654–5657. [CrossRef]
37. Zavascki, A.P.; Goldani, L.Z.; Li, J.; Nation, R.L. Polymyxin B for the treatment of multidrug-resistant pathogens: A critical review. *J. Antimicrob. Chemother.* **2007**, *60*, 1206–1215. [CrossRef] [PubMed]
38. Cock, I.E. The medicinal properties and phytochemistry of plants of the genus *Terminalia* (Combretaceae). *Inflammopharmacology* **2015**, *23*, 203–229. [CrossRef]
39. Kumari, S.; Joshi, A.B.; Gurav, S.; Bhandarkar, A.V.; Agarwal, A.; Deepak, M.; Gururaj, G.M. A pharmacognostic, phytochemical, and pharmacological review of *Terminalia bellirica. J. Pharmacogn. Phytochem.* **2017**, *6*, 368–376.

40. Bag, A.; Bhattacharyya, S.K.; Chattopadhyay, R.R. The development of *Terminalia chebula* Retz. (Combretaceae) in clinical research. *Asian Pac. J. Trop. Biomed.* **2013**, *3*, 244. [CrossRef]
41. Embaby, M.A.; El-Raey, M.A.; Zaineldain, M.; Almaghrabi, O.; Marrez, D.A. Synergistic effect and efflux pump inhibitory activity of *Ficus nitida* phenolic extract with tetracycline against some pathogenic bacteria. *Toxin Rev.* **2021**, *40*, 1187–1197. [CrossRef]
42. Adamczak, A.; Ożarowski, M.; Karpiński, T.M. Antibacterial activity of some flavonoids and organic acids widely distributed in plants. *J. Clin. Med.* **2020**, *9*, 109. [CrossRef]
43. Zhang, Z.; Xu, Q.; Wang, Y.; Qu, S.; Tan, J.; Tang, Y.; Li, P.; Zheng, X. Exploiting the synergistic antibacterial activity of shikimic acid and ceftiofur against methicillin-resistant *Staphylococcus aureus*. *World J. Microbiol. Biotechnol.* **2024**, *40*, 1–11. [CrossRef]
44. Yang, X.; Gao, X.; Ou, J.; Chen, G.; Ye, L. Antimicrobial activity and mechanism of anti-MRSA of phloroglucinol derivatives. *DARU J. Pharm. Sci.* **2024**, *32*, 177–187. [CrossRef]
45. Shen, D.; Duan, S.; Hu, Y.; Liang, J.; Tang, Y. Antibacterial activity and synergistic antibiotic mechanism of trialdehyde phloroglucinol against methicillin-resistant *Staphylococcus aureus*. *Phytother. Res.* **2023**, *37*, 490–504. [CrossRef]
46. Mittal, N.; Tesfu, H.H.; Hogan, A.M.; Cardona, S.T.; Sorensen, J.L. Synthesis and antibiotic activity of novel acylated phloroglucinol compounds against methicillin-resistant *Staphylococcus aureus*. *J. Antibiot.* **2019**, *72*, 253–259. [CrossRef] [PubMed]
47. Wei, C.; Cui, P.; Liu, X. Antibacterial activity and mechanism of madecassic acid against *Staphylococcus aureus*. *Molecules* **2023**, *28*, 1895. [CrossRef] [PubMed]
48. Haraguchi, H.; Kataoka, S.; Okamoto, S.; Hanafi, M.; Shibata, K. Antimicrobial triterpenes from *Ilex integra* and the mechanism of antifungal action. *Phytother. Res.* **1999**, *13*, 151–160. [CrossRef]
49. Zhang, J.; Li, L.; Kim, S.H.; Hagerman, A.E.; Lü, J. Anti-cancer, anti-diabetic and other pharmacologic and biological activities of penta-galloyl-glucose. *Pharm. Res.* **2009**, *26*, 2066–2080. [CrossRef]
50. Cho, J.Y.; Sohn, M.J.; Lee, J.; Kim, W.G. Isolation and identification of pentagalloylglucose with broad-spectrum antibacterial activity from *Rhus trichocarpa* Miquel. *Food Chem.* **2010**, *123*, 501–506. [CrossRef]
51. Masota, N.E.; Ohlsen, K.; Schollmayer, C.; Meinel, L.; Holzgrabe, U. Isolation and characterization of galloylglucoses effective against multidrug-resistant strains of *Escherichia coli* and *Klebsiella pneumoniae*. *Molecules* **2022**, *27*, 5045. [CrossRef]
52. Pfundstein, B.; El Desouky, S.K.; Hull, W.E.; Haubner, R.; Erben, G.; Owen, R.W. Polyphenolic compounds in the fruits of Egyptian medicinal plants (*Terminalia bellerica*, *Terminalia chebula* and *Terminalia horrida*): Characterization, quantitation and determination of antioxidant capacities. *Phytochemistry* **2010**, *71*, 1132–1148. [CrossRef]
53. Avula, B.; Wang, Y.H.; Wang, M.; Shen, Y.H.; Khan, I.A. Simultaneous determination and characterization of tannins and triterpene saponins from the fruits of various species of *Terminalia* and *Phyllantus emblica* using a UHPLC-UV-MS Method: Application to triphala. *Planta Med.* **2013**, *29*, 181–188. [CrossRef] [PubMed]
54. Manosroi, A.; Jantrawut, P.; Ogihara, E.; Yamamoto, A.; Fukatsu, M.; Yasukawa, K.; Tokuda, H.; Suzuki, N.; Manosroi, J.; Akihisa, T. Biological activities of phenolic compounds and triterpenoids from the Galls of *Terminalia chebula*. *Chem. Biodivers.* **2013**, *10*, 1448–1463. [CrossRef]
55. Bag, A.; Chattopadhyay, R.R. Efflux-pump inhibitory activity of a gallotannin from *Terminalia chebula* fruit against multidrug-resistant uropathogenic *Escherichia coli*. *Nat. Prod. Res.* **2014**, *28*, 1280–1283. [CrossRef]
56. Bag, A.; Chattopadhyay, R.R. Synergistic antibiofilm efficacy of a gallotannin 1,2,6-tri-O-galloyl-β-D-glucopyranose from *Terminalia chebula* fruit in combination with gentamicin and trimethoprim against multidrug resistant uropathogenic *Escherichia coli* biofilms. *PLoS ONE* **2017**, *12*, e0178712. [CrossRef]
57. Hricovíniová, Z.; Mascaretti, Š.; Hricovíniová, J.; Čížek, A.; Jampílek, J. New unnatural gallotannins: A way toward green antioxidants, antimicrobials and antibiofilm agents. *Antioxidants* **2021**, *10*, 1288. [CrossRef]
58. Abbas, M.A.; Lee, E.B.; Boby, N.; Biruhanu, B.T.; Park, S.C. A pharmacodynamic investigation to assess the synergism of orbifloxacin and propyl gallate against *Escherichia coli*. *Front. Pharmacol.* **2022**, *13*, 989395. [CrossRef]
59. Tamang, M.D.; Bae, J.; Park, M.; Jeon, B. Potentiation of β-Lactams against Methicillin-Resistant *Staphylococcus aureus* (MRSA) Using octyl gallate, a food-grade antioxidant. *Antibiotics* **2022**, *11*, 266. [CrossRef]
60. Gesek, J.; Jakimiuk, K.; Atanasov, A.G.; Tomczyk, M. Sanguiins—Promising molecules with broad biological potential. *Int. J. Mol. Sci.* **2021**, *22*, 12972. [CrossRef]
61. Aguilera-Correa, J.J.; Fernández-López, S.; Cuñas-Figueroa, I.D.; Pérez-Rial, S.; Alakomi, H.L.; Nohynek, L.; Oksman-Caldentey, K.M.; Salminen, J.P.; Esteban, J.; Cuadros, J.; et al. Sanguiin H-6 fractionated from cloudberry (*Rubus chamaemorus*) seeds can prevent the methicillin-resistant *Staphylococcus aureus* biofilm development during wound infection. *Antibiotics* **2021**, *10*, 1481. [CrossRef]
62. Zhu, H.L.; Chen, G.; Chen, S.N.; Wang, Q.R.; Wan, L.; Jian, S.P. Characterization of polyphenolic constituents from *Sanguisorba officinalis* L. and its antibacterial activity. *Eur. Food Res. Technol.* **2019**, *245*, 1487–1498. [CrossRef]
63. Hossain, M.A.; Park, H.C.; Park, S.W.; Park, S.C.; Seo, M.G.; Her, M.; Kang, J. Synergism of the combination of traditional antibiotics and novel phenolic compounds against *Escherichia coli*. *Pathogens* **2020**, *9*, 811. [CrossRef]
64. Bassyouni, R.H.; Dwedar, R.A.; Farahat, M.G.; Kamel, Z.; Elwekel, M. Protective effect of hamamelitannin against biofilm production by methicillin-resistant staphylococci Isolated from blood of patients at intensive care units. *Microbiol. Res. J. Int.* **2015**, *10*, 1–8. [CrossRef]
65. Dhingra, A.K.; Chopra, B.; Grewal, A.S.; Guarve, K. Pharmacological properties of chebulinic acid and related ellagitannins from nature: An emerging contemporary bioactive entity. *Pharmacol. Res. Mod. Chin. Med.* **2022**, *5*, 100163. [CrossRef]

66. Yang, Z.N.; Su, B.J.; Wang, Y.Q.; Liao, H.B.; Chen, Z.F.; Liang, D. Isolation, absolute configuration, and biological activities of chebulic acid and brevifolincarboxylic acid derivatives from *Euphorbia hirta*. *J. Nat. Prod.* **2020**, *83*, 985–995. [CrossRef]
67. Li, K.; Lin, Y.; Li, B.; Pan, T.; Wang, F.; Yuan, R.; Ji, J.; Diao, Y.; Wang, S. Antibacterial constituents of *Fructus Chebulae Immaturus* and their mechanisms of action. *BMC Complement. Altern. Med.* **2016**, *16*, 1–10. [CrossRef]
68. Tasduq, S.A.; Singh, K.; Satti, N.K.; Gupta, D.K.; Suri, K.A.; Johri, R.K. *Terminalia chebula* (fruit) prevents liver toxicity caused by sub-chronic administration of rifampicin, isoniazid and pyrazinamide in combination. *Hum. Exp. Toxicol.* **2006**, *25*, 111–118. [CrossRef]
69. Lima, V.N.; Oliveira-Tintino, C.D.M.; Santos, E.S.; Morais, L.P.; Tintino, S.R.; Freitas, T.S.; Geraldo, Y.S.; Pereira, R.L.; Cruz, R.P.; Menezes, I.R.; et al. Antimicrobial and enhancement of the antibiotic activity by phenolic compounds: Gallic acid, caffeic acid and pyrogallol. *Microb. Pathog.* **2016**, *99*, 56–61. [CrossRef]
70. Jenic, D.; Waller, H.; Collins, H.; Erridge, C. Reversal of tetracycline resistance by cepharanthine, cinchonidine, ellagic Acid and propyl gallate in a multi-drug resistant *Escherichia coli*. *Nat. Prod. Bioprospect.* **2021**, *11*, 345–355. [CrossRef]
71. Quave, C.L.; Estévez-Carmona, M.; Compadre, C.M.; Hobby, G.; Hendrickson, H.; Beenken, K.E.; Smeltzer, M.S. Ellagic acid derivatives from *Rubus ulmifolius* inhibit *Staphylococcus aureus* biofilm formation and improve response to antibiotics. *PLoS ONE* **2012**, *7*, e28737. [CrossRef]
72. Anek, P.; Kumpangcum, S.; Roytrakul, S.; Khanongnuch, C.; Saenjum, C.; Phannachet, K. Antibacterial activities of phenolic compounds in Miang extract: Growth inhibition and change in protein expression of extensively drug-Resistant *Klebsiella pneumoniae*. *Antibiotics* **2024**, *13*, 536. [CrossRef]
73. Vitko, N.P.; Richardson, A.R. Laboratory maintenance of methicillin-resistant *Staphylococcus aureus* (MRSA). *Curr. Protoc. Microbiol.* **2013**, *28*, 9C.2.1–9C.2.14. [CrossRef]
74. Doern, C.D. When does 2 plus 2 equal 5? A review of antimicrobial synergy testing. *J. Clin. Microbiol.* **2014**, *52*, 4124–4128. [CrossRef]

MDPI AG
Grosspeteranlage 5
4052 Basel
Switzerland
Tel.: +41 61 683 77 34

Antibiotics Editorial Office
E-mail: antibiotics@mdpi.com
www.mdpi.com/journal/antibiotics

www.ingramcontent.com/pod-product-compliance
Lightning Source LLC
Chambersburg PA
CBHW061547210926
51850CB00009B/2021
9783725848911